DIMENSIONAL ANALYSIS

CALCULATING DOSAGES SAFELY

SECOND EDITION

Brief Contents

DIMENSIONAL ANALYSIS

CALCULATING DOSAGES SAFELY

SECOND EDITION

Tracy Horntvedt, RN, MSN, BA

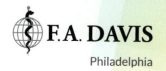

F.A. DAVIS

Philadelphia

F. A. Davis Company
1915 Arch Street
Philadelphia, PA 19103
www.fadavis.com

Printed in the United States of America

Last digit indicates print number: 10 9 8 7 6 5 4 3 2 1

Publisher: Megan Klim
Senior Content Project Manager: Elizabeth Hart
Design and Illustrations Manager: Carolyn O'Brien
Senior Manager, Digital Licensing & Content: Sandra A. Glennie

As new scientific information becomes available through basic and clinical research, recommended treatments and drug therapies undergo changes. The author(s) and publisher have done everything possible to make this book accurate, up to date, and in accord with accepted standards at the time of publication. The author(s), editors, and publisher are not responsible for errors or omissions or for consequences from application of the book, and make no warranty, expressed or implied, in regard to the contents of the book. Any practice described in this book should be applied by the reader in accordance with professional standards of care used in regard to the unique circumstances that may apply in each situation. The reader is advised always to check product information (package inserts) for changes and new information regarding dose and contraindications before administering any drug. Caution is especially urged when using new or infrequently ordered drugs.

Library of Congress Cataloging-in-Publication Data

Names: Horntvedt, Tracy, author.
Title: Calculating dosages safely : a dimensional analysis approach / Tracy
    Horntvedt.
Description: Second. | Philadelphia, PA : F.A. Davis Company, [2019] |
    Includes bibliographical references and index.
Identifiers: LCCN 2018018148 (print) | LCCN 2018018985 (ebook) | ISBN
    9780803689794 | ISBN 9780803661899 (pbk.)
Subjects: | MESH: Drug Dosage Calculations | Nursing Care—methods |
    Problems and Exercises
Classification: LCC RS57 (ebook) | LCC RS57 (print) | NLM QV 18.2 | DDC
    615.1/401513—dc23
LC record available at https://lccn.loc.gov/2018018148

Dedication

To my family and friends who have provided their love and support: Thank you from the bottom of my heart.

To nursing students everywhere: Bless you for wanting to take care of people. It is such a joy and privilege to be a nurse! Thank you!

Preface

Introduction

The second edition of *Dimensional Analysis: Calculating Dosages Safely* provides a systematic approach to solving both simple and complex dosage problems. The dimensional analysis method organizes data methodically and allows students to examine developing calculations for errors. It is an ideal method to build confidence, speed, and competency in dosage calculations. The second edition of this book serves to correct the errors contained within the first edition, address electronic documentation, and update safety information.

This text also emphasizes safe medication practices. Although accuracy in calculating dosages is extremely important, healthcare providers who administer medications also need to be able to read drug labels, interpret medication orders, apply principles of safe drug administration to their practice, document administered drugs accurately, and understand the considerations that must be made when administering drugs to special populations.

Organization

Calculating Dosages Safely: A Dimensional Analysis Approach is organized in a simple-to-complex manner, where each chapter is designed to build on concepts learned in earlier chapters. The text is divided into four units:

Unit 1: Arithmetic Review and Dimensional Analysis includes basic arithmetic concepts such as working with whole numbers, fractions, decimals, percents, and introduces the principles of dimensional analysis.

Unit 2: Medication Administration covers concepts of medication administration such as systems of measurements, converting between systems of measurement, safety considerations, medication orders, reading labels and dosing devices, calculating dosages based on body weight and body surface area, intravenous delivery systems, and calculating intravenous flow rates.

Unit 3: Special Topics addresses enteral tube feedings, insulin and heparin administration, critical care dosage calculations, and lifespan considerations in dosage calculations.

Unit 4: Answers to Chapter Post-Test contains the answers to each chapter's post-test.

The three appendices at the end of the book provide extra assistance on using a calculator, interpreting Roman numerals, and converting the civilian clock to military time.

Features

Calculating Dosages Safely: A Dimensional Analysis Approach offers the following features:

- **Arithmetic Skills Assessment:** This pre-test is designed to highlight strengths and weaknesses, allowing students to focus on areas of remediation before starting study on dosage calculations.
- **Arithmetic Review:** Chapters 1, 2, and 3 are for students who want or need to review basic arithmetic skills.
- **Glossaries:** Each chapter contains a glossary of terms used in math or medication administration.
- **Learning Objectives:** Expected learning outcomes for the student are specified.
- **Icons:** Note and Alert icons are designed to bring attention to important points:
  - The **Note** icon directs attention to information that may highlight a concept or contain a shortcut hint.
  - The **Alert** icon directs attention to information that is vital for safe medication practice, including avoiding errors in dosage calculation.
- **Examples:** Each topic includes adequate examples that walk the student through the problem in a step-by-step manner.
- **Labels:** Real and simulated drug labels help students become comfortable with gathering the information needed to reconstitute powdered medications or calculate dosages accurately.
- **Practice:** Each chapter is interspersed with short practice quizzes that assess the student's skill level with the topics just learned.
- **Case Studies:** Selected chapters feature case studies that reflect actual clinical practice experiences in calculating dosages, using clinical protocols, and administering medications.
- **Key Points:** Each chapter contains a list of the most important points contained within the chapter.
- **Chapter Post-Tests:** Chapter post-tests assess skills learned in that chapter.
- **Unit Post-Tests:** Unit post-tests assess skills learned in the entire unit.
- **Comprehensive Post-Test:** The comprehensive post-test assesses skills learned throughout the entire book.

DavisPlus Materials

Student Resources

- **Basic Math Interactive Exercise** provides review of fractions, decimals, and roman numerals.
- **Speed Challenge Chapter Quizzes** challenge students' ability to calculate dosages quickly and accurately.
- **Syringe Pull Exercises** test the accuracy of drawing up medications in a syringe.
- **Dosage Calculation Tools** for quick calculation of BMI, temperature, and more.
- **Links** to additional web-based resources:
  - Practice opportunities for basic arithmetic skills through games
  - Organizations related to safe medication practices, such as the U.S. Food and Drug Administration and the Institute for Safe Medication Practices
  - YouTube videos and animations showing demonstrations of skills related to medication administration

Instructor Resources

- **Instructors Guide** with sample syllabi
- **Powerpoint presentations** covering each chapter of instruction
- **Instructor test bank** with over 250 questions.
- **Speed Challenge Answer Key** provides answers for the student quizzes.

Using This Book

Many student nurses say that making a medication error is their biggest fear. Medication errors happen every day in healthcare facilities and are a major reason for extended hospital stays, patient injury, and even death. *Dimensional Analysis: Calculating Dosages Safely* was designed and written to provide you with skill and confidence to calculate simple and complex dosage problems.

After reading the introduction, browse through a chapter and become familiar with the layout.

1. Each chapter starts with a glossary. Read through it to familiarize yourself with terms that may be new to you.

2. Read through the learning objectives. The learning objectives introduce the topics to be covered and outline the goals to be achieved after reading the chapter and completing the practice questions and case studies.

3. Read each section carefully, paying special attention to notes and alerts. Review the examples provided until you clearly understand the concept.

4. Take the Practice quiz after each section of instruction.
   Before calculating your answer, review your work to make sure that you have accounted for all relevant information in the problem, and review your equation to make sure that no errors have been made. After calculating the answer, critically evaluate it to see if it reasonable and logical. Compare your answers to those in the answer key. Since accuracy is of utmost importance in dosage calculations, carefully review any wrong answers. Ask for help if you do not understand where an error exists.

5. Complete the Case Study if one is included at the end of the chapter. The case studies are designed to reflect "real-life" clinical experiences with medication administration and dosage calculations.

6. Read through the Key Points to review important concepts discussed within the chapter.

7. Take the chapter post-test to assess how well you understand the material presented in the chapter, and your ability to calculate dosages accurately.

8. Take the chapter Speed Challenge test on Davis*Plus*. The goal is to complete the quiz with 100% accuracy within 20 minutes.

9. After completing all chapters in a unit, take the unit post-test. Assess any wrong answers carefully.

10. After completing all chapters, take the comprehensive post-test in the book. If additional practice is desired, take the comprehensive post-test included the five comprehensive speed challenge quizzes on DavisPlus.

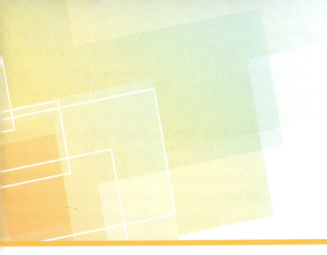

Reviewers

Millie Carroll, MSN, RN
Nursing Faculty
Snead State Community College
Boaz, Alabama

Connie Houser, MSN,
  RNC-OB, CNE
ADN Instructor
Central Carolina Technical College
Sumter, South Carolina

Linda S. Smith, PhD, RN, CLNC
Vice President, Research
Data Design, Inc.
Horseshoe Bend, Arkansas
Nursing Faculty
Ozarka College
Melbourne, Arkansas

Acknowledgments

I would like to acknowledge those at F. A. Davis Company who guided me through the writing process and answered my many questions. Many thanks to Elizabeth Hart and Jacalyn Sharp for their encouragement and assistance.

I would also like to thank the following manufacturers for allowing me to use their product images in this text:

- Abbott Nutrition, Columbus, OH
- AbbVie, Inc., North Chicago, IL
- America Regent Laboratories, Shirley, NY
- APP Pharmaceuticals LLC, Schaumburg, IL
- Baxter Healthcare Corporation, Round Lake, IL
- Bayer Pharmaceutical Products, West Haven, CT
- Bedford Laboratories, a Division of Ben Venue Laboratories, Inc., Bedford, OH
- Tyco Healthcare Group LP d/b/a Covidien, Mansfield, MA
- Eli Lilly, Indianapolis, IN
- Hospira, Inc., Lake Forest, IL
- Novo Nordisk, Inc., Princeton, NJ
- Omnicell, Mountain View, CA
- Ovation Pharmceuticals, Deerfield, IL

Thank you to those who reviewed the chapters and offered insight and suggestions for improvement.

Table of Contents

Arithmetic Skills Assessment *(answers in Unit 4)*

This Arithmetic Skills Assessment is designed to pinpoint your weak areas in arithmetic skills.

Follow the instructions in each section, completing the assessment without using a calculator. Do not round the answer unless directed. If you miss more than two questions in any area, particularly the first three questions in a section, review the corresponding chapter in Unit 1, Arithmetic Review.

Add these whole numbers.

1. $36 + 79$

2. $340 + 9308$

3. $1726 + 9372$

4. $26 + 493 + 31 + 3630$

Subtract these whole numbers.

5. $89 - 65$

6. $272 - 44$

7. $3691 - 723$

8. $7432 - 6889$

Multiply these whole numbers.

9. 8×5

10. 15×7

11. 23×40

12. 602×82

Divide these whole numbers.

13. $44 \div 2$

14. $75 \div 15$

15. $348 \div 16$

16. $1210 \div 25$

Add these fractions and reduce to the lowest terms.

17. $\frac{1}{2} + \frac{3}{4}$

18. $\frac{2}{3} + \frac{5}{8}$

19. $1\frac{3}{5} + 8\frac{4}{9}$

20. $3\frac{7}{16} + 7\frac{9}{16}$

Subtract these fractions and reduce to the lowest terms.

21. $\frac{8}{15} - \frac{3}{15}$

22. $\frac{2}{3} - \frac{2}{9}$

23. $1\frac{1}{4} - \frac{3}{8}$

24. $23\frac{13}{14} - 6\frac{1}{7}$

Multiply these fractions and reduce to the lowest terms.

25. $\frac{1}{3} \times \frac{5}{6}$

26. $1\frac{5}{7} \times \frac{8}{9}$

27. $9\frac{3}{8} \times \frac{3}{5}$

28. $1\frac{1}{4} \times 3\frac{1}{3}$

Divide these fractions and reduce to the lowest terms.

29. $\frac{6}{7} \div \frac{5}{7}$

30. $\frac{9}{12} \div \frac{3}{24}$

31. $2\frac{1}{2} \div 1\frac{2}{5}$

32. $2\frac{3}{8} \div \frac{5}{7}$

Add these decimals.

33. 1.1 + 3.6

34. 10.3 + 82.9

35. 0.09 + 1.42

36. 0.082 + 827.41 + 5.29

Subtract these decimals.

37. 1.1 − 0.9

38. 4 − 3.25

39. 61.2 − 59.45

40. 340 − 11.79

Multiply these decimals.

41. 0.5 × 1.2

42. 8 × 8.2

43. 10.25 × 9.6

44. 30.22 × 10.92

Divide these decimals.

45. 1.1 ÷ 0.1

46. 5.25 ÷ 1.5

47. 24.36 ÷ 4.8

48. 10,400 ÷ 25

Round these numbers.

49. 21.144 to the nearest tenth

50. 73.51 to the nearest tenth

51. 152.785 to the nearest hundredth

52. 3.0845 to the nearest thousandth

Write these fractions and decimal numbers as instructed. Reduce fractions to lowest terms.

53. $\frac{4}{10}$ as a decimal number

54. 63.6 as a fraction

55. 8.17 as a fraction

56. $\frac{1}{4}$ as a decimal number

Write these percents as instructed.

57. 89.2% as a decimal

58. 2.3% as a fraction

59. 0.9% as a decimal

60. 0.56 as a percent

UNIT 1

Arithmetic Review and Dimensional Analysis

Chapter 1

Whole Numbers

Glossary

Dividend: The number that is to be divided into parts.

Difference: The amount that remains after one number is subtracted from another.

Divisor: The number by which the dividend is to be divided.

Equation: A mathematical statement (for example: $5 + 3 = 8$).

Product: The answer reached when two numbers are multiplied.

Quotient: The answer reached when dividing one number (the dividend) by another number (the divisor).

Sum: The amount obtained after adding one number to another.

Whole number: A number that does not contain fractions, decimals, or negative numbers.

Objectives

After completing this chapter, the learner will be able to—

1. Define *whole number.*
2. Add whole numbers.
3. Subtract whole numbers.
4. Multiply whole numbers.
5. Divide whole numbers.

Types of Numbers

Numbers can be classified in several different ways. They can be expressed as integers, rational numbers, irrational numbers, real numbers, prime numbers, factors, whole numbers, fractions, or decimals (see Box 1-1). Adding, subtracting, multiplying, and dividing numbers must be completed in a certain order (see Box 1-2 and Box 1-3). This chapter reviews adding, subtracting, multiplying, and dividing whole numbers.

▇ Box 1-1 Types of Numbers

Integers
Integers are positive and negative whole numbers.
    Examples: 3, 2, 1, 0, −1, −2, −3, …

Rational Numbers
Rational numbers include integers and fractions.
    Examples: $-1, -0.5, -\dfrac{1}{2}, \dfrac{4}{5}, 0.7, 1, 2, \ldots$

Irrational Numbers
Irrational numbers are those that have nonrepeating decimal places.
    Example: $\pi = 3.14159\ldots$

Real Numbers
Real numbers encompass both rational and irrational numbers.

Prime Numbers
A prime number can be evenly divided by only 1 and itself.
    Examples: 1, 3, 5, 7, 11, …

Factors
Factors are numbers that divide evenly into another number.
    Example: The factors of 20 are 1, 2, 4, 5, and 10.

Whole Numbers
Whole numbers do not contain fractions, decimals, or negative numbers.
    Examples: 4, 8, 25, 102, 1429, …

Fractions
Fractions are numbers that are part of a whole number.
    Examples: $\dfrac{2}{3}, \dfrac{4}{5}, \dfrac{3}{10}, \dfrac{9}{17}, \ldots$

Decimals
Decimals are numbers that represent a part of a whole number, and/or may be a combination of a whole number and a part of a number.
    Examples: 0.25, 3.1, 10.164, 184.3, …

■ Box 1-2   **Properties of Numbers**

Commutative Property of Numbers
This property applies to operations of addition and multiplication only. The order of operations can be changed without affecting the final answer.

$$a + b = b + a$$
$$a \times b = b \times a$$

Example: 2 + 3 = 5
3 + 2 = 5
Example: 2 × 3 = 6
3 × 2 = 6

Associative Property of Numbers
This property also applies to operations of addition and multiplication only. Operations may be grouped differently without affecting the final answer.

$$(a + b) + c = a + (b + c)$$
$$(a \times b) \times c = a \times (b \times c)$$

Example: (2 + 3) + 4 = 9
2 + (3 + 4) = 9
Example: (2 × 3) × 4 = 24
2 × (3 × 4) = 24

Distributive Property of Numbers
This property shows how equations with multiplication and addition operations can be broken into smaller pieces.

$$a \times (b + c) = (a \times b) + (a \times c)$$

Example: 10 × (2 + 3) = 50
(10 × 2) + (10 × 3) = 50

■ Box 1-3   **Order of Mathematical Operations**

1. Perform operations that are inside the parentheses first.
2. Perform the operations that require multiplying or dividing first, starting from left to right.
3. Perform the operations that require adding or subtracting next, starting from left to right.

Whole Numbers

Whole numbers are also called natural numbers or counting numbers. They include the number 0 and all positive numbers, such as *1, 2, 3, 4,* and so on. Adding, subtracting, and multiplying whole numbers result in answers that are whole numbers. Dividing whole numbers may result in a fraction or decimal. Figure 1-1 shows the place values of numbers up to the seventh (or millions) place.

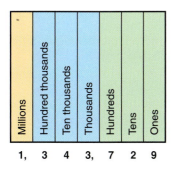

Figure 1-1 Place Value of Whole Numbers. These are the place values for the whole number 1,343,729.

Adding Whole Numbers

The symbol for addition is the plus sign +. The answer to an addition problem is called the **sum** or **total**. To add whole numbers, follow the directions in Examples 1–5.

Example 1: 3 + 2

$$\begin{array}{r} 3 \\ + \ 2 \\ \hline \end{array}$$

1. Line up the numbers so that the digits in the ones place line up under each other.

$$\begin{array}{r} 3 \\ + \ 2 \\ \hline 5 \end{array}$$

2. Add the numbers in the column.

Note: If the sum of the column exceeds **10**, record the number in the ones column and carry the tens digit to the column to the left.

Example 2: 10 + 15

$$\begin{array}{r} 10 \\ + \ 15 \\ \hline \end{array}$$

1. In this example, each number has two digits. Write the numbers so that the digits in the ones and tens columns line up under each other.

$$\begin{array}{r} 10 \\ + \ 15 \\ \hline 25 \end{array}$$

2. Add each column of numbers.

Example 3: 29 + 43

1. In this example, the sum of the ones column exceeds *10 (9 + 3 = 12)*. Write 2 in the ones column and carry the 1 to the next column.

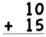

$$\begin{array}{r} 1 \quad\ \\ 29 \\ + \ 43 \\ \hline 72 \end{array}$$

2. Add the numbers in the tens column, including the carried digit.

For Examples 4 and 5, refer to the directions in Examples 1–3.

Example 4: 198 + 322 + 16

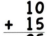

$$\begin{array}{r} 1\ 1\quad\ \\ 198 \\ + \ 322 \\ + \ \ \ 16 \\ \hline 536 \end{array}$$

Example 5: 5 + 4002 + 635 + 33

$$\begin{array}{r} 1\quad\quad\ \\ 5 \\ + \ 4002 \\ + \ \ 635 \\ + \ \ \ \ 33 \\ \hline 4675 \end{array}$$

Note: To line up numbers greater than *999*, omit all commas.

Practice Adding Whole Numbers

(answers on page 13)

Add these whole numbers.

1. 3 + 8 = _____

2. 2 + 51 = _____

3. 12 + 36 = _____

4. 99 + 171 = _____

5. 132 + 837 = _____

6. 6386 + 1927 = _____

7. 928 + 385 + 73 = _____

8. 17 + 839 + 2893 = _____

9. 4 + 29 + 738 + 8302 = _____

10. 93,756 + 280,655 = _____

Subtracting Whole Numbers

The symbol for subtraction is the minus sign − . The answer to a subtraction problem is called the **difference**. To subtract whole numbers, refer to the directions in Examples 1–5:

Example 1:   9 − 7

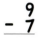

1. Place the larger number on top and the smaller number on the bottom.

$$
\begin{array}{r} 9 \\ -\ 7 \\ \hline 2 \end{array}
$$

2. Subtract the bottom number from the top number.

Example 2:   82 − 41

> **Note:** Work from the right (ones column) to the left when subtracting numbers with more than one digit.

$$
\begin{array}{r} 82 \\ -\ 41 \\ \hline 41 \end{array}
$$

Example 3:   923 − 839

1. In this example, the digit in the top ones column is smaller than the digit in the bottom ones column (that is, the *3* in *923* is smaller than the *9* in *839*). To subtract *9* from *3*, borrow 10 units from the (tens) column to the left of the *3*.

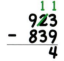

2. Borrowing 10 units from the middle (tens) column turns the *3* into *13* and reduces the *2* in the middle (tens) column to *1*. Subtract *9* from *13* and record the answer *4* in the ones column.

3. Subtract the digits in the middle (tens) column. Notice that 3 must now be subtracted from the 1. Again, borrow 10 units from the (hundreds) column to the left, a step that reduces *9* to *8*. Subtract *3* from *11* and record the answer *8* in the middle (tens) column

> **Note:** When you subtract *8* from the remaining *8* in the far left (hundreds) column, the result is zero. The problem is complete.

Example 4: 1,205 − 799

1. In this example, the digit in the tens column is 0, so you cannot borrow from the tens column. Therefore, you must borrow 100 units from the hundreds column, leaving 90 of the units in the tens column (written as 9) and giving 10 units to the ones column.

2. Subtract the numbers in the ones, tens, and hundreds columns.

For Example 5, refer to the directions in Examples 1–4.

Example 5: 9,375,295 − 10,638

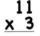
$$\begin{array}{r} \overset{4\,1\,8\,1}{9375295} \\ -\ \ 10638 \\ \hline 9364657 \end{array}$$

Practice Subtracting Whole Numbers
(answers on page 13)

Subtract these whole numbers.

1. 7 − 3 = _____

2. 21 − 17 = _____

3. 39 − 24 = _____

4. 76 − 51 = _____

5. 402 − 184 = _____

6. 936 − 688 = _____

7. 2957 − 562 = _____

8. 8126 − 2953 = _____

9. 10,003 − 9255 = _____

10. 483,276 − 319,028 = _____

Multiplying Whole Numbers

Multiplication of whole numbers is indicated by the signs × or *. The answer to a multiplication problem is called the **product**. To multiply whole numbers, refer to the directions in Examples 1–5.

Example 1: 11 × 3

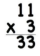
$$\begin{array}{r} 11 \\ \times\ 3 \\ \hline \end{array}$$

1. Place the larger number *(11)* on the top line. Write the *3* under the *11*; line up the digits in the ones column.

$$\begin{array}{r} 11 \\ \times\ 3 \\ \hline 33 \end{array}$$

2. Multiply each 1 in *11* by *3*, being careful to keep the columns in line.

Example 2: 12 × 9

$$\begin{array}{r} 12 \\ \times\ 9 \\ \hline \end{array}$$

1. Set up the equation as described in Example 1.

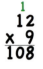
$$\begin{array}{r} \overset{1}{12} \\ \times\ 9 \\ \hline 108 \end{array}$$

2. Multiply the *2* in *12* by the *9*. Since *9* × *2* equals the double-digit *18*, place the *8* in the ones column and carry the *1* to the tens column. Add the *1* to the product obtained from multiplying the *1* in *12* by the *9*.

For Example 3, refer to the directions in Examples 1 and 2.

Example 3:   23 × 7

```
  2
 23
x  7
161
```

Example 4:   25 × 36

```
  25
x 36
```
1. Set up the equation as described in Example 1.

```
   3
  25
x 36
 150
```
2. In this example, *25* is multiplied by 36, a two-digit number. First, multiply the *5* in *25* by *6*, carrying the *3* to the tens column. Then multiply the *2* in *25* by *6* and add the carried *3* to this product.

```
   1
   3
  25
x 36
 150
 750  ← Placeholder
```
3. Before multiplying *25* by *3*, place a *0* in the ones column. This *0* acts as a placeholder. The placeholder serves as a reminder to move the product to the next column to the left.

```
   1
   3
  25
x 36
 150
 750
 900
```
4. Add the numbers in the ones, tens, and hundreds columns.

Example 5:   101 × 17

```
 101
x 17
```
1. Set up the equation as explained in Example 1.

```
  101
x  17
  707
 1010  ← Placeholder
```
2. Multiply *101* by *7*, then insert a *0* as a placeholder before multiplying *101* by *1*.

```
  101
x  17
  707
 1010
 1717
```
3. Add the columns.

Note: For help with multiplying and dividing zeros, see Box 1-4.

■ Box 1-4   Multiplying and Dividing Zeros

$0 \times 0 = 0$

$0 \times 1 = 0$

$\dfrac{0}{1} = 0$

$\dfrac{1}{0}$ undefined (there is no mathematical meaning)

Example 6:   798 x 251

$$\begin{array}{r} 798 \\ \times\ 251 \\ \hline \end{array}$$ 1. Set up the equation.

$$\begin{array}{r} 798 \\ \times\ 251 \\ \hline 798 \end{array}$$ 2. Multiply *798* by *1*.

$$\begin{array}{r} 44 \\ 798 \\ \times\ 251 \\ \hline 798 \\ 39900 \end{array}$$ ←— Placeholder   3. Insert a *0* as a placeholder in the ones column, then multiply *798* by *5*.

$$\begin{array}{r} 1\ 1 \\ 44 \\ 798 \\ \times\ \ \ 251 \\ \hline 798 \\ 39900 \\ 159600 \end{array}$$ ←— Two Placeholders   4. Insert *0*'s as placeholders in the ones and tens columns. Multiply *798* by *2*.

$$\begin{array}{r} 1\ 1 \\ 44 \\ 798 \\ \times\ \ \ 251 \\ \hline 798 \\ 39900 \\ 159600 \\ \hline 200298 \end{array}$$ 5. Add the columns.

Note: See Box 1-5 for shortcuts to multiplying numbers with trailing zeros.

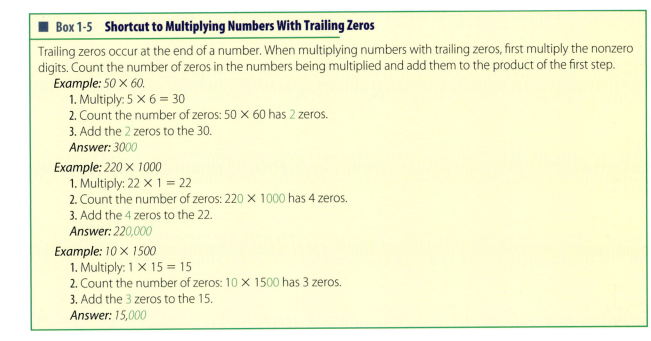

■ **Box 1-5** **Shortcut to Multiplying Numbers With Trailing Zeros**

Trailing zeros occur at the end of a number. When multiplying numbers with trailing zeros, first multiply the nonzero digits. Count the number of zeros in the numbers being multiplied and add them to the product of the first step.

Example: 50 × 60.
  1. Multiply: 5 × 6 = 30
  2. Count the number of zeros: 50 × 60 has 2 zeros.
  3. Add the 2 zeros to the 30.
Answer: 3000

Example: 220 × 1000
  1. Multiply: 22 × 1 = 22
  2. Count the number of zeros: 220 × 1000 has 4 zeros.
  3. Add the 4 zeros to the 22.
Answer: 220,000

Example: 10 × 1500
  1. Multiply: 1 × 15 = 15
  2. Count the number of zeros: 10 × 1500 has 3 zeros.
  3. Add the 3 zeros to the 15.
Answer: 15,000

Practice Multiplying Whole Numbers

(answers on page 13)

Multiply these whole numbers.

1. 13 × 4 = _____

2. 3 × 16 = _____

3. 10 × 7 = _____

4. 57 × 3 = _____

5. 92 × 5 = _____

6. 132 × 8 = _____

7. 420 × 80 = _____

8. 300 × 21 = _____

9. 984 × 125 = _____

10. 471 × 273 = _____

Dividing Whole Numbers

Division of whole numbers may be indicated by several different signs: the division sign ÷, the slash /, the fraction bar ⁻, or the long division sign ‾. The numbers in a division problem have specific names. For example, in the problem 15 ÷ 5 = 3, 15 is the **dividend**, 5 is the **divisor**, and the answer 3 is the **quotient**. To divide whole numbers, refer to the directions in Examples 1–5.

Example 1: 42 ÷ 3

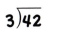

1. Draw the long division sign ‾ on your paper. Write the divisor *3* to the left of the long division sign and the dividend *42* inside the long division sign.

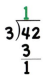

2. Divide the dividend by the divisor, working from left to right. Write the answer on top of the long division sign, keeping the digits aligned in the correct columns. In this example, *3* goes into *4* once. Write the *3* below the *4* in the dividend and subtract the numbers. This problem has a remainder of *1*.

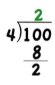

3. The remainder *1* cannot be divided equally by the divisor *3,* so the next number in the dividend (*2*) must be brought down.

$$
\begin{array}{r}
14 \\
3\overline{)42} \\
\underline{3} \\
12 \\
\underline{12} \\
0
\end{array}
$$

4. Divide the *12* by the divisor *3.* In this case, 12 ÷ 3 = 4. Write *4* on top of the long division sign, and subtract *12* from the *12.* The result is *0,* and the problem is complete: 42 ÷ 3 = 14

Example 2:   100 ÷ 4

$$
\begin{array}{r}
2 \\
4\overline{)100} \\
\underline{8} \\
2
\end{array}
$$

1. Set up the long division equation, and divide the dividend by the divisor. In this example, *4* does not go into the *1* in *100* equally. However, *4* does go into *10* twice, with a remainder of *2.*

$$
\begin{array}{r}
25 \\
4\overline{)100} \\
\underline{8} \\
20 \\
\underline{20} \\
0
\end{array}
$$

2. Bring down the next digit in *100* (in this case, a 0) because *4* does not go into *2.*

Example 3:   5,515 ÷ 250

$$
\begin{array}{r}
2 \\
250\overline{)5515} \\
\underline{500} \\
51
\end{array}
$$

1. Set up the long division equation and divide the dividend by the divisor. Notice in this example that *250* does not go into *5* or *55,* but it will go into *551* with a remainder of *51.*

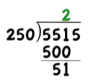

2. Bring down the next number in the dividend, the *5.* Divide *515* by *250,* writing the remainder in the row below.

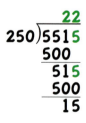

3. Observe that *15* is not divisible by the divisor *250,* and there are no more numbers to bring down from the dividend. Therefore, *5,515* cannot be divided equally by *250.* As a result, the answer (the quotient) to this problem will include a decimal, or partial number. To calculate the partial number, add a decimal point after the dividend and add a zero. Add a decimal point to the quotient as well to signal the beginning of the decimal answer.

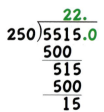

> ■ **Box 1-6 Shortcut to Dividing Numbers With Trailing Zeros**
>
> When the divisor and the dividend end with one or more zeros, the equation can be reduced to make it smaller and more manageable. Simply cancel the same number of zeros from the divisor and dividend.
>   *Example:* $6,000 \div 500 = 60 \div 5 = 12$
>   *Example:* $10,000 \div 1,000 = 10 \div 1 = 10$

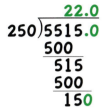

4. Bring down the zero to the remainder, and again try to divide the remainder by the divisor.

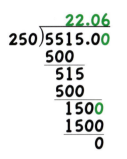

5. Notice that *150* is still too small to be divided by *250*. Add another zero to the dividend, and bring it down to the remainder. Divide the remainder by the divisor $1500 \div 250 = 6$. This step is the end of the calculation. See Box 1-6.

Note: Occasionally, division answers result in repeating decimals, such as 2.313131.... The numbers 31 repeat themselves over and over again. In this case, write the number this way: $2.\overline{31}$. The bar over the 3 and 1 indicates that this sequence of numbers repeats itself indefinitely.

Practice Dividing Whole Numbers

(answers on page 13)

Divide these whole numbers.

1. $36 \div 6 =$ _____

2. $63 \div 3 =$ _____

3. $152 \div 8 =$ _____

4. $75 \div 15 =$ _____

5. $126 \div 12 =$ _____

6. $186 \div 3 =$ _____

7. $932 \div 8 =$ _____

8. $7431 \div 10 =$ _____

9. $10,500 \div 250 =$ _____

10. $16,032 \div 334 =$ _____

Key Points

1. Whole numbers include the number 0 and all positive numbers such as 1, 2, 3, and 4.
2. The addition of numbers is shown by a + sign and results in a sum.
3. The subtraction of numbers is shown by a − sign and results in a difference.
4. The multiplication of numbers is shown by a x or * sign and results in a product.
5. The division of numbers is shown by a ÷ sign, a long division sign $\overline{)}$, or a fraction bar −. The number to be divided is called the dividend. The number doing the dividing is the divisor, and the answer is the quotient.

Chapter Post-Test

(answers in Unit 4)

Add these whole numbers.

1. $8 + 2 =$ _____

2. $14 + 26 =$ _____

3. $104 + 69 =$ _____

4. $1927 + 3018 =$ _____

5. $23,529 + 7275 =$ _____

Subtract these whole numbers.

6. $9 - 7 =$ _____

7. $82 - 33 =$ _____

8. $926 - 272 =$ _____

9. $5552 - 3800 =$ _____

10. $101,736 - 75,229 =$ _____

Multiply these whole numbers.

11. $8 \times 9 =$ _____

12. $11 \times 7 =$ _____

13. $23 \times 13 =$ _____

14. $68 \times 21 =$ _____

15. $190 \times 32 =$ _____

Divide these whole numbers.

16. $6 \div 3 =$ _____

17. $21 \div 7 =$ _____

18. $76 \div 2 =$ _____

19. $150 \div 15 =$ _____

20. $1872 \div 36 =$ _____

Answers to Practice Questions

Adding Whole Numbers

1.
```
    1
    3
  + 8
  ────
   11
```

2.
```
    2
 + 51
 ────
   53
```

3.
```
   12
 + 36
 ────
   48
```

4.
```
   11
   99
+ 171
─────
  270
```

5.
```
  132
+ 837
─────
  969
```

6.
```
  111
 6386
+1927
─────
 8313
```

7.
```
   11
  928
+ 385
+  73
─────
 1386
```

8.
```
  111
   17
+ 839
+2893
─────
 3749
```

9.
```
  1 2
    4
 +  29
 + 738
 +8302
 ─────
  9073
```

Subtracting Whole Numbers

1.
```
    7
  - 3
  ───
    4
```

2.
```
   11
   2̸1
 - 17
 ────
    4
```

3.
```
   39
 - 24
 ────
   15
```

4.
```
   76
 - 51
 ────
   25
```

5.
```
  3 9 1
   4̸0̸2̸
 - 184
 ─────
   218
```

6.
```
    1
  8 2 1
   9̸3̸6̸
  - 688
  ─────
    248
```

7.
```
   8 1
  2̸9̸57
 -  562
 ──────
   2395
```

8.
```
    1
  7 0 1
  8̸1̸26
 - 2953
 ──────
   5173
```

9.
```
  0 9 9 9 1
  1̸0̸0̸0̸3
  - 9255
  ──────
     748
```

Multiplying Whole Numbers

1.
```
    1
   13
 ×  4
 ────
   52
```

2.
```
    1
   16
 ×  3
 ────
   48
```

3.
```
   10
 ×  7
 ────
   70
```

4.
```
    2
   57
 ×  3
 ────
  171
```

5.
```
    1
   92
 ×  5
 ────
  460
```

6.
```
   21
  132
 ×  8
 ─────
 1056
```

7.
```
     1
   420
 ×  80
 ─────
 33600
```

8.
```
   300
 ×  21
 ─────
  6300
```

9.
```
      1
    4 2
    984
 ×  125
 ──────
   4920
  19680
  98400
 ───────
 123000
```

Dividing Whole Numbers

1.
```
      6
   6)36
     36
     ──
      0
```

2.
```
     21
   3)63
     6
     ──
     03
      3
     ──
      0
```

3.
```
     19
   8)152
     8
     ──
     72
     72
     ──
      0
```

4.
```
      5
   15)75
      75
      ──
       0
```

5.
```
      10.5
   12)126.0
      12
      ───
       060
        60
       ───
         0
```

6.
```
      62
   3)186
     18
     ──
      06
       6
      ──
       0
```

13

Answers to Practice Questions—cont'd

Adding Whole Numbers	Subtracting Whole Numbers	Multiplying Whole Numbers	Dividing Whole Numbers

Adding Whole Numbers

10.
```
  1 111
   93756
+ 280655
  374411
```

Subtracting Whole Numbers

10.
```
   71 61
  48 3276
- 319028
  164248
```

Multiplying Whole Numbers

10.
```
      1
      4
      2
    471
x   273
   1413
  32970
  94200
 128583
```

Dividing Whole Numbers

7.
```
      116.5
   8)932.0
     8
     13
      8
     52
     48
      40
      40
       0
```

8.
```
      743.1
  10)7431.0
     70
     43
     40
      31
      30
      10
      10
       0
```

9.
```
        42
  250)10500
     1000
      500
      500
        0
```

10.
```
        48
  334)16032
     1336
     2672
     2672
        0
```

Glossary

Common denominator: A number that may be evenly divided by all denominators in a set of fractions.

Denominator: The bottom number in a fraction. The denominator represents the total number of parts in the whole.

Factors: Numbers that are multiplied to make another number.

Fraction: A quantity that is a part of a whole number.

Improper fraction: A fraction with a numerator that is greater than or equal to the denominator.

Mixed fraction: A numerical expression that contains both a whole number and a fraction.

Numerator: The top number in a fraction. The numerator represents the number of parts of a whole.

Proper fraction: A fraction with a numerator that is less than the denominator.

Objectives

After completing this chapter, the learner will be able to—
1. Define *fraction*.
2. Describe the various types of fractions.
3. Reduce a fraction to its lowest terms.
4. Add fractions.
5. Subtract fractions.
6. Multiply fractions.
7. Divide fractions.

Types of Fractions

A **fraction** describes a quantity that is part of a whole. For example, one piece of a pie that is cut into 8 separate pieces can be denoted by the fraction $\frac{1}{8}$ (see Figure 2-1). One month is $\frac{1}{12}$ of a year. One penny is $\frac{1}{100}$ of a dollar. See Box 2-1 for different types of fractions.

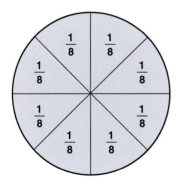

Figure 2-1 If you took one piece of this pie, you would have ⅛ of a pie, leaving the remaining ⅞ of the pie.

■ **Box 2-1 Types of Fractions**

Proper Fraction
A fraction with a numerator that is less than the denominator. The value of a proper fraction is less than 1.

Examples: $\frac{1}{2}, \frac{3}{5}, \frac{1}{20}, \frac{130}{137}, \ldots$

Improper Fraction
A fraction with a numerator that is equal to or greater than the denominator. The value of an improper fraction is greater than or equal to 1.

Examples: $\frac{5}{2}, \frac{11}{3}, \frac{101}{100}, \frac{4}{4}, \ldots$

Mixed Fraction
A fraction that has both whole numbers and fractions.

Examples: $1\frac{1}{2}, 8\frac{2}{3}, 10\frac{9}{10}, 125\frac{7}{8}, \ldots$

Fractions are written with the **numerator** on top and the **denominator** on the bottom.

$$\frac{\text{numerator}}{\text{denominator}}$$

The numerator corresponds to the available number of pieces of the whole. The denominator represents the total number of pieces that the whole is divided into.

Reducing Fractions to the Lowest Terms

When a fraction is written in the smallest numbers possible, it has been reduced to its lowest terms.

Note: If the numerator and denominator are even numbers, both may be reduced by the number 2.

Example 1: Reduce $\frac{10}{30}$ to the lowest terms.

1. Find the greatest common number (called a **factor**) that divides evenly into both the numerator and denominator. In this case, the greatest possible factor that can be divided evenly into both *10* and *30* is *10*. Note that *10* and *30* can also be evenly divided by *2* and *5*. That is, *2* and *5* may be used to reduce the fraction $\frac{10}{30}$, but additional steps would then be needed to reach the lowest terms.

$$\frac{10 \div 10}{30 \div 10} = \frac{1}{3}$$

2. Divide the numerator and denominator by the greatest common factor, *10*.

3. The fraction $\frac{1}{3}$ cannot be reduced further, so it is in the lowest terms.

Example 2: Reduce $\frac{150}{375}$ to the lowest terms.

1. Find a common factor. Both *150* and *375* are evenly divisible by *5, 15, 25,* and *75*. Since *75* is the greatest common factor, use it to reduce the fraction.

$$\frac{150 \div 75}{375 \div 75} = \frac{2}{5}$$

2. Divide the numerator and denominator by *75*.

3. The fraction $\frac{2}{5}$ cannot be reduced further, so it is in the lowest terms.

Example 3: Reduce $\frac{31}{56}$ to the lowest terms.

Since *31* is not divisible by any numbers other than *1* and *31*, and *56* cannot be evenly divided by *31*, the fraction $\frac{31}{56}$ is already in the lowest terms.

Practice Reducing Fractions

(answers on page 29)

Reduce these fractions to the lowest terms.

1. $\frac{14}{16} =$ _____

2. $\frac{25}{50} =$ _____

3. $\frac{4}{6} =$ _____

4. $\frac{5}{15} =$ _____

5. $\frac{3}{5} =$ _____

6. $\frac{16}{24} =$ _____

7. $\frac{17}{51} =$ _____

8. $\frac{100}{1000} =$ _____

9. $\frac{26}{39} =$ _____

10. $\frac{550}{750} =$ _____

Adding Fractions

Adding fractions may involve several steps, especially if the denominators are different or if one of the fractions is a mixed fraction.

Adding Fractions With Identical Denominators

To add fractions with identical denominators, follow the directions in Examples 1 and 2.

Example 1: $\frac{1}{4} + \frac{1}{4}$

$\frac{1 + 1}{4} = \frac{2}{4}$ 1. Add the numerators. The common denominator is *4*.

$\frac{2 \div 2}{4 \div 2} = \frac{1}{2}$ 2. Reduce the resulting fraction to the lowest terms.

Example 2: $\frac{3}{8} + \frac{5}{8}$

$\frac{3 + 5}{8} = \frac{8}{8}$ 1. Add the numerators.

$\frac{8 \div 8}{8 \div 8} = \frac{1}{1} = 1$ 2. Reduce the fraction to the lowest terms. The greatest common factor is *8*. Divide the numerator and denominator by *8*.

Adding Fractions With Different Denominators

Adding fractions with different denominators involves "raising" fractions to higher terms in order to have a **common denominator**, a number that can be divided evenly by all denominators in a set of fractions. After a common denominator has been determined, the fractions can be added and reduced to the lowest terms.

Example 1: $\frac{2}{7} + \frac{1}{4}$

To find the common denominator for $\frac{2}{7}$ and $\frac{1}{4}$:

$$\frac{2}{7} = \frac{2 \times 4}{7 \times 4} = \frac{8}{28}$$

1. Multiply the numerator and denominator by 4 (the denominator of $\frac{1}{4}$).

   The fraction $\frac{2}{7}$ is equivalent to $\frac{8}{28}$.

$$\frac{1}{4} = \frac{1 \times 7}{4 \times 7} = \frac{7}{28}$$

2. Multiply the numerator and denominator of $\frac{1}{4}$ by 7, (the denominator of $\frac{2}{7}$).

   The fraction $\frac{1}{4}$ is equivalent to $\frac{7}{28}$.

$$\frac{8 + 7}{28} = \frac{15}{28}$$

3. Add $\frac{8}{28}$ and $\frac{7}{28}$.

4. Reduce the resulting fraction to the lowest terms. The fraction $\frac{15}{28}$ cannot be reduced further, so it is in the lowest terms.

Example 2: $\frac{1}{3} + \frac{3}{8}$

To find the common denominator for $\frac{1}{3}$ and $\frac{3}{8}$:

$$\frac{1 \times 8}{3 \times 8} = \frac{8}{24}$$

1. Multiply the numerator and denominator of $\frac{1}{3}$ by 8 (the denominator of $\frac{3}{8}$).

$$\frac{3 \times 3}{8 \times 3} = \frac{9}{24}$$

2. Multiply the numerator and denominator of $\frac{3}{8}$ by 3 (the denominator of $\frac{1}{3}$).

   The common denominator of $\frac{1}{3}$ and $\frac{3}{8}$ is 24.

$$\frac{8 + 9}{24} = \frac{17}{24}$$

3. Add $\frac{8}{24}$ and $\frac{9}{24}$.

4. Reduce the resulting fraction to the lowest terms. The fraction $\frac{17}{24}$ cannot be reduced further.

Adding Mixed Fractions

Mixed fractions have both whole numbers and fractions. Thus, adding them requires several steps. To add mixed fractions, follow the directions in Examples 1 and 2.

Example 1: $1\frac{2}{3} + 2\frac{1}{5}$

$1 + 2 = 3$

1. Add the whole numbers together.

$\frac{2}{3} = \frac{2 \times 5}{3 \times 5} = \frac{10}{15}$

$\frac{1}{5} = \frac{1 \times 3}{5 \times 3} = \frac{3}{15}$

2. Find the common denominator for $\frac{2}{3}$ and $\frac{1}{5}$ (as described in the sections above). Raise each fraction to higher terms using the common denominator *15*.

$\frac{10 + 3}{15} = \frac{13}{15}$

3. Add the fractions $\frac{10}{15}$ and $\frac{3}{15}$.

4. Reduce $\frac{13}{15}$ to the lowest terms. The fraction $\frac{13}{15}$ cannot be reduced further, so it is in the lowest terms.

$3 + \frac{13}{15} = 3\frac{13}{15}$

5. Add the whole number from step 1 and the fraction calculated in step 4.

Example 2: $10\frac{3}{4} + 8\frac{5}{6}$

$10 + 8 = 18$

1. Add the whole numbers.

$\frac{3}{4} = \frac{3 \times 3}{4 \times 3} = \frac{9}{12}$

$\frac{5}{6} = \frac{5 \times 2}{6 \times 2} = \frac{10}{12}$

2. Find the common denominator for $\frac{3}{4}$ and $\frac{5}{6}$. The lowest common denominator for *4* and *6* is *12*. Raise each fraction to higher terms using the common denominator *12*.

$\frac{9 + 10}{12} = \frac{19}{12}$

3. Add the fractions $\frac{9}{12}$ and $\frac{10}{12}$.

4. Reduce to the lowest terms. The improper fraction $\frac{19}{12}$ can be reduced to $1\frac{7}{12}$.

$18 + 1\frac{7}{12} = 19\frac{7}{12}$

5. Add the whole number from step 1 to the mixed fraction calculated in step 4.

Note: If one denominator in a pair of fractions is a factor of the other denominator, use the greater denominator as the common denominator.

Example 3: $2\frac{1}{2} + 3\frac{3}{4}$

In this example, the denominator of the first fraction is a factor of the denominator of the second fraction. Since 2 is a factor of 4, use *4* as the common denominator in this example.

2 + 3 = 5

1. Add the whole numbers.

$$\frac{1}{2} = \frac{1 \times 2}{2 \times 2} = \frac{2}{4}$$

2. Raise the fraction $\frac{1}{2}$ to higher terms using *4* as the common denominator.

$$\frac{2 + 3}{4} = \frac{5}{4}$$

3. Add the fractions $\frac{2}{4}$ and $\frac{3}{4}$.

$$\frac{5}{4} = 1\frac{1}{4}$$

4. Reduce the improper fraction $\frac{5}{4}$ to the lowest terms.

$$5 + 1\frac{1}{4} = 6\frac{1}{4}$$

5. Add the whole number from step 1 to the mixed fraction calculated in step 4.

Practice Adding Fractions

(answers on page 30)

Add these fractions.

1. $\frac{1}{4} + \frac{3}{4} =$ _____

2. $3\frac{9}{10} + 7\frac{1}{10} =$ _____

3. $\frac{6}{7} + \frac{4}{9} =$ _____

4. $\frac{11}{12} + \frac{1}{2} =$ _____

5. $\frac{5}{6} + \frac{17}{18} =$ _____

6. $\frac{2}{5} + \frac{5}{8} =$ _____

7. $1\frac{1}{3} + 2\frac{14}{15} =$ _____

8. $\frac{29}{30} + 2\frac{1}{15} =$ _____

9. $10\frac{8}{22} + 6\frac{9}{11} =$ _____

10. $2\frac{11}{14} + 1\frac{39}{42} =$ _____

Subtracting Fractions

The process of subtracting fractions depends on the denominators in the fractions (are they identical or different) and on whether the fractions are mixed.

Subtracting Fractions With Identical Denominators

To subtract fractions with identical denominators, follow the directions in Examples 1 and 2.

Example 1: $\frac{5}{8} - \frac{3}{8}$

$$\frac{5 - 3}{8} = \frac{2}{8}$$

1. Subtract the smaller fraction from the larger fraction.

$$\frac{2}{8} = \frac{2 \div 2}{8 \div 2} = \frac{1}{4}$$

2. Reduce $\frac{2}{8}$ to the lowest terms.

Example 2: $\frac{13}{16} - \frac{7}{16}$

$$\frac{13 - 7}{16} = \frac{6}{16}$$

1. Subtract the smaller fraction from the larger fraction.

$$\frac{6}{16} = \frac{6 \div 2}{16 \div 2} = \frac{3}{8}$$

2. Reduce $\frac{6}{16}$ to the lowest terms.

Subtracting Fractions With Different Denominators

Subtracting fractions and adding fractions with different denominators require similar steps. To subtract, follow the directions in Examples 1 and 2.

Example 1: $\frac{4}{5} - \frac{3}{7}$

To find the common denominator for $\frac{4}{5}$ and $\frac{3}{7}$:

$$\frac{4 \times 7}{5 \times 7} = \frac{28}{35}$$

1. Multiply the numerator and denominator of $\frac{4}{5}$ by 7 (the denominator of $\frac{3}{7}$).

$$\frac{3 \times 5}{7 \times 5} = \frac{15}{35}$$

2. Multiply the numerator and denominator of $\frac{3}{7}$ by 5 (the denominator of $\frac{4}{5}$).

$$\frac{28 - 15}{35} = \frac{13}{35}$$

3. Subtract $\frac{15}{35}$ from $\frac{28}{35}$.

4. Reduce to the lowest terms. The fraction $\frac{13}{35}$ cannot be reduced further.

Example 2: $\frac{15}{16} - \frac{7}{8}$

$\frac{7 \times 2}{8 \times 2} = \frac{14}{16}$

1. Find the common denominator for $\frac{15}{16}$ and $\frac{7}{8}$. In this case, *16* is the common denominator for these fractions because *16* is evenly divisible by *8*. Therefore, only $\frac{7}{8}$ needs to be raised to higher terms. Multiply the numerator and denominator of $\frac{7}{8}$ by *2*.

$\frac{15 - 14}{16} = \frac{1}{16}$

2. Subtract $\frac{14}{16}$ from $\frac{15}{16}$.

3. Reduce to the lowest terms. The fraction $\frac{1}{16}$ cannot be reduced further, so it is in the lowest terms.

Subtracting Mixed Fractions

To subtract mixed fractions, follow the directions in Examples 1 and 2.

Example 1: $4\frac{3}{4} - 2\frac{5}{8}$

$\frac{(4 \times 4) + 3}{4} = \frac{16 + 3}{4} = \frac{19}{4}$

$\frac{(8 \times 2) + 5}{8} = \frac{16 + 5}{8} = \frac{21}{8}$

1. Convert $4\frac{3}{4}$ and $2\frac{5}{8}$ to improper fractions:

   1a. Multiply the denominator of each fraction by its whole number.
   1b. Add the numerator.
   1c. Place this sum over the denominator.

$\frac{19}{4} = \frac{19 \times 2}{4 \times 2} = \frac{38}{8}$

2. Find the common denominator for $\frac{19}{4}$ and $\frac{21}{8}$. In this case, *8* is the common denominator because *4* goes into *8* twice. Convert $\frac{19}{4}$ into a fraction with a denominator of *8*.

$\frac{38 - 21}{8} = \frac{17}{8}$

3. Subtract $\frac{21}{8}$ from $\frac{38}{8}$.

$\frac{17}{8} = 2\frac{1}{8}$

4. Reduce $\frac{17}{8}$ to the lowest terms.

Example 2: $21\frac{23}{25} - 14\frac{83}{100}$

$\frac{(25 \times 21) + 23}{25} = \frac{525 + 23}{25} = \frac{548}{25}$

$\frac{(100 \times 14) + 83}{100} = \frac{1400 + 83}{100} = \frac{1483}{100}$

1. Convert $21\frac{23}{25}$ and $14\frac{83}{100}$ to improper fractions.

$$\frac{548}{25} = \frac{548 \times 4}{25 \times 4} = \frac{2192}{100}$$

2. Find the common denominator for $\frac{548}{25}$ and $\frac{1483}{100}$. In this case, *100* is the common denominator because *25* goes into *100* four times. Convert $\frac{548}{25}$ to a fraction with a denominator of *100*.

$$\frac{2192}{100} - \frac{1483}{100} = \frac{709}{100}$$

3. Subtract $\frac{1483}{100}$ from $\frac{2192}{100}$.

$$\frac{709}{100} = 7\frac{9}{100}$$

4. Reduce $\frac{709}{100}$ to the lowest terms.

Practice Subtracting Fractions
(answers on page 31)

Subtract these fractions.

1. $\frac{7}{9} - \frac{5}{9} = $ _____

2. $1\frac{3}{11} - \frac{1}{11} = $ _____

3. $\frac{1}{2} - \frac{1}{3} = $ _____

4. $\frac{23}{25} - \frac{3}{5} = $ _____

5. $1 - \frac{1}{3} = $ _____

6. $5\frac{2}{9} - 2\frac{8}{9} = $ _____

7. $10\frac{23}{26} - 9\frac{17}{52} = $ _____

8. $2\frac{14}{21} - 1\frac{1}{4} = $ _____

9. $3\frac{2}{17} - 2 = $ _____

10. $15\frac{1}{6} - 15\frac{1}{8} = $ _____

Multiplying Fractions

To multiply fractions, follow the directions in Examples 1–4.

Example 1: $\frac{1}{3} \times \frac{1}{3}$

$$\frac{1 \times 1}{3 \times 3} = \frac{1}{9}$$

1. Multiply the numerators, then multiply the denominators.

2. Reduce to the lowest terms. The fraction $\frac{1}{9}$ cannot be reduced further, so it is in the lowest terms.

Note: $\frac{1}{9}$ is smaller than the original fraction, $\frac{1}{3}$. Multiplying fractions results in a number that is smaller than either of the original fractions. See Figures 2-2 and 2-3.

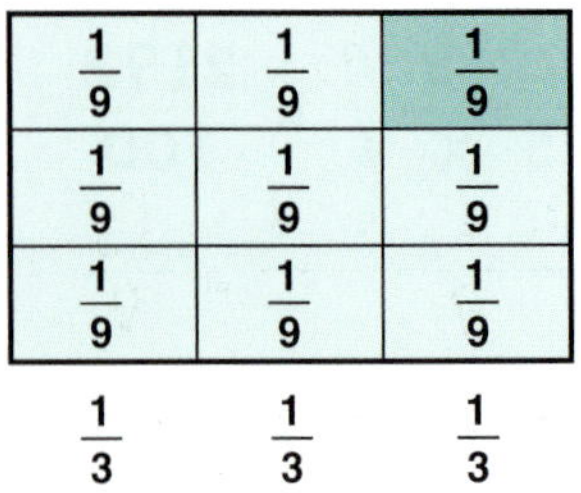
1/9 1/9 1/9
1/9 1/9 1/9
1/9 1/9 1/9
1/3 1/3 1/3

Figure 2-2 One square of this block represents ⅓ of ⅓, or ⅑.

Example 2: $\frac{4}{5} \times \frac{2}{5}$

$$\frac{4 \times 2}{5 \times 5} = \frac{8}{25}$$

1. Multiply the numerators and denominators of each fraction.

2. Reduce to the lowest terms. The fraction $\frac{8}{25}$ cannot be reduced further, so it is in the lowest terms.

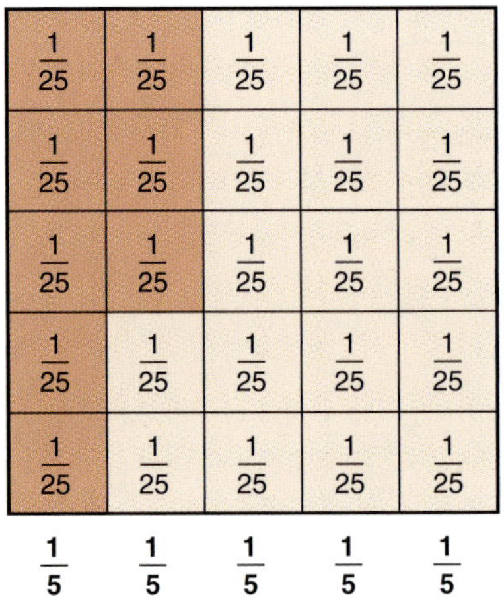
1/25 1/25 1/25 1/25 1/25
1/25 1/25 1/25 1/25 1/25
1/25 1/25 1/25 1/25 1/25
1/25 1/25 1/25 1/25 1/25
1/25 1/25 1/25 1/25 1/25
1/5 1/5 1/5 1/5 1/5

Figure 2-3 Eight squares of this block represents ⅘ of ⅖, or 8⁄25.

Example 3: $2\frac{2}{3} \times \frac{7}{10}$

$$2\frac{2}{3} = \frac{(3 \times 2) + 2}{3} = \frac{8}{3}$$

1. In this example, a mixed fraction is multiplied by a simple fraction. Convert the mixed number to an improper fraction before multiplying.

$$\frac{8}{3} \times \frac{7}{10} = \frac{56}{30}$$

2. Multiply the numerators and denominators of each fraction.

$$\frac{56}{30} = 1\frac{26}{30} = 1\frac{13}{15}$$

3. Reduce to the lowest terms.

Example 4: $1\frac{4}{9} \times 3\frac{1}{7}$

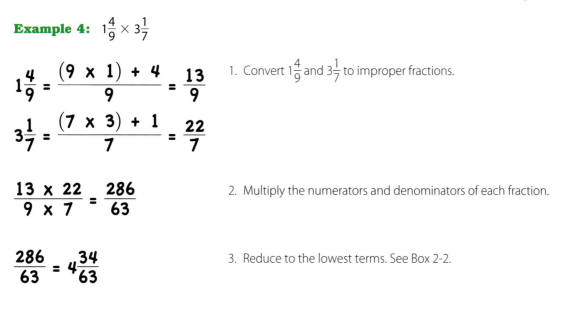

$1\frac{4}{9} = \dfrac{(9 \times 1) + 4}{9} = \dfrac{13}{9}$

$3\frac{1}{7} = \dfrac{(7 \times 3) + 1}{7} = \dfrac{22}{7}$

1. Convert $1\frac{4}{9}$ and $3\frac{1}{7}$ to improper fractions.

$\dfrac{13 \times 22}{9 \times 7} = \dfrac{286}{63}$

2. Multiply the numerators and denominators of each fraction.

$\dfrac{286}{63} = 4\frac{34}{63}$

3. Reduce to the lowest terms. See Box 2-2.

■ Box 2-2   Canceling Fractions

Canceling fractions reduces large fractions, making them easier to multiply. Find a factor that is common to both the numerator and denominator. Reduce the fraction by dividing the numerator and denominator by the common factor.

Example: $\dfrac{25}{28} \times \dfrac{1}{5} \times \dfrac{4}{7}$

Long method

$\dfrac{25}{28} \times \dfrac{1}{5} \times \dfrac{4}{7} = \dfrac{25 \times 1 \times 4}{28 \times 5 \times 7} = \dfrac{100}{980} = \dfrac{10}{98} = \dfrac{5}{49}$

Canceling method

$\dfrac{\overset{5}{\cancel{25}}}{\underset{7}{\cancel{28}}} \times \dfrac{1}{5} \times \dfrac{\overset{1}{\cancel{4}}}{7} = \dfrac{5}{7} \times \dfrac{1}{1} \times \dfrac{1}{7} = \dfrac{5}{49}$

Practice Multiplying Fractions

(answers on page 32)

Multiply these fractions.

1. $\dfrac{1}{3} \times \dfrac{1}{4} =$ _____

2. $\dfrac{3}{5} \times \dfrac{2}{3} =$ _____

3. $\dfrac{5}{7} \times \dfrac{8}{9} =$ _____

4. $\dfrac{3}{11} \times \dfrac{1}{9} =$ _____

5. $\dfrac{12}{13} \times \dfrac{1}{3} =$ _____

6. $\dfrac{2}{15} \times \dfrac{8}{13} =$ _____

7. $3\frac{4}{5} \times \dfrac{1}{2} =$ _____

8. $10\frac{3}{4} \times 5\frac{5}{8} =$ _____

9. $\dfrac{1}{5} \times \dfrac{10}{11} \times \dfrac{7}{12} =$ _____

10. $1\frac{2}{3} \times 2\frac{7}{8} \times \dfrac{1}{10} =$ _____

Dividing Fractions

Dividing fractions is like multiplying fractions, except dividing requires the extra step of inverting the divisor of one of the fractions. To divide, follow the directions in Examples 1–4.

Example 1: $\frac{3}{4} \div \frac{1}{3}$

$\frac{3}{4} \times \frac{3}{1} =$

1. Change the division sign to a multiplication sign and invert the divisor of the second fraction.

$\frac{3 \times 3}{4 \times 1} = \frac{9}{4}$

2. Multiply the numerators and denominators.

$\frac{9}{4} = 2\frac{1}{4}$

3. Reduce to the lowest terms.

Example 2: Divide $\frac{3}{10}$ by $\frac{1}{2}$.

$\frac{3}{10} \times \frac{2}{1} =$

1. Change the division sign to a multiplication sign and invert the divisor.

$\frac{3 \times 2}{10 \times 1} = \frac{6}{10}$

2. Multiply the numerators and denominators.

$\frac{6}{10} = \frac{3}{5}$

3. Reduce to the lowest terms.

Example 3: $\frac{15}{16} \div \frac{4}{9}$

$\frac{15}{16} \times \frac{9}{4} =$

1. Change the division sign into a multiplication sign and invert the divisor.

$\frac{15 \times 9}{16 \times 4} = \frac{135}{64}$

2. Multiply the numerators and denominators.

$\frac{135}{64} = 2\frac{7}{64}$

3. Reduce to the lowest terms.

Example 4: $3\frac{1}{8} \div 1\frac{5}{24}$

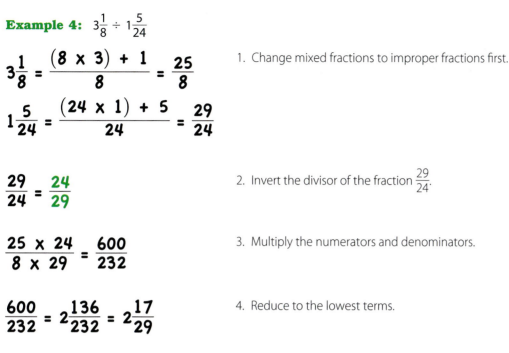

$3\frac{1}{8} = \dfrac{(8 \times 3) + 1}{8} = \dfrac{25}{8}$

1. Change mixed fractions to improper fractions first.

$1\frac{5}{24} = \dfrac{(24 \times 1) + 5}{24} = \dfrac{29}{24}$

$\dfrac{29}{24} = \dfrac{24}{29}$

2. Invert the divisor of the fraction $\frac{29}{24}$.

$\dfrac{25 \times 24}{8 \times 29} = \dfrac{600}{232}$

3. Multiply the numerators and denominators.

$\dfrac{600}{232} = 2\dfrac{136}{232} = 2\dfrac{17}{29}$

4. Reduce to the lowest terms.

Practice Dividing Fractions

(answers on page 33)

Divide these fractions.

1. $\dfrac{1}{4} \div \dfrac{1}{4} = $ _____

2. $\dfrac{6}{7} \div \dfrac{2}{3} = $ _____

3. $\dfrac{6}{11} \div \dfrac{1}{3} = $ _____

4. $\dfrac{8}{13} \div \dfrac{3}{4} = $ _____

5. $\dfrac{25}{27} \div \dfrac{3}{5} = $ _____

6. $\dfrac{73}{100} \div \dfrac{20}{31} = $ _____

7. $1 \div \dfrac{7}{8} = $ _____

8. $2\dfrac{34}{51} \div \dfrac{3}{17} = $ _____

9. $3\dfrac{5}{9} \div 1\dfrac{9}{10} = $ _____

10. $\dfrac{13}{16} \div 2 = $ _____

Key Points

1. A fraction represents parts of a whole and is written with a numerator on top and a denominator on the bottom.

2. Fractions come in three types.

   a. Proper fractions have numerators that are less than the denominators. The value of a proper fraction is less than 1.

   b. Improper fractions have numerators that are greater than or equal to the denominators. The value of an improper fraction is equal to or greater than 1.

   c. A mixed fraction contains both a whole number and a fraction.

3. Reducing a fraction to the lowest terms involves finding a factor that divides evenly into both the numerator and denominator.

4. Adding fractions requires finding a common denominator for the fractions, adding the numerators, and then reducing the result to the lowest terms.

5. Subtracting fractions requires finding a common denominator for the fractions, subtracting the smaller fraction from the larger one, and then reducing the result to the lowest terms.

6. Multiplying fractions requires multiplying the numerators of the fractions, multiplying the denominators, and then reducing the result to the lowest terms.

7. Dividing fractions requires changing the division sign to a multiplication sign, inverting the divisor, multiplying the numerators and denominators, and then reducing the result to the lowest terms.

Chapter Post-Test

(answers in Unit 4)

Reduce these fractions to the lowest terms.

1. $\frac{2}{4} = $ _____

2. $\frac{25}{40} = $ _____

3. $\frac{6}{9} = $ _____

4. $\frac{125}{100} = $ _____

5. $\frac{75}{90} = $ _____

Add these fractions.

6. $\frac{1}{3} + \frac{3}{5} = $ _____

7. $\frac{9}{10} + \frac{1}{5} = $ _____

8. $\frac{4}{9} + \frac{13}{18} = $ _____

9. $1\frac{7}{16} + 2\frac{3}{8} = $ _____

10. $\frac{4}{7} + \frac{20}{21} = $ _____

Subtract these fractions.

11. $\frac{7}{9} - \frac{2}{9} = $ _____

12. $\frac{3}{4} - \frac{1}{6} = $ _____

13. $1\frac{14}{15} - \frac{3}{5} = $ _____

14. $8\frac{2}{3} - 7\frac{5}{6} = $ _____

15. $3\frac{4}{7} - 1\frac{23}{28} = $ _____

Multiply these fractions.

16. $\frac{2}{3} \times \frac{1}{2} = $ _____

17. $\frac{5}{6} \times \frac{4}{5} = $ _____

18. $1\frac{4}{7} \times \frac{7}{9} = $ _____

19. $3\frac{6}{7} \times \frac{3}{4} = $ _____

20. $\frac{5}{8} \times 2\frac{7}{12} = $ _____

Divide these fractions.

21. $\frac{1}{2} \div \frac{1}{4} = $ _____

22. $\frac{5}{6} \div \frac{1}{3} = $ _____

23. $\frac{9}{13} \div \frac{3}{5} = $ _____

24. $1\frac{4}{7} \div \frac{1}{8} = $ _____

25. $2\frac{8}{9} \div 1\frac{2}{3} = $ _____

Answers to Practice Questions

Reducing Fractions

1. $\dfrac{14 \div 2}{16 \div 2} = \dfrac{7}{8}$

2. $\dfrac{25 \div 25}{50 \div 25} = \dfrac{1}{2}$

3. $\dfrac{4 \div 2}{6 \div 2} = \dfrac{2}{3}$

4. $\dfrac{5 \div 5}{15 \div 5} = \dfrac{1}{3}$

5. $\dfrac{3}{5}$ (This fraction is in the lowest terms.)

6. $\dfrac{16 \div 8}{24 \div 8} = \dfrac{2}{3}$

7. $\dfrac{17 \div 17}{51 \div 17} = \dfrac{1}{3}$

8. $\dfrac{100 \div 100}{1000 \div 100} = \dfrac{1}{10}$

9. $\dfrac{26 \div 13}{39 \div 13} = \dfrac{2}{3}$

10. $\dfrac{550 \div 50}{750 \div 50} = \dfrac{11}{15}$

Adding Fractions

1. $\dfrac{1 + 3}{4} = \dfrac{4}{4} = 1$

2. $3 + 7 + \dfrac{9}{10} + \dfrac{1}{10} = 3 + 7 + \dfrac{10}{10} = 11$

3. $\dfrac{6 \times 9}{7 \times 9} + \dfrac{4 \times 7}{9 \times 7} = \dfrac{54}{63} + \dfrac{28}{63} = \dfrac{82}{63} = 1\dfrac{19}{63}$

4. $\dfrac{11 \times 2}{12 \times 2} + \dfrac{1 \times 12}{2 \times 12} = \dfrac{22}{24} + \dfrac{12}{24} = \dfrac{34}{24} = 1\dfrac{5}{12}$ or

   $\dfrac{11}{12} + \dfrac{1 \times 6}{2 \times 6} = \dfrac{11}{12} + \dfrac{6}{12} = \dfrac{17}{12} = 1\dfrac{5}{12}$

5. $\dfrac{5 \times 18}{6 \times 18} + \dfrac{17 \times 6}{18 \times 6} = \dfrac{90}{108} + \dfrac{102}{108} = \dfrac{192}{108} = 1\dfrac{7}{9}$ or

   $\dfrac{5 \times 3}{6 \times 3} + \dfrac{17}{18} = \dfrac{15}{18} + \dfrac{17}{18} = \dfrac{32}{18} = 1\dfrac{7}{9}$

6. $\dfrac{2 \times 8}{5 \times 8} + \dfrac{5 \times 5}{8 \times 5} = \dfrac{16}{40} + \dfrac{25}{40} = \dfrac{41}{40} = 1\dfrac{1}{40}.$

7. $1 + 2 + \dfrac{1 \times 15}{3 \times 15} + \dfrac{14 \times 3}{15 \times 3} = 3 + \dfrac{15}{45} + \dfrac{42}{45} = 3 + \dfrac{57}{45} = 4\dfrac{12}{45} = 4\dfrac{4}{15}$ or

   $1 + 2 + \dfrac{1 \times 5}{3 \times 5} + \dfrac{14}{15} = 3 + \dfrac{5}{15} + \dfrac{14}{15} = 3 + \dfrac{19}{15} = 4\dfrac{4}{15}$

8. $2 + \dfrac{29}{30} + \dfrac{1 \times 2}{15 \times 2} = 2 + \dfrac{29}{30} + \dfrac{2}{30} = 2 + \dfrac{31}{30} = 3\dfrac{1}{30}$

9. $10 + 6 + \dfrac{8}{22} + \dfrac{9 \times 2}{11 \times 2} = 16 + \dfrac{26}{22} = 17\dfrac{4}{22} = 17\dfrac{2}{11}$

10. $2 + 1 + \dfrac{11 \times 3}{14 \times 3} + \dfrac{39}{42} = 3 + \dfrac{72}{42} = 4\dfrac{30}{42} = 4\dfrac{5}{7}$

Subtracting Fractions

1. $\dfrac{2}{9}$

2. $\dfrac{14}{11} - \dfrac{1}{11} = \dfrac{13}{11} = 1\dfrac{2}{11}$

3. $\dfrac{1 \times 3}{2 \times 3} - \dfrac{1 \times 2}{3 \times 2} = \dfrac{3}{6} - \dfrac{2}{6} = \dfrac{1}{6}$

4. $\dfrac{23}{25} - \dfrac{3 \times 5}{5 \times 5} = \dfrac{23}{25} - \dfrac{15}{25} = \dfrac{8}{25}$

5. $\dfrac{1 \times 3}{1 \times 3} - \dfrac{1}{3} = \dfrac{3}{3} - \dfrac{1}{3} = \dfrac{2}{3}$

6. $\dfrac{47}{9} - \dfrac{26}{9} = \dfrac{21}{9} = 2\dfrac{3}{9} = 2\dfrac{1}{3}$

7. $\dfrac{283}{26} - \dfrac{485}{52} = \dfrac{283 \times 2}{26 \times 2} - \dfrac{485}{52} = \dfrac{566}{52} - \dfrac{485}{52} = \dfrac{81}{52} = 1\dfrac{29}{52}$

8. $\dfrac{56}{21} - \dfrac{5}{4} = \dfrac{56 \times 4}{21 \times 4} - \dfrac{5 \times 21}{4 \times 21} = \dfrac{224}{84} - \dfrac{105}{84} = \dfrac{119}{84} = 1\dfrac{35}{84} = 1\dfrac{5}{12}$

9. $\dfrac{53}{17} - \dfrac{34}{17} = \dfrac{19}{17} = 1\dfrac{2}{17}$

10. $\dfrac{91}{6} - \dfrac{121}{8} = \dfrac{91 \times 8}{6 \times 8} - \dfrac{121 \times 6}{8 \times 6} = \dfrac{728}{48} - \dfrac{726}{48} = \dfrac{2}{48} = \dfrac{1}{24}$

Multiplying Fractions

1. $\dfrac{1 \times 1}{3 \times 4} = \dfrac{1}{12}$

2. $\dfrac{3 \times 2}{5 \times 3} = \dfrac{6}{15} = \dfrac{2}{5}$

3. $\dfrac{5 \times 8}{7 \times 9} = \dfrac{40}{63}$

4. $\dfrac{3 \times 1}{11 \times 9} = \dfrac{3}{99} = \dfrac{1}{33}$

5. $\dfrac{12 \times 1}{13 \times 3} = \dfrac{12}{39} = \dfrac{4}{13}$

6. $\dfrac{2 \times 8}{15 \times 13} = \dfrac{16}{195}$

7. $\dfrac{19}{5} \times \dfrac{1}{2} = \dfrac{19 \times 1}{5 \times 2} = \dfrac{19}{10} = 1\dfrac{9}{10}$

8. $\dfrac{43}{3} \times \dfrac{45}{8} = \dfrac{43 \times 45}{4 \times 8} = \dfrac{1935}{32} = 60\dfrac{15}{32}$

9. $\dfrac{1 \times 10 \times 7}{5 \times 11 \times 12} = \dfrac{70}{660} = \dfrac{7}{66}$

10. $\dfrac{5}{3} \times \dfrac{23}{8} \times \dfrac{1}{10} = \dfrac{5 \times 23 \times 1}{3 \times 8 \times 10} = \dfrac{115}{240} = \dfrac{23}{48}$

Dividing Fractions

1. $\dfrac{1 \times 4}{4 \times 1} = \dfrac{4}{4} = 1$

2. $\dfrac{6 \times 3}{7 \times 2} = \dfrac{18}{14} = 1\dfrac{2}{7}$ or $\dfrac{6}{7} \times \dfrac{\overset{3}{\cancel{3}}}{\underset{1}{\cancel{2}}} = \dfrac{9}{7} = 1\dfrac{2}{7}$

3. $\dfrac{6 \times 3}{11 \times 1} = \dfrac{18}{11} = 1\dfrac{7}{11}$

4. $\dfrac{8 \times 4}{13 \times 3} = \dfrac{32}{39}$

5. $\dfrac{25 \times 5}{27 \times 3} = \dfrac{125}{81} = 1\dfrac{44}{81}$

6. $\dfrac{73 \times 31}{100 \times 20} = \dfrac{2263}{2000} = 1\dfrac{263}{2000}$

7. $\dfrac{1 \times 8}{1 \times 7} = \dfrac{8}{7} = 1\dfrac{1}{7}$

8. $\dfrac{136 \times 17}{51 \times 3} = \dfrac{2312}{153} = 15\dfrac{1}{9}$ or $\dfrac{136}{\underset{3}{\cancel{51}}} \times \dfrac{\overset{1}{\cancel{17}}}{3} = \dfrac{136}{3} \times \dfrac{1}{3} = \dfrac{136}{9} = 15\dfrac{1}{9}$

9. $\dfrac{32 \times 10}{9 \times 19} = \dfrac{320}{171} = 1\dfrac{149}{171}$

10. $\dfrac{13 \times 1}{16 \times 2} = \dfrac{13}{32}$

Chapter 3
Decimals and Percents

⟲ Glossary

Decimal: A number that represents a fraction of a number. A combination of a whole number and a fraction of a number that is separated by the decimal point.
Percent: A number that is a fraction of 100, expressed by the % symbol.
Place value: The value of a digit based upon its position in a number.

Objectives

After completing this chapter, the learner will be able to—
1. Define *decimal*.
2. Round decimals.
3. Add decimals.
4. Subtract decimals.
5. Multiply decimals.
6. Divide decimals.
7. Convert between fractions and decimals.

Decimal Numbers

Decimals, like fractions, are an alternative method of writing numbers that are less than one. Like whole numbers, decimal numbers have **place value**. The place value of a decimal is expressed as ten**ths**, hundred**ths**, thousand**ths**, ten thousand**ths**, and so on. See Figure 3-1 and Box 3-1.

Example 1:   *1.3* is equivalent to $1\frac{3}{10}$.

Example 2:   *0.85* is equivalent to $\frac{85}{100}$, which can be reduced to $\frac{17}{20}$.

Example 3:   *342.8068* is equivalent to $342\frac{8068}{10,000}$, which can be reduced to $342\frac{2017}{2500}$.

Hundreds	Tens	Ones	Tenths	Hundredths	Thousandths	Ten thousandths
4	8	3 .	9	2	7	8

Figure 3-1 The place value of the decimal number 483.9278 is as shown.

■ Box 3-1   Decimal/Fraction Equivalents

$$0.1 = \frac{1}{10}$$

$$0.01 = \frac{1}{100}$$

$$0.001 = \frac{1}{1000}$$

$$0.0001 = \frac{1}{10,000}$$

$$0.00001 = \frac{1}{100,000}$$

$$0.000001 = \frac{1}{1,000,000}$$

Rounding Decimal Numbers

Rounding is a method of approximating the value of a number. The fraction portion of the decimal number is most commonly rounded. How far to round *to* depends upon the degree of accuracy needed. For example, a person may weigh 182.583 pounds. However, we rarely need that accurate of a weight. An approximation (or estimate) of that person's weight is 182.6 pounds (rounding to the tenth of a pound) or 183 pounds (rounding to the nearest whole pound).

To round decimal numbers, follow the directions in Examples 1–5.

Example 1:   Round 1.4 to the nearest whole number.

1.4   1. Find the decimal place to round to—in this example, the whole number—and underline that number. In this example, the nearest whole number in *1.4* is *1*; underline the *1*.

1   2. Look at the number to the right of the underlined number. If the number is 5 or greater, round up. If the number is less than 5, round down. In this example, the number to the right of *1* is *4*, which is less than *5*. Round down to *1*.

For Examples 2–5, refer to the directions in Example 1.

Example 2:   Round 9.9 to the nearest whole number.

9.9   1. Find and underline the whole number, which is *9*.

10   2. The number to the right of the underlined *9* is *9*; round up to *10*.

Example 3:   Round 23.35 to the nearest tenth.

23.35   1. Find and underline the number in the tenths place, which is *3*.

23.4   2. The number to the right of the underlined *3* is *5*; round up to *23.4*.

Example 4: Round 4.7382 to the nearest hundredth.

4.73̲82   1. Find and underline the number in the hundredths place.

4.74   2. The number to the right of the underlined *3* is *8*; round up to *4.74.*

> **Note:** The 2 in the ten-thousandths place is disregarded in Example 2 because it is not *immediately* to the right of the 3 (the hundredths place).

Example 5: Round 632.97 to the nearest tenth.

632.9̲7   1. Find and underline the number in the tenths place, which is *9.*

633   2. The number to the right of the underlined number is *7;* round up to *633.*

> **Note:** When the number to be rounded up is a *9,* change the *9* to *0* and add *1* to the number immediately to the left. In this example, the number to the immediate left is a whole number. Therefore, *632.97* is rounded to *633.*

Practice Rounding Decimal Numbers

(answers on page 51)

Round these decimals as indicated.

1. Round 4.8 to the nearest whole number. _____

2. Round 12.1 to the nearest whole number. _____

3. Round 7.478 to the nearest whole number. _____

4. Round 83.381 to the nearest tenth. _____

5. Round 9.01 to the nearest tenth. _____

6. Round 0.054 to the nearest tenth. _____

7. Round 93.999 to the nearest hundredth. _____

8. Round 221.332 to the nearest hundredth. _____

9. Round 82.8126 to the nearest thousandth. _____

10. Round 101.69824 to the nearest ten-thousandth. _____

Adding Decimal Numbers

Adding decimals is similar to adding whole numbers; be certain to line up the numbers properly. To add decimal numbers, follow the directions in Examples 1–5.

Example 1: 4.8 + 7.9

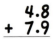

1. Write the numbers to be added in a column with the decimal points aligned.

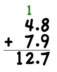

2. Working from right to left, add the numbers in the far right (ones) column first, carrying any digits greater than 10.

For Examples 2–5, refer to the directions in Example 1.

Example 2:   0.398 + 2.1

Note: Add trailing zeros where needed to align the decimal points correctly.

$$
\begin{array}{r}
0.398 \\
+\ 2.100 \\
\hline
2.498
\end{array}
$$

Example 3:   100.3856 + 0.67

$$
\begin{array}{r}
{}^{1}\ {}^{1} \\
100.3856 \\
+\ \ \ 0.6700 \\
\hline
101.0556
\end{array}
$$

Example 4:   25 + 0.001 + 8.3

$$
\begin{array}{r}
{}^{1} \\
25.000 \\
+\ 0.001 \\
+\ 8.300 \\
\hline
33.301
\end{array}
$$

Example 5:   0.50025 + 12.3 + 1.37 + 224.836

$$
\begin{array}{r}
{}^{2}\ {}^{1} \\
0.50025 \\
+\ \ \ \ 12.30000 \\
+\ \ \ \ \ 1.37000 \\
+\ 224.83600 \\
\hline
239.00625
\end{array}
$$

Practice Adding Decimal Numbers

(answers on page 51)

Add these decimals.

1. 0.2 + 4.6 = _____

2. 9.1 + 2.5 = _____

3. 8.5 + 2 = _____

4. 10.79 + 7.3 = _____

5. 53.005 + 14.7 = _____

6. 65.02 + 21.38 = _____

7. 75.902 + 29.10 = _____

8. 3.85 + 231.4 = _____

9. 0.78 + 1.2 + 3 = _____

10. 43.846 + 56.2 + 8.2 = _____

Subtracting Decimal Numbers

To subtract decimal numbers, follow the directions in Examples 1–5.

Example 1: 10.5 – 3.2

$$\begin{array}{r} 10.5 \\ -\ 3.2 \end{array}$$

1. Write the numbers to be subtracted in a column with the larger number on top, aligning the decimal points.

$$\begin{array}{r} 10.5 \\ -\ 3.2 \\ \hline 7.3 \end{array}$$

2. Starting with the far right column and working to the left, subtract the numbers.

For Examples 2–5, refer to the directions in Example 1.

Example 2: 9.4 – 2.7

Note: In this example, the needed digits are borrowed from the column to the left.

$$\begin{array}{r} \overset{8\ \ 1}{9.4} \\ -\ 2.7 \\ \hline 6.7 \end{array}$$

Example 3: 0.084 – 0.03

Note: To align numbers easily, add trailing zeros.

$$\begin{array}{r} 0.084 \\ -\ 0.030 \\ \hline 0.054 \end{array}$$

Example 4: 100.649 – 38.75

$$\begin{array}{r} \overset{\quad 1}{\overset{0\,9\,9\ 5\,1}{100.649}} \\ -\ 38.750 \\ \hline 61.899 \end{array}$$

Example 5: 293.1 – 0.956

$$\begin{array}{r} \overset{\quad 1}{\overset{2\ 0\,9\,1}{293.100}} \\ -\ 0.956 \\ \hline 292.144 \end{array}$$

Practice Subtracting Decimal Numbers

(answers on page 52)

Subtract these decimals.

1. 7.9 – 4.3 = _____

2. 10.3 – 9.5 = _____

3. 100.2 – 87.4 = _____

4. 3.05 – 1.09 = _____

5. 12.28 – 2.49 = _____

6. 163.03 – 0.92 = _____

7. 52.295 – 33.381 = _____

8. 67.739 – 56.4 = _____

9. 82.8 – 65.323 = _____

10. 2.8367 – 1.8368 = _____

Multiplying Decimal Numbers

Example 1:   2.1 × 0.5

$$\begin{array}{r} 21 \\ \times\ \ 5 \\ \hline 105 \end{array}$$

1. Multiply the numbers, ignoring the decimal point.

1.05

2. To determine the number of decimal places in the answer, refer to the original problem. Looking at all of the numbers to be multiplied, count all of the decimal places to the right of the decimal point. In this example, notice that *2.1* has one decimal place, and *0.5* has one decimal place. Therefore, the answer has two decimal places. Insert the decimal point.

For Examples 2–5, refer to the directions in Example 1.

Example 2:   1.7 × 3.8

$$\begin{array}{r} 17 \\ \times\ 38 \\ \hline 136 \\ 510 \leftarrow \\ \hline 646 \end{array}$$

1. Multiply the numbers.

Note: Remember to add a zero when multiplying two numbers that each have two digits. For numbers with 3 digits, add 2 zeros, and so forth.

6.46

2. Insert the decimal point.

Example 3:   11.3 × 9.21

$$\begin{array}{r} 113 \\ \times\ \ 921 \\ \hline 113 \\ 2260 \\ 101700 \\ \hline 104073 \end{array}$$

1. Multiply the numbers.

104.073

2. Insert the decimal point.

Example 4:   0.009 × 7.35

$$
\begin{array}{r}
735 \\
\times\ \ 9 \\
\hline
6615
\end{array}
$$

1. Multiply the numbers.

Note: In this example, ignore the leading zeros in the first number and place the smaller number on the bottom.

0.06615
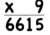
  5 4 3 2 1

2. Insert the decimal point.

Note: In this example, *0.009* has three decimal places and *7.35* has two decimal places. Therefore, the answer has five decimal places. You must add a leading zero to the 4-digit number.

Example 5:   1.501 × 10.435

$$
\begin{array}{r}
10435 \\
\times\ \ \ \ \ 1501 \\
\hline
10435 \\
000000 \\
5217500 \\
10435000 \\
\hline
15662935
\end{array}
$$

1. Multiply the numbers.

15.662935
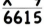
   6 5 4 3
   2 1

2. Insert the decimal point.

Practice Multiplying Decimal Numbers

(answers on page 52)

Multiply these decimals. Do not round your answers.

1. 3.5 × 2 = _____

2. 0.8 × 4.2 = _____

3. 1.6 × 1.9 = _____

4. 4.2 × 3.36 = _____

5. 10.7 × 8.1 = _____

6. 20 × 6.75 = _____

7. 0.39 × 0.56 = _____

8. 1.151 × 2.05 = _____

9. 0.755 × 6.33 = _____

10. 0.002 × 10.005 = _____

Dividing Decimal Numbers

Except for an added step or two, dividing decimal numbers is similar to dividing whole numbers. To divide decimal numbers, follow the directions in Examples 1–5.

Example 1:   1.25 ÷ 0.5

1. Set up the equation in long division format, and change the divisor to a whole number by moving the decimal point to the far right.

Note: In this example, *0.5* is the divisor (the number doing the dividing); *1.25* is the dividend (the number being divided).

$$0.5\overline{)1.25}$$

2. Count the number of spaces the divisor's decimal point moved, and move the dividend's decimal point to the right the same number of spaces.

Note: Add zeros to the end of the dividend, if needed.

$$5\overline{)1.25} = 5\overline{)12.5}$$

3. Complete the long division, aligning the decimal points.

Alert! Be certain to place the quotient's decimal point directly over the dividend's decimal point.

$$
\begin{array}{r}
2.5 \\
5\overline{)12.5} \\
\underline{10} \\
2\,5 \\
\underline{2\,5} \\
0
\end{array}
$$

For Examples 2–5, refer to the directions in Example 1.

Example 2:   6.8 ÷ 2.3

$$2.3\overline{)6.8}$$

1. Change the divisor to a whole number.

$$23\overline{)6.8} = 23\overline{)68}$$

2. Move the decimal point in the dividend.

3. Complete the long division.

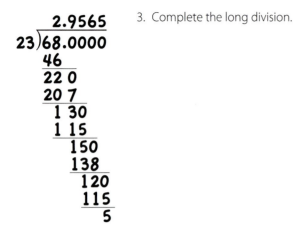

```
       2.9565
   23)68.0000
      46
      22 0
      20 7
       1 30
       1 15
         150
         138
         120
         115
           5
```

> **Note:** Zeros must be added to the dividend if the quotient is not going to be a whole number. Carry out the decimal point as far as required. In this case, the decimal point is carried to the ten-thousandths place, though we could calculate the answer to at least the millionths place.

Example 3: $24 \div 4.32$

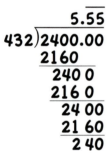

1. Change the divisor to a whole number.

2. Move the decimal point in the dividend, adding zeros as needed.

3. Complete the long division.

```
          5.55
   432)2400.00
       2160
        240 0
        216 0
         24 00
         21 60
          2 40
```

Example 4: $69.33 \div 3.33$

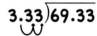

1. Change the divisor to a whole number.

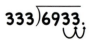

2. Move the decimal point in the dividend.

$$\begin{array}{r} \overline{20.819} \\ 333\overline{)6933.000} \\ 666 \\ \hline 273 \\ 0 \\ \hline 273\ 0 \\ 266\ 4 \\ \hline 6\ 60 \\ 3\ 33 \\ \hline 3\ 270 \\ 2\ 997 \\ \hline 273 \end{array}$$

3. Complete the long division.

Example 5:   96.848 ÷ 0.002

$$0.002\overline{)96.848}$$

1. Change the divisor to a whole number.

$$2\overline{)96.848}$$

2. Move the decimal point in the dividend, adding zeros as needed.

$$\begin{array}{r} 48424 \\ 2\overline{)96848} \\ 8 \\ \hline 16 \\ 16 \\ \hline 08 \\ 8 \\ \hline 04 \\ 4 \\ \hline 08 \\ 8 \\ \hline 0 \end{array}$$

3. Complete the long division.

Practice Dividing Decimal Numbers

(answers on page 53)

Divide these decimal numbers, calculating to the thousandths place if necessary.

1. 12.4 ÷ 0.3 = _____

2. 8.1 ÷ 0.9 = _____

3. 4.6 ÷ 2.2 = _____

4. 3.3 ÷ 1.1 = _____

5. 15.25 ÷ 2.5 = _____

6. 188.425 ÷ 5.75 = _____

7. 100.82 ÷ 25.6 = _____

8. 0.625 ÷ 0.125 = _____

9. 1.0386 ÷ 10.8 = _____

10. 3 ÷ 0.66 = _____

Changing Decimals to Fractions—and Fractions to Decimals

Numbers containing decimals are simply fractions written in a different way. Converting decimals into fractions, and fractions into decimals, is easy.

Changing Decimals to Fractions

To change decimals to fractions, follow the directions in Examples 1–3.

Example 1: Change 0.9 to a fraction.

$$0.\underset{1}{\overset{\frown}{9}} = 9$$

1. Move the decimal point to the right until the decimal number becomes a whole number. Count the number of places moved. In this example, move the decimal point to the right one place to change *0.9* to *9*.

$$\frac{9}{1}$$

2. Draw a line under the whole number, and write *1* as a denominator.

$$\frac{9}{10}$$

3. To the right of the *1*, add zeros equal to the number of places the decimal point moved.

4. Reduce to the lowest terms. $\frac{9}{10}$ is the lowest terms.

For Examples 2 and 3, refer to the directions in Example 1.

Example 2: Change 0.38 to a fraction.

$$0.\underset{1\ \ 2}{\overset{\frown\frown}{38}} = 38$$

1. Move the decimal point to the right two places.

$$\frac{38}{1}$$

2. Draw a line under *38* and write a *1* as a denominator.

$$\frac{38}{100}$$

3. Add zeros to the right of the *1*.

$$\frac{38}{100} = \frac{19}{50}$$

4. Reduce to the lowest terms.

Example 3: Change 7.9284 to a fraction.

$$7.\underset{1\ 2\ 3\ 4}{\overset{\frown\frown\frown\frown}{9284}} = 79284$$

1. Move the decimal point to the right.

$$\frac{79,284}{1}$$

2. Draw a line under *79,284* and write *1* as a denominator.

$$\frac{79,284}{10,000}$$

3. Add zeros to the right of the *1*.

$$\frac{79,284}{10,000} = 7\frac{9284}{10,000} = 7\frac{2321}{2500}$$

4. Reduce to the lowest terms.

Changing Fractions to Decimals

To change fractions to decimals, follow the directions in Examples 1–3.

Example 1: Change $\frac{2}{3}$ to a decimal, rounding to the hundredths place.

```
     0.66̄6
  3)2.000
    1 8
      20
      18
       20
       18
        2
```

1. Divide the numerator by the denominator.

$0.66̄6 = 0.67$

2. Round the answer to the hundredth place.

Example 2: Change $\frac{1}{4}$ to a decimal, rounding to the hundredths place.

```
     0.25
  4)1.00
    8
    20
    20
     0
```

1. Divide the numerator by the denominator.

$0.25 = 0.25$

2. Round the answer to the hundredths place. 0.25 is rounded to the hundredths place.

Example 3: Change $2\frac{30}{55}$ to a decimal, rounding to the tenths place.

```
      0.54
 55)30.00
    27 5
     2 50
     2 20
       30
```

1. Divide the numerator by the denominator. Notice that this problem contains a mixed fraction. For now, ignore the whole number; you will return it at the end of the conversion.

$2.54 = 2.5$

2. Round the answer to the tenths place. Return the whole number. (Don't forget!)

Practice Changing Fractions and Decimals

(answers on page 54)

Convert these numbers into decimals or fractions as indicated. Round decimal answers to the nearest hundredths place if needed and reduce fractions to the lowest terms.

1. Convert $\frac{1}{2}$ into a decimal. _____

2. Convert $\frac{3}{5}$ into a decimal. _____

3. Convert $\frac{7}{9}$ into a decimal. _____

4. Convert $\frac{3}{8}$ into a decimal. _____

5. Convert $\frac{3}{4}$ into a decimal. _____

6. Convert 0.7 into a fraction. _____

7. Convert 0.875 into a fraction. _____

8. Convert 0.592 into a fraction. _____

9. Convert 0.009 into a fraction. _____

10. Convert 0.4 into a fraction. _____

Percents

Percents are similar to fractions and decimals in that they define a part of a whole number—in particular, part of 100. For example, if someone has 100 apples, and 50 of them are red; then 50% of the apples are red. Another way to express the relationship is to say that $\frac{1}{2}$ of the apples are red.

Changing Fractions to Percents

To change a fraction to a percent, follow the directions in Examples 1–3.

Example 1: Change $\frac{3}{4}$ to a percent.

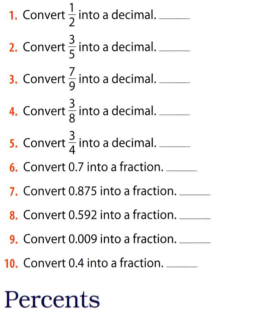

$$\begin{array}{r} 0.75 \\ 4\overline{)3.00} \end{array}$$

1. Divide the numerator by the denominator.

0.75 x 100 = 75%   2. Multiply the product by *100* and add the percent sign (%).

Example 2: Change $\frac{2}{5}$ to a percent.

$$\begin{array}{r} 0.4 \\ 5\overline{)2.0} \end{array}$$

1. Divide.

0.4 x 100 = 40%   2. Multiply by *100*; add %.

Example 3: Change $\frac{7}{9}$ to a percent.

$$\begin{array}{r} 0.7\overline{7} \\ 9\overline{)7.00} \end{array}$$

1. Divide.

$$0.77 \times 100 = 77\%$$

2. Multiply by *100*; add %.

Changing Percents to Fractions

To change a percent to a fraction, follow the directions in Examples 1–3.

Example 1: Change 89% to a fraction.

89   1. Drop the percent sign.

$$\frac{89}{100}$$ 2. Divide the number by 100 and reduce the fraction to the lowest terms.

For Examples 2 and 3, refer to the directions in Example 1.

Example 2: Change 42% to a fraction.

$$42\% = \frac{42}{100} = \frac{21}{50}$$

Example 3: Change 69.8% to a fraction.

Note: In this example, dividing 69.8 by 100 leaves a fraction of $\frac{69.8}{100}$. To eliminate the decimal point in the numerator, move the decimal point to the right one place, and add a zero to the denominator. Reduce the fraction to the lowest terms.

$$69.8\% = \frac{69.8}{100} = \frac{698}{1000} = \frac{349}{500}$$

Changing Decimals to Percents

To change a decimal to a percent, follow the directions in Example 1.

Example 1: Change 2.9 into a percent.

2.90.   1. Move the decimal point to the right two places. Add zeros at the end if needed.

290%   2. Add the percent sign (%).

For Examples 2 and 3, refer to the directions in Example 1.

Example 2: Change 0.8927 to a percent.

$$0.8927 = 89.27\%$$

Example 3: Change 0.09 to a percent.

$$0.09 = 9\%$$

Changing Percents to Decimals

To express percents as decimals, follow the directions in Example 1.

Example 1: Change 23% to a decimal. Move the decimal point to the left two places.

$$23\% = 0.23$$

For Examples 2 and 3, refer to the directions in Example 1.

Example 2: Change 33.7% to a decimal.

$$33.7\% = 0.337$$

Example 3: Change 123% to a decimal.

$$123\% = 1.23$$

Practice Changing Decimals and Percents

(answers on page 54)

Complete these problems.

1. Change $\frac{8}{9}$ to a decimal, rounding to the nearest hundredth. _____

2. Change $\frac{1}{3}$ to a decimal, rounding to the nearest tenth. _____

3. Change 0.51 to a fraction. _____

4. Change 0.723 to a fraction. _____

5. Change $\frac{24}{25}$ to a percent. _____

6. Change $\frac{14}{15}$ to a percent. _____

7. Change 0.009 to a percent. _____

8. Change 0.601 to a percent. _____

9. Change 59% to a fraction. _____

10. Change 21.6% to a fraction. _____

Key Points

1. Decimals describe numbers that are less than one.
2. Decimals have place values, which are expressed as tenths, hundredths, thousandths, and so on.
3. Rounding decimals up or down depends on the number directly to the right of the target place value. If the number to the right is less than 5, the target place value is rounded down. If the number to the right is 5 or greater, the target place value is rounded up.
4. Adding decimals is the same as adding whole numbers except that all of the decimal points must align. Adding then follows the rules for addition of whole numbers.
5. Subtracting decimals is the same as subtracting whole numbers except that all of the decimal points must align.
6. Multiplying decimals is only slightly different from multiplying whole numbers: Initially the decimal point is ignored; then, the decimal places are counted and the decimal point is inserted in the appropriate place.
7. Dividing decimals is basically a long division problem in which the divisor is changed to a whole number, the dividend is changed correspondingly, and zeros added as necessary. The decimal points must be aligned in the dividend and quotient. Converting decimals to fractions involves moving the decimal point.
8. Changing a fraction to a decimal involves dividing the numerator of the fraction by the denominator.

Chapter Post-Test

(answers in Unit 4)

Round these decimals as indicated.

1. Round 6.5 to the nearest whole number. _____

2. Round 42.09 to the nearest whole number. _____

3. Round 99.01 to the nearest tenth. _____

4. Round 75.51 to the nearest tenth. _____

5. Round 107.233 to the nearest hundredth. _____

Add these decimals.

6. 3.7 + 7.2 = _____

7. 14.01 + 2.6 = _____

8. 44.922 + 62.31 = _____

9. 0.572 + 6 + 10.22 = _____

10. 29.9 + 0.005 + 103.8 = _____

Subtract these decimals.

11. 8.2 – 7.9 = _____

12. 16.29 – 13.25 = _____

13. 43.76 – 0.28 = _____

14. 0.904 – 0.233 = _____

15. 193.6284 – 189.933 = _____

Multiply these decimals (do not round your answers).

16. 2 × 0.4 = _____

17. 8.5 × 1.5 = _____

18. 10 × 5.389 = _____

19. 12.2 × 11.61 = _____

20. 0.75 × 0.387 = _____

Divide these decimals (do not round your answers).

21. 36.8 ÷ 4 = _____

22. 2.21 ÷ 1.3 = _____

23. 10.575 ÷ 2.35 = _____

24. 56.235 ÷ 6.9 = _____

25. 0.2888 ÷ 0.76 = _____

Convert these numbers as indicated.

26. Change 0.563 to a percent.

27. Change $\frac{3}{7}$ to a percent, rounding to the nearest tenth if necessary.

28. Change 534% to a decimal.

29. Change 9% to a fraction.

30. Change $\frac{4}{5}$ to a percent, rounding to the nearest tenth if necessary.

Answers to Practice Questions

Rounding Decimal Numbers

1. 5
2. 12
3. 7
4. 83.4
5. 9.0 or 9
6. 0.1
7. 94.00 or 94
8. 221.33
9. 82.813
10. 101.6982

Adding Decimal Numbers

1.
```
   0.2
 + 4.6
   4.8
```

2.
```
   9.1
 + 2.5
  11.6
```

3.
```
   8.5
 + 2.0
  10.5
```

4.
```
  10.79
 + 7.30
  18.09
```

5.
```
   53.005
 + 14.700
   67.705
```

6.
```
   65.02
 + 21.38
   86.40
```

7.
```
   75.902
 + 29.100
  105.002
```

8.
```
     3.85
 + 231.40
   235.25
```

9.
```
   0.78
 + 1.20
 + 3.00
   4.98
```

10.
```
   43.846
 + 56.200
 +  8.200
  108.246
```

Subtracting Decimal Numbers

1.
```
    7.9
  - 4.3
    3.6
```

2.
```
  0  9  1
  1  0. 3
  -  9. 5
     0. 8
```

3.
```
  0  9  9  1
  1  0  0. 2
  -  8  7. 4
     1  2. 8
```

4.
```
     2  9  1
     3. 0  5
   - 1. 0  9
     1. 9  6
```

5.
```
        1
     1  1  1
  1  2. 2  8
  -  2. 4  9
     9. 7  9
```

6.
```
        2  1
  1  6  3. 0  3
  -     0. 9  2
  1  6  2. 1  1
```

7.
```
        1
     4  1  1
     5  2. 2  9  5
   - 3  3. 3  8  1
     1  8. 9  1  4
```

8.
```
    67.739
  - 56.400
    11.339
```

9.
```
  7 1  7 9 1
  8 2. 8 0 0
  - 6 5. 3 2 3
    1 7. 4 7 7
```

10.
```
        1 1 1
     1  7 2 5 1
     2. 8 3 6 7
   - 1. 8 3 6 8
     0. 9 9 9 9
```

Multiplying Decimal Numbers

1.
```
    3.5
  x   2
    7.0
```

2.
```
    4.2
  x 0.8
    3.36
```

3.
```
     1.6
  x  1.9
     1 4 4
  x 1 6 0
     3.0 4
```

4.
```
    3.3 6
  x     4.2
      6 7 2
  1 3 4 4 0
  1 4.1 1 2
```

5.
```
    1 0.7
  x    8.1
      1 0 7
    8 5 6 0
    8 6.6 7
```

6.
```
    6.75
  x   20
      000
  13500
  135.00
```

7.
```
    0.39
  x 0.56
      234
    1950
  0.2184
```

8.
```
    1.151
  x  2.05
     5755
    00000
   230200
  2.35955
```

9.
```
    0.7 5 5
  x     6.33
      2 2 6 5
    2 2 6 5 0
  4 5 3 0 0 0
  4.7 7 9 1 5
```

10.
```
    10.005
 x   0.002
  0.020010
```

Dividing Decimal Numbers

1.
```
      41.333
  3)124.000
    12
     04
      3
     10
      9
     10
      9
     10
      9
      1
```

2.
```
     9
  9)81
    81
     0
```

3.
```
     2.090
 22)46.000
    44
    20
     0
    200
    198
     20
```

4.
```
     3
 11)33
    33
     0
```

5.
```
     6.1
 25)152.5
    150
     25
     25
      0
```

6.
```
       32.769
 575)18842.500
     1725
     1592
     1150
     4425
     4025
     4000
     3450
     5500
     5175
      325
```

7.
```
       3.938
 256)1008.200
     768
     2402
     2304
      980
      768
     2120
     2048
       72
```

8.
```
       5
 125)625
     625
       0
```

9.
```
      0.096
 108)10.386
     9 72
      666
      648
       18
```

10.
```
      4.545
 66)300.000
    264
    360
    330
    300
    264
    360
    330
     30
```

Changing Fractions and Decimals

1.
$$\begin{array}{r} 0.5 \\ 2\overline{)1.0} \\ \underline{1\ 0} \\ 0 \end{array}$$

2.
$$\begin{array}{r} 0.6 \\ 5\overline{)3.0} \\ \underline{3\ 0} \\ 0 \end{array}$$

3.
$$\begin{array}{r} 0.7\overline{7} \\ 9\overline{)7.00} \\ \underline{63} \\ 70 \\ \underline{63} \\ 70 \\ \underline{63} \\ 7 \end{array}$$

4.
$$\begin{array}{r} 0.375 = 0.38 \\ 8\overline{)3.000} \\ \underline{24} \\ 60 \\ \underline{56} \\ 40 \\ \underline{40} \\ 0 \end{array}$$

5.
$$\begin{array}{r} 0.75 \\ 4\overline{)3.00} \\ \underline{28} \\ 20 \\ \underline{20} \\ 0 \end{array}$$

6. $\dfrac{7}{10}$

7. $\dfrac{875}{1000} = \dfrac{7}{8}$

8. $\dfrac{592}{1000} = \dfrac{74}{125}$

9. $\dfrac{9}{1000}$

10. $\dfrac{4}{10} = \dfrac{2}{5}$

Changing Decimals and Percents

1.
$$\begin{array}{r} 0.88\overline{8} \\ 9\overline{)8.000} \end{array} \text{ rounded to } 0.89$$

2.
$$\begin{array}{r} 0.3\overline{3} \\ 3\overline{)1.00} \end{array} \text{ rounded to } 0.3$$

3. $\dfrac{51}{100}$

4. $\dfrac{723}{1000}$

5.
$$\begin{array}{r} 0.96 \\ 25\overline{)24.00} \end{array}$$

$0.96 \times 100\% = 96\%$

6.
$$\begin{array}{r} 0.9\overline{3} \\ 15\overline{)14.00} \end{array}$$

$0.93 \times 100\% = 93\%$

7. $0.009 = 0.9\%$

8. $0.601 = 60.1\%$

9. $59\% = \dfrac{59}{100}$

10. $21.6\% = \dfrac{216}{1000} = \dfrac{27}{125}$

Chapter 4
Dimensional Analysis

☿ Glossary

Conversion factor: A common equivalent needed to convert quantities between different systems of measurement, such as between minutes to hours, ounces to milliliters, or pounds to kilograms.

Dimensional analysis: A method of problem-solving that studies the dimensions or relationships between physical properties.

Given quantity: A specified amount of material, ingredient, or physical property.

Units of measure: The quantity of a physical property being measured. Examples: Distance is a physical property that can be measured in a quantity of feet, miles, or kilometers. Speed is a physical property that can be measured in feet per second or miles per hour.

Objectives

After completing this chapter, the learner will be able to—
1. Define *dimensional analysis*.
2. Solve simple math problems using dimensional analysis.
3. Solve complex math problems using dimensional analysis.

What Is Dimensional Analysis?

Dimensional analysis (also known as the factor-label or the unit-factor method) is an equation-solving technique commonly used in science to understand complex physical states. It is a useful tool for solving problems in which the properties or dimensions of two or more quantities are related to each other but are expressed in different units of measure. One of the quantities must be converted to the other by using a common equivalent or conversion factor.

Dimensional analysis is particularly helpful in calculating medication dosages. Medications are ordered and supplied in a wide range of dosage units, such as teaspoons, milliliters, micrograms, milligrams, units, or milliequivalents. Traditional methods of calculating dosages rely on memorizing formulas or performing multiple-step ratio and proportion computations. By following the steps of dimensional analysis, healthcare professionals can solve simple and complex dosage calculation problems easily and accurately.

Dimensional Analysis for Simple Math Problems

Dimensional analysis offers the ability to compute answers to problems in a format of five easy-to-understand, easy-to-use steps. See Box 4-1.

1. Establish the Answer's Units of Measure

The first step in dimensional analysis is to determine the unit of measure needed for the answer. The unit of measure is the amount of the physical property being measured, such as feet per minute, tablets per dose, or miles per hour. To find the units of measure, read the problem carefully. What must be determined? How should the final answer be expressed?

■ **Box 4-1 Summary of Dimensional Analysis Steps**

1. Establish the answer's units of measure.
2. Insert the given quantities.
3. Determine the necessary conversion factor.
4. Calculate the answer.
5. Critically evaluate the answer.

Let's start with an example: We follow speed limit laws when driving our cars. A speed limit describes the relationship between how far we can drive (the number of miles) in a given amount of time (one hour). In the United States, rates of speed (speed limits) are expressed as *miles per hour, miles/hour*, or *mph*.

But what if we wanted to know a car's rate of speed if the car traveled 2 miles in 10 minutes? Calculating the miles-per-minute speed (2 miles per 10 minutes or 1 mile per 5 minutes) is easy, but calculating the miles-per-hour speed requires the conversion of *miles per minute* to *miles per hour*.

To begin a dimensional analysis equation, write the final answer's units of measure on the left side of the paper. Notice that the format looks somewhat like a fraction.

Note: Even though the dimensional analysis equation resembles a fraction, the ratio expresses a relationship, not a fraction.

$$\frac{\text{miles}}{\text{hour}}$$

Immediately after writing the answer's units of measure, place an *equal sign* to the right of the ratio and draw a line to the right of the equal sign.

$$\frac{\text{miles}}{\text{hour}} = \underline{\qquad}$$

Note: Avoid writing the units of measure in these formats: *mph* or *miles/hour*. Keeping the units orderly will help later in the process.

2. Insert the Given Quantities

The second step is to insert the given quantities into the equation. A **given quantity** is the amount of material or physical property specified in the problem. Sometimes the given quantities are easy to determine, such as a speed limit (60 miles per 1 hour) or an amount of medication in a capsule (300 milligrams in 1 capsule). Sometimes, one of the given quantities is only implied. For example, for a child who is 43 inches tall, we wouldn't say, "There are 43 inches in this 1 child." Yet the relationship exists, and it needs to be defined when setting up a dimensional analysis equation.

In our example, the given quantities are *2 miles* and *10 minutes*. Insert the given quantity that refers to miles in the numerator position to the right of the equal sign. **The numerators on both sides of the equal sign must be identical!**

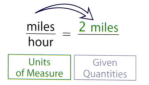

Next, find the second given quantity (the quantity that is related to the numerator), and write it in the denominator position to the right of the equal sign. In this case, the quantity is *10 minutes*. Notice that the relationship between the two given quantities is expressed as a ratio.

The relationship between the two quantities would be the same even if the ratio was reversed:
$\frac{10 \text{ minutes}}{2 \text{ miles}}$.

$$\underbrace{\frac{\text{miles}}{\text{hour}}}_{\substack{\text{Units}\\\text{of Measure}}} = \underbrace{\frac{2 \text{ miles}}{10 \text{ minutes}}}_{\substack{\text{Given}\\\text{Quantities}}}$$

   Then, place a multiplication sign to the right of the given quantity and draw another line to the right of it. Notice that the ratio *miles/minute* is not the format of the units of measure—this is a clue that additional calculations are needed.

$$\underbrace{\frac{\text{miles}}{\text{hour}}}_{\substack{\text{Units}\\\text{of Measure}}} = \underbrace{\frac{2 \text{ miles}}{10 \text{ minutes}}}_{\substack{\text{Given}\\\text{Quantities}}} \times \underline{\hspace{2cm}}$$

3. Determine the Necessary Conversion Factor

A **conversion factor** is a common equivalent needed to convert between different systems of measurement. In this example, we want to convert minutes into hours because our final answer is expressed in miles/hour, not miles/minute. The needed conversion factor is 60 minutes in 1 hour. Since the units of measure (the final answer) is to be expressed as miles/hour, place 60 minutes on top of the line and 1 hour below the line. The minutes unit will cancel out.

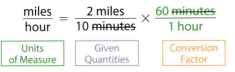

$$\underbrace{\frac{\text{miles}}{\text{hour}}}_{\substack{\text{Units}\\\text{of Measure}}} = \underbrace{\frac{2 \text{ miles}}{10 \text{ minutes}}}_{\substack{\text{Given}\\\text{Quantities}}} \times \underbrace{\frac{60 \text{ minutes}}{1 \text{ hour}}}_{\substack{\text{Conversion}\\\text{Factor}}}$$

> **Alert!** Remember that the quantities expressed in the dimensional analysis pathway are not true fractions. Numerical fractions cannot be manipulated; for example, 2/10 is not the same quantity as 10/2. The numerators and denominators in the dimensional analysis pathway may be placed in either position, depending upon the need to cancel units.

4. Calculate the Answer

Examine the equation. Are the remaining units to the right of the first equal sign the same as the units in the unknown quantity? If so, the equation is complete. Finish the calculation.

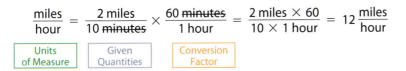

$$\underbrace{\frac{\text{miles}}{\text{hour}}}_{\substack{\text{Units}\\\text{of Measure}}} = \underbrace{\frac{2 \text{ miles}}{10 \text{ minutes}}}_{\substack{\text{Given}\\\text{Quantities}}} \times \underbrace{\frac{60 \text{ minutes}}{1 \text{ hour}}}_{\substack{\text{Conversion}\\\text{Factor}}} = \frac{2 \text{ miles} \times 60}{10 \times 1 \text{ hour}} = 12 \frac{\text{miles}}{\text{hour}}$$

5. Critically Evaluate the Answer

To assess your work, ask these questions:

- Is the equation set up properly?
- Is the conversion factor correct?
- Is the math right? Recheck the calculations for computational errors. Make sure that all units have been canceled properly.
- Does the answer seem reasonable? Is it plausible?

In the example given, the car traveled 2 miles in 10 minutes. A car going 60 miles per hour will cover 1 mile in 1 minute (60 miles/60 minutes). If it takes 10 minutes for the car to travel 2 miles, then it seems logical that it is going very slowly; thus, our answer of 12 miles per hour is reasonable.

Example 1:

A nurse takes the pulse of a client for 15 seconds and counts 18 beats. She must record the pulse in the client's chart in beats per minute. Calculate the client's pulse rate in beats per minute.

$$\frac{\text{beats}}{\text{minute}}$$

1. Establish the answer's units of measure.

2. Insert the given quantities in the numerator and denominator. Prepare for the conversion factor if needed.

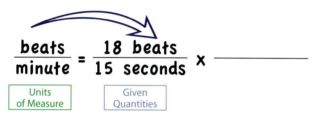

$$\underbrace{\frac{\text{beats}}{\text{minute}}}_{\text{Units of Measure}} = \underbrace{\frac{18\ \text{beats}}{15\ \text{seconds}}}_{\text{Given Quantities}} \times \underline{\qquad\qquad}$$

3. Determine the necessary conversion factor. The answer must be expressed in *minutes* for the final answer. Therefore, the correct conversion factor is 60 seconds per 1 minute.

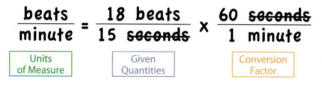

$$\underbrace{\frac{\text{beats}}{\text{minute}}}_{\text{Units of Measure}} = \underbrace{\frac{18\ \text{beats}}{15\ \cancel{\text{seconds}}}}_{\text{Given Quantities}} \times \underbrace{\frac{60\ \cancel{\text{seconds}}}{1\ \text{minute}}}_{\text{Conversion Factor}}$$

> **Note:** After the *seconds* units are canceled, the remaining units on the right side of the equation match the units of measure on the left side of the equation. The answer can now be calculated.

4. Calculate the answer.

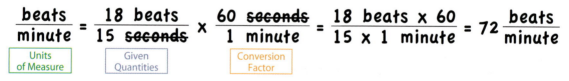

$$\underbrace{\frac{\text{beats}}{\text{minute}}}_{\text{Units of Measure}} = \underbrace{\frac{18\ \text{beats}}{15\ \cancel{\text{seconds}}}}_{\text{Given Quantities}} \times \underbrace{\frac{60\ \cancel{\text{seconds}}}{1\ \text{minute}}}_{\text{Conversion Factor}} = \frac{18\ \text{beats} \times 60}{15 \times 1\ \text{minute}} = 72\ \frac{\text{beats}}{\text{minute}}$$

5. Critically evaluate the answer. Was the equation set up correctly? Is the conversion factor right? Is the math correct? Does a pulse of 72 beats per minute seem reasonable? Answer: Yes, the number of beats is within the normal range of 60 to 100 beats per minute.

Example 2:

A 38-year-old man has a headache. He looks at the label on a bottle of acetaminophen to find that the recommended dosage for adults is 650 mg. The tablets in the bottle contain 325 milligrams each. How many tablets should the man take?

1. Establish the answer's units of measure. The question requires calculating the number of tablets that the man will take. In fact, the unstated assumption within this problem is that the tablets will be administered with *each dose*. Remember, dimensional analysis is concerned with relationships between properties. Expressing this relationship in fraction form can help keep the units of measure correctly aligned.

$$\frac{\text{tablets}}{\text{dose}}$$

Units of Measure

2. Insert the given quantity in the numerator and denominator, and prepare for the conversion factor, if needed. Remember that the numerator of the first given quantity must be identical to the numerator of the units of measure. Therefore, write _1 tablet_ in the numerator position. Each tablet contains 325 milligrams of acetaminophen, so write the strength of the tablet (325 mg) as the denominator.

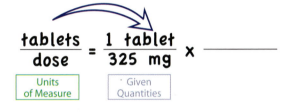

$$\frac{\text{tablets}}{\text{dose}} = \frac{1 \text{ tablet}}{325 \text{ mg}} \times \underline{\qquad}$$

Units of Measure   · Given Quantities

3. Determine the necessary conversion factor, if needed. In this example, no conversion factor is needed because the recommended dosage of acetaminophen (650 mg) is expressed in the same units as the supply (325 mg). When the milligram units are canceled, the remaining units match the unknown quantity. No further work is needed.

$$\frac{\text{tablets}}{\text{dose}} = \frac{1 \text{ tablet}}{325 \; \cancel{\text{milligrams}}} \times \frac{650 \; \cancel{\text{milligrams}}}{\text{dose}}$$

Units of Measure   Given Quantities   Given Quantity

4. Calculate the answer.

$$\frac{\text{tablets}}{\text{dose}} = \frac{1 \text{ tablet}}{325 \; \cancel{\text{milligrams}}} \times \frac{650 \; \cancel{\text{milligrams}}}{\text{dose}}$$

Units of Measure   Given Quantities   Given Quantity

$$= \frac{1 \text{ tablet} \times 650}{325 \text{ dose}} = 2 \frac{\text{tablets}}{\text{dose}}$$

5. Critically evaluate the answer. Was the equation set up correctly? Is the math correct? Is the answer reasonable? Yes, taking 2 acetaminophen tablets is reasonable for an adult male.

Steps for Complex Problems

Complex problems require multiple conversion factors or sets of variables. The basic steps of dimensional analysis remain the same, but the equation becomes longer.

Example 1:

A coffee growing company makes a profit of $2 per pound of coffee beans picked. Coffee bean pickers can pick 1 ton of beans per day. How many days of picking are necessary for the company to make $100,000 profit?

1. Establish the answer's units of measure. In this example, we need to determine the number of picking days necessary to make a certain profit. We might show the relationship this way:

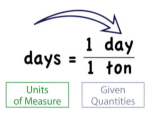

$$\frac{\text{days of picking}}{\$100,000 \text{ profit}}$$

> Units of Measure

To keep the equation from being cumbersome, simplify the wording.

days

> Units of Measure

2. Insert the given quantities. Because a complex equation may have more than one given quantity, select the set of values with the same wording as the answer's units of measure.

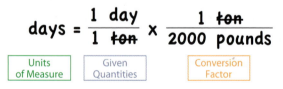

$$\text{days} = \frac{1 \text{ day}}{1 \text{ ton}}$$

> Units of Measure   Given Quantities

3. Determine the necessary conversion factors to convert tons to pounds.

$$\text{days} = \frac{1 \text{ day}}{1 \text{ \sout{ton}}} \times \frac{1 \text{ \sout{ton}}}{2000 \text{ pounds}}$$

> Units of Measure   Given Quantities   Conversion Factor

After canceling the *tons*, *pounds* remains in the equation. This fact signals that another set of values—found in the question— is necessary to cancel the *pounds*. Notice that 1 pound of coffee beans brings a profit of $2.

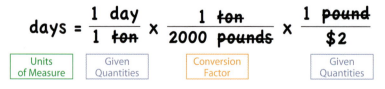

$$\text{days} = \frac{1 \text{ day}}{1 \text{ \sout{ton}}} \times \frac{1 \text{ \sout{ton}}}{2000 \text{ \sout{pounds}}} \times \frac{1 \text{ \sout{pound}}}{\$2}$$

> Units of Measure   Given Quantities   Conversion Factor   Given Quantities

After *pounds* are canceled, *day/$* remain. The *$* units needs to be canceled so that *days* is the only remaining unit in the equation. This is accomplished by inserting the last given quantity $100,000.

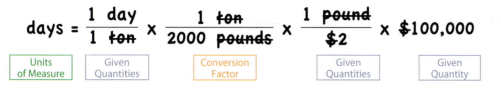

| Units of Measure | Given Quantities | Conversion Factor | Given Quantities | Given Quantity |

Note: Given quantities that stand "alone," such as $100,000 can also be written as $\frac{\$100,000}{1}$. Writing quantities in a ratio format can help keep numerators and denominators aligned when you're doing your calculations.

4. Calculate the answer.

$$= \frac{day \times 100{,}000}{2000 \times 2} = 25 \text{ days}$$

5. Critically evaluate the answer. Was the equation set up correctly? Is the math correct? Is the answer reasonable? Yes, it is because the pickers can pick *1* ton of beans per day, which earns a profit of $4000 ($2/pound x 2000 pounds). If the pickers pick for 25 days, the company will make $100,000 (25 days x $4000/day).

Example 2:

A speed walker using a pedometer measures her walking speed in feet per minute. If she wants to walk 6 miles in 1 hour, at what feet/minute speed will she have to walk?

1. Establish the answer's units of measure.

$$\frac{\textbf{feet}}{\textbf{minute}}$$

| Units of Measure |

2 and 3. Insert the given quantities and determine the conversion factor. Notice that the problem has no quantities expressed in feet per minute. However, 6 miles is a related quantity. A conversion factor is required to convert miles into feet.

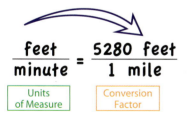

$$\frac{\textbf{feet}}{\textbf{minute}} = \frac{\textbf{5280 feet}}{\textbf{1 mile}}$$

| Units of Measure | Conversion Factor |

Insert the given quantities.

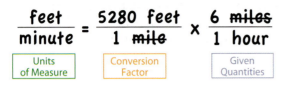

$$\frac{feet}{minute} = \frac{5280\ feet}{1\ \cancel{mile}} \times \frac{6\ \cancel{miles}}{1\ hour}$$

| Units of Measure | Conversion Factor | Given Quantities |

After the miles units are canceled, *feet/hour* remain. An additional conversion factor is needed to change hours into minutes.

$$\frac{feet}{minute} = \frac{5280\ feet}{1\ \cancel{mile}} \times \frac{6\ \cancel{miles}}{1\ \cancel{hour}} \times \frac{1\ \cancel{hour}}{60\ minutes}$$

| Units of Measure | Conversion Factor | Given Quantity | Conversion Factor |

4. Calculate the answer.

$$= \frac{5280\ feet \times 6}{60\ minutes} = 528\frac{feet}{minute}$$

5. Critically evaluate the answer. Was the equation set up correctly? Is the math correct? Is the answer reasonable? Yes, it is because the *6* in the numerator can be reduced to *1,* and the *60* in the denominator can be reduced to *10.* Therefore, *5280* divided by *10* is 528 feet.

Example 3:

A cook has been approached by the town mayor to make chili for the town's annual Fourth of July party. The cook estimates that 400 people will be eating the chili. The original recipe, which serves 25 people, calls for 4 tablespoons of hot sauce. How many quarts of hot sauce will the cook need to make the chili for the party? The cook knows that 1 quart is equivalent to 4 cups, and 1 cup contains 16 tablespoons (tbsp).

1. Establish the answer's units of measure.

quarts

| Units of Measure |

2 and 3. Insert the given quantities and the conversion factor.

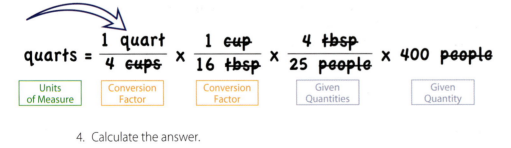

$$quarts = \frac{1\ quart}{4\ \cancel{cups}} \times \frac{1\ \cancel{cup}}{16\ \cancel{tbsp}} \times \frac{4\ \cancel{tbsp}}{25\ \cancel{people}} \times 400\ \cancel{people}$$

| Units of Measure | Conversion Factor | Conversion Factor | Given Quantities | Given Quantity |

4. Calculate the answer.

$$= \frac{1\ quart \times 4 \times 400\ quarts}{4 \times 16 \times 25} = 1\ quart$$

5. Critically evaluate the answer. Was the equation set up correctly? Is the math correct? Is the answer reasonable? Yes, it is because a batch of chili serving 400 people will require 16 times the ingredients of the recipe serving 25. If the original recipe contains 4 tablespoons of hot sauce, then the chili for the Fourth of July party will require 16 times that amount, or 64 tablespoons. Thus, 64 tablespoons divided by 16 tablespoons/cup equals 4 cups, which is equal to 1 quart.

Practice Dimensional Analysis

(answers on pages 66–67)

Calculate these units of measure using dimensional analysis principles. Round the answer to the nearest whole number unless otherwise specified.

1. A baker is making a wedding cake. The original recipe calls for 3 tablespoons of baking powder. The baker has lost the utensil that measures tablespoons, but still has a teaspoon. The baker knows that 1 tablespoon contains 3 teaspoons. How many teaspoons of baking powder will the baker put into the recipe?

2. A nurse is counting the respirations of a client. She counts 9 breaths in 30 seconds. What is the client's respiratory rate per minute?

3. A parent is filling out a government form for his son. The form asks for the child's height in centimeters. The parent knows that the child is 38 inches tall. How tall is the child in centimeters? Tip: One inch is equivalent to 2.5 centimeters.

4. A long-distance runner ran 15 miles in 180 minutes yesterday. How fast did the runner run in miles per hour?

5. A parent consults a pediatrician about the amount of ibuprofen to give her infant for a fever. The pediatrician advises the parent to administer 2 droppersful of ibuprofen elixir to the infant. The bottle of ibuprofen elixir comes with a dropper that holds 50 milligrams of ibuprofen. How many milligrams of ibuprofen is the infant getting if the parent administers the dosage recommended by the physician?

6. Two university students are measuring the time it takes for a rock to fall 25 feet. On the first try, it takes the rock 3 seconds to fall to the ground. What was the rate of descent of the rock expressed in feet per minute?

7. A nursing student is counting the minutes until graduation. There are 14 weeks left. How many minutes are there until graduation day?

8. Nine high school students pool their money to buy pizza. They collect enough to buy 3 large pizzas. Each pizza is cut into 12 pieces. If the pizzas are divided evenly, how many pieces will each student get?

9. An airplane is flying at a speed of 550 miles per hour from Seattle to London, a distance of 4950 miles. How many hours will the flight take to reach London?

10. A recycling company makes $500 per ton of aluminum scrap collected. If the company collects 250 pounds of aluminum scrap per day, how many days are needed to make $1500? Tip: One ton equals 2000 pounds.

Key Points

1. Dimensional analysis is a mathematical problem-solving method that is systematic, logical, and well suited to problems involving quantities that are related to each other.
2. The five steps to solving equations using dimensional analysis are as follows:
   1. Establish the answer's units of measure.
   2. Insert the given quantities.
   3. Determine the necessary conversion factor.
   4. Calculate the answer.
   5. Critically evaluate the answer.

Chapter Post-Test

(answers in Unit 4)

Calculate these units of measure using dimensional analysis principles. Round to the nearest whole number unless otherwise specified.

1. A popcorn concessionaire has 25 pounds of popcorn kernels. If he uses 1/4 pound of kernels for every bag he sells, how many bags of popcorn can he make?

2. A local coffee bar offers customers 5 bonus points for each tall latte purchased. After 80 points are collected, customers are eligible for a free latte. How many tall vanilla lattes would a customer have to buy to get a free one?

3. If a satellite can travel 200 feet per second, how many hours will it take the satellite to travel 10,000 miles?

4. A cookie manufacturer wants to claim that its chocolate chip cookies have the most chips in each cookie. To make this claim, each cookie must have at least 25 chocolate chips. A 1-pound bag of chocolate chips contains 500 chips. How many cookies can the company make using 10 pounds of chocolate chips?

5. A town is celebrating its 100th birthday. The town council wants to make an ice cream sundae for the town's 500 residents. If each resident eats 4 ounces of ice cream, how many pounds of ice cream will the town need to purchase? Tip: One pound contains 16 ounces.

6. A certain brand of toilet uses 5 quarts of water for every flush. If the average household flushes the toilet 12 times per day, how many gallons of water are used each day for flushing? Tip: One gallon contains four quarts. Round the answer to the nearest tenth.

7. A clothing store sells an average of 4 pairs of jeans at $45 per pair, for every hour it is open. If the store is open 7 days per week for 10 hours each day, how much money does the store make in 2 weeks? Round the answer to the nearest penny.

8. A bottle of medicine contains 16 fluid ounces of medication. If 1 dose of the medicine is equal to 1 teaspoon, and there are approximately 6 teaspoons in 1 ounce, what is the total number of doses in the bottle?

9. A nursing student is measuring the heart rate of a patient. If the student counts 18 beats in 15 seconds, what is the heart rate of the patient per minute?

10. A college student buys 2 cases of chicken-flavored ramen noodles at a discount grocery store. Each case contains 48 packages of noodles. If the student eats 2 packages of noodles each day, how many days will the noodles last?

11. A group of hospital volunteers is trying to raise $1000 to buy a video game system for the hospital's pediatric unit. The volunteers are selling cookies for $3 per dozen. How many cookies will the group need to sell in order to raise the $1000?

12. A couple of travelers are planning a road trip on the old U.S. Route 66. The trip encompasses 2448 miles. If the travelers want to finish the trip in 7 days, how many miles per day must they travel?

13. If the travelers in question 12 drive an average of 60 miles per hour, how many hours per day must they drive? Round the answer to the nearest tenth.

14. Four college students are planning a 1652-mile trip for spring break. The car they are driving gets 25 miles to the gallon, and gasoline prices average $2.63 per gallon. How much money will each student need for gas if they want to split the cost evenly? Round the answer to the nearest penny.

15. An import buyer has a $10,000 budget to purchase pottery in Mexico. Each piece of pottery costs 100 pesos. One American dollar is equivalent to 13 pesos. How many pieces of pottery can the buyer purchase without going over the $10,000 budget?

16. A caterer is preparing tea for a wedding reception. If 1 cup of tea uses 10 grams of tea leaves, how many grams of tea leaves are needed to make 2 gallons of tea? Tip: 4 cups equal a quart, and 4 quarts equal a gallon.

17. A bicycle courier can cycle at a speed of 15 miles per hour. If the courier must travel a distance of 0.25 miles between stops, how many minutes will it take him?

18. A runner wants to be able to run 400 meters in 50 seconds. What miles-per-hour speed must the runner attain to accomplish this goal? The runner knows that there are 1609 meters in a mile.

19. A grocery store sells bananas for $0.70 per pound. If the store sells 1/2 ton of bananas, how much money will the store receive? Round the answer to the nearest penny.

20. A subway train makes 1 stop every 3 minutes. If the train runs for 22 hours each day, how many stops does the train make in one day?

21. The estimated cost of raising a child from birth to age 18 is $124,800. What is the average cost per month of raising that child? Round the answer to the nearest hundredth.

22. A pharmacy technician is filling a bottle of liquid medicine for a customer. If the customer is supposed to take 30 doses of the medicine, and each dose contains 5 milliliters of medicine, how many milliliters of medicine should the technician put into the bottle?

23. A bakery sells individual slices of apple pie. If each pie contains 1 pound of apples, and each pie is cut into 8 slices, how many ounces of apples does each slice contain? Tip: 1 pound = 16 ounces.

24. A furniture store receives $300 profit per bedroom suite sold. If the company sells an average of 2 bedroom suites per day, how many days will it take for them to make a $60,000 profit?

25. A student is curious as to how many times his heart beats in one day. If his heart beats 65 times each minute, how many times will his heart beat in 24 hours?

Answers to Practice Questions

Dimensional Analysis

1. 9 teaspoons

$$\text{teaspoon} = \frac{3 \text{ teaspoons}}{1 \text{ } \cancel{\text{tablespoon}}} \times 3 \text{ } \cancel{\text{tablespoons}} = \frac{3 \text{ teaspoons} \times 3}{1} = 9 \text{ teaspoons}$$

2. 18 breaths/minute

$$\frac{\text{breaths}}{\text{minute}} = \frac{9 \text{ breaths}}{30 \text{ } \cancel{\text{seconds}}} \times \frac{60 \text{ } \cancel{\text{seconds}}}{1 \text{ minute}} = \frac{9 \text{ breaths} \times 60}{30 \times 1 \text{ minute}} = \frac{540 \text{ breaths}}{30 \text{ minutes}} = 18 \frac{\text{breaths}}{\text{minute}}$$

3. 95 centimeters

$$\text{centimeters} = \frac{2.5 \text{ centimeters}}{1 \text{ } \cancel{\text{inch}}} \times 38 \text{ } \cancel{\text{inches}}$$

$$= 2.5 \times 38 \text{ centimeters} = 95 \text{ centimeters}$$

4. 5 miles/hour

$$\frac{\text{miles}}{\text{hour}} = \frac{15 \text{ miles}}{180 \text{ } \cancel{\text{minutes}}} \times \frac{60 \text{ } \cancel{\text{minutes}}}{1 \text{ hour}} = \frac{15 \text{ miles} \times 60}{180 \text{ hours}} = 5 \frac{\text{miles}}{\text{hour}}$$

5. 100 milligrams/dose

$$\frac{\text{milligrams}}{\text{dose}} = \frac{50 \text{ milligrams}}{1 \text{ } \cancel{\text{dropperful}}} \times \frac{2 \text{ } \cancel{\text{droppersful}}}{1 \text{ dose}} = \frac{50 \text{ milligrams} \times 2}{1 \text{ dose}} = 100 \frac{\text{milligrams}}{\text{dose}}$$

6. 500 feet/minute

$$\frac{\text{feet}}{\text{minute}} = \frac{25 \text{ feet}}{3 \text{ } \cancel{\text{seconds}}} \times \frac{60 \text{ } \cancel{\text{seconds}}}{1 \text{ minute}} = \frac{25 \text{ feet} \times 60}{3 \text{ minutes}} = 500 \frac{\text{feet}}{\text{minute}}$$

7. 141,120 minutes

$$\text{minutes} = \frac{60 \text{ minutes}}{1 \text{ } \cancel{\text{hour}}} \times \frac{24 \text{ } \cancel{\text{hours}}}{1 \text{ day}} = \frac{7 \text{ } \cancel{\text{days}}}{1 \text{ } \cancel{\text{week}}} \times 14 \text{ } \cancel{\text{weeks}}$$

$$= \frac{60 \text{ minutes} \times 24 \times 7 \times 14}{1} = 141,120 \text{ minutes}$$

8. 4 pieces/student

$$\frac{\text{pieces pizza}}{\text{student}} = \frac{12 \text{ pieces}}{1 \text{ pizza}} \times \frac{3 \text{ pizzas}}{9 \text{ students}} = \frac{12 \text{ pieces} \times 3}{9 \text{ students}} = 4 \frac{\text{pieces}}{\text{student}}$$

9. 9 hours

$$\text{hours} = \frac{1 \text{ hour}}{550 \text{ miles}} \times 4950 \text{ miles} = \frac{1 \text{ hour} \times 4950}{550} = 9 \text{ hours}$$

10. 24 days

$$\text{days} = \frac{1 \text{ day}}{250 \text{ pounds}} \times \frac{2000 \text{ pounds}}{1 \text{ ton}} \times \frac{1 \text{ ton}}{\$500} \times \$1500$$

$$= \frac{1 \text{ day} \times 2000 \times 1500}{250 \times 500} = 24 \text{ days}$$

Unit 1 Post-Test

(answers in Unit 4)

After studying Unit 1 "Arithmetic Review and Dimension Analysis," answer these questions, reducing fractions to the lowest terms. Do not round decimal answers unless specified in the question.

1. $4 + 203.6 =$ _____

2. Convert $\frac{6}{7}$ into a decimal. Round to the nearest tenth place. _____

3. $\frac{1}{5} + \frac{5}{7} =$ _____

4. $86 - 42 =$ _____

5. Convert 79.9% into a decimal. _____

6. A freight train is traveling from Seattle to Portland, a distance of 225 miles. It is traveling at a speed of 50 miles per hour. How long will the train take to get to Portland? Round to the nearest half hour. _____

7. $7.6 \times 0.3 =$ _____

8. $\frac{3}{5} \times \frac{5}{6} =$ _____

9. $96.63 - 62.02 =$ _____

10. Convert 12.3% into a fraction. _____

11. $\frac{3}{5} \times \frac{8}{9} =$ _____

12. $5899 + 342 =$ _____

13. There are 1736 yards in one mile and 3 feet in 1 yard. If a hiker walks 3.45 miles, how many feet has he traveled? Round to the nearest tenth foot. _____

14. Round 45.88 to the nearest tenth. _____

15. $\frac{2}{9} \div \frac{1}{3} =$ _____

16. Convert 29.79% into a decimal. _____

17. Convert 0.753 into a percent. _____

18. $3\frac{1}{2} - \frac{7}{8} =$ _____

19. $\frac{3}{7} \div \frac{2}{3} =$ _____

20. Convert $\frac{1}{2}$ into a percent. _____

21. Round 79.82 to the nearest whole number. _____

22. Convert 55.1% into a fraction. _____

23. A group of school children have been collecting dimes to purchase a book for their classroom. The book costs $54.70. How many dimes will the children need to collect to buy the book? _____

24. $88 \times 2.1 =$ _____

25. $637.42 - 567.119 =$ _____

26. $4.4 \div 2.2 =$ _____

27. Convert 0.034 into a fraction. _____

28. $3\frac{2}{3} - 2\frac{1}{6} =$ _____

29. Round 0.919 to the nearest hundredth. _____

30. $34 + 902 + 382 =$ _____

31. Convert 0.52 into a fraction. _____

32. $1207 - 853 =$ _____

33. Round 6.7892 to the nearest thousandth. _____

34. $6\frac{11}{12} - 3\frac{1}{12} =$ _____

35. $23 - 14 =$ _____

36. $32.16 \div 4.8 =$ _____

37. A pilot knows that she can fly 8.3 miles on 1 gallon of fuel. One gallon of fuel costs $2.25. If she wants to fly 428 miles, how much will it cost her to fill up her airplane with fuel? Round to the nearest penny. _____

38. $\frac{9}{10} + \frac{7}{8} =$ _____

39. Convert $\frac{3}{8}$ into a decimal. _____

40. $61{,}622 - 4335 =$ _____

41. $4 + 7.18 + 3.273 + 0.15 =$ _____

42. $\frac{5}{12} + \frac{17}{24} =$ _____

43. $62 \times 115 =$ _____

44. An elevator can hold a maximum of 12 people or 1500 pounds. Can this elevator hold 11 people who weigh an average of 160 pounds each?

_____

45. $225 \div 15 =$ _____

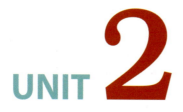

UNIT 2

Medication Administration

Chapter 5
Measures and Equivalents

Objectives

After completing this chapter, the learner will be able to—
1. Describe the history of metric and household measurement systems.
2. Write metric measures using the proper rules of notation.
3. Identify metric and household equivalencies.
4. Explain the unique characteristics of International Units and milliequivalents.

Metric Measures

As international commerce and scientific discovery grew, so did the need for a reliable, uniform system of measurement. In 1791, after much effort to select units of measure that were logical and practical, French scientists declared the meter and the kilogram as the fundamental units of measure for length and mass (weight), known as the metric system.

In 1960, the metric system was updated in response to the need for more precise measuring units. This new system was called the Système International d'Unités, or the International System of Units (SI for short). The SI is managed by the Bureau International des Poids et Mesures (BIPM), or the International Bureau of Weights and Measures, in Paris, France, and meets periodically to assess the need for changes. With the signing of the Treaty of the Meter in 1875, the United States demonstrated a commitment to the metric system, although complete conversion to metrics has been slow in gaining acceptance outside the U.S. scientific arena. However, the metric system is the preferred method for prescribing and dispensing medication in the United States.

Basic Units and Notation Rules

The basic units of the SI (metric system) for length, weight, and liquid volume are the meter (m), the kilogram (kg), and the liter (L). These units are based on the powers of 10, which means that all multiples and subunits of basic metric units can be multiplied or divided by 10. For example, if a liter is divided into 10 units, the resulting unit is $\frac{1}{10}$ L and is called a deciliter (dL), and a meter that is divided into 1000 units is $\frac{1}{1000}$ m, or millimeter (mm). On the other hand, if a meter is multiplied by 1000, the resulting unit is a kilometer (km). Common metric system unit abbreviations (called **unit symbols** in SI terminology) and equivalencies are listed in Table 5-1. Table 5-2 shows the metric system prefixes used for very large and small measurements.

Table 5-1	**Common Metric System Units and Symbols**		
Measurement	Unit	Symbol/Abbreviation	Equivalent Measures
Length	millimeter	mm	
	centimeter	cm	10 mm = 1 cm
	meter	m	100 cm = 1 m
	kilometer	km	1000 m = 1 km
Mass (weight)	microgram	μg or mcg	
	milligram	mg	1000 mcg = 1 mg
	gram	g	1000 mg = 1 g
	kilogram	kg	1000 g = 1 kg
	metric ton	t	1000 kg = 1 t
Volume	milliliter	mL	
	deciliter	dL	1000 mL = 1 L
	liter	L	10 dL = 1 L

Table 5-2	**Metric Prefixes**	
Prefix	Symbol	Multiplier
Mega (10^6)	M	1,000,000
Kilo (10^3)	k	1000
Hecto (10^2)	h	100
Deka (10^1)	da	10
Deci (10^{-1})	d	0.1
Centi (10^{-2})	c	0.01
Milli (10^{-3})	m	0.001
Micro (10^{-6})	μ	0.000001

Metric abbreviations should be written following metric system rules of notation (see Table 5-3). However, please note that the Institute for Safe Medication Practices (ISMP) discourages the use of the "micro" symbol μ, since it can be confused with the letter *m* in handwritten form. For example, the symbol μ*g* is the symbol for microgram. However, in the medical field, *mcg* is the preferred abbreviation for microgram.

Table 5-3	SI Metric System Rules of Notation		
Rule		Correct	Incorrect
Write unit symbols in the singular form.		8.1 cm	8.1 cms or cm's
		4.5 mg	4.5 mgs or mg's
Do not add any additional letters to a symbol.		9 g	9 gm or 9 grm
		1 mg	1 mgm
Be aware of letters that must be capitalized in the symbol.		m	M
		kg	Kg
		mL	Ml
		g	G
Do not use a period after a unit symbol unless it is the last word in a sentence.		7.2 kg	7.2 kg.
		4.9 L	4.9 L.
		The length of the boat was 16 m.	
Use a space to separate the number from the symbol.		29 km	29km
		399 mm	399mm

Practice Measures and Equivalents

(answers on page 78)

Multiple choice. Select the best answer.

1. Which of the following agencies is responsible for managing the International System of Units?
   a. The U.S. Food and Drug Administration
   b. The International Bureau of Weights and Measures
   c. The Institute for Safe Medication Practices
   d. The World Health Organization

Write the correct notation for these quantities.

2. 4.1 liters _____

3. 2.5 kilometers _____

4. 69.4 kilograms _____

5. 231 micrograms _____

6. 532 grams _____

7. 10 milliliters _____

8. 775 centimeters _____

Identify these equivalent measures.

9. 1000 mcg = _____ mg

10. 10 mm = _____ cm

11. 1 kg = _____ g

12. 10 dL = _____ L

13. 1 L = _____ mL

14. 1 km = _____ m

15. 100 cm = _____ m

Household Measures

Household measures (also known as the United States customary system, or customary weights and measures) originated from the British Imperial Units system. Household measurements are becoming obsolete for prescribing, compounding, and administering medications. However, familiarity with the household system is necessary in clinical practice to calculate patient intake or to convert a patient's weight from pounds to kilograms.

Basic Units and Notation Rules

The basic units of the household system include the ounce (oz) and pound (lb) for weight; the inch (in), foot (ft), yard (yd), and mile (mi) for length; and the teaspoon (tsp), tablespoon (Tbsp), ounce (fl oz, or oz), cup (c), pint (pt), quart (qt), and gallon (gal) for liquids. Approximate metric equivalents of household measures are listed in Tables 5-4, 5-5, and 5-6. Notation rules for household measures are similar to those for metric notations. The number should be written to the left of the unit symbol, leaving a space between the number and the unit.

Table 5-4	Approximate Household and Metric Weight Equivalents	
Household		**Metric**
1 oz		28 g
1 lb		454 g
2.2 lb		1 kg

Table 5-5	Approximate Household and Metric Fluid Volume Equivalents	
Household		**Metric**
1 tsp		5 mL
1 Tbsp		15 mL
1 fl oz		30 mL
1 c		240 mL
1 pt		480 mL
1 qt		960 mL
1 gal		3.8 L

Table 5-6	Approximate Household and Metric Length Equivalents	
Household		**Metric**
1 in		2.5 cm
1 ft		30 cm
1 yd		0.9 m
1 mi		1.6 km

International Units

International Units measure the biological activity or potency of a drug, not a drug's weight. To determine the International Unit measure of a new drug, the World Health Organization compares the new drug with a similar drug with a known International Unit value. For example, the International Unit measure of a new antibiotic may be determined by testing its ability to inhibit bacterial growth compared with an established antibiotic. Types of medications that are measured using International Units include vaccines, antitoxins, vitamins, and certain blood products, like coagulation factors.

Medications labeled in the United States and registered with the United States Pharmacopeia may read USP units instead of International Units (IU). The United States Pharmacopeia is a nongovernmental institution that sets the standard for drug quality. In most cases, the biological activity of a drug labeled as an International Unit is identical to one labeled as a USP unit.

Basic Units and Notation Rules

The International Unit is the only form of this system of measure. Equivalencies between IUs and other units of measure, such as metric or household systems, do not exist. Medications that are ordered in units will be packaged and dispensed as units per tablet or units per milliliter.

Milliequivalents

A milliequivalent measures the ability of a substance to mix with another substance. Examples of medications that are measured in milliequivalents include calcium chloride, potassium chloride, sodium bicarbonate, and sodium chloride.

Basic Units and Notation Rules

Milliequivalents are abbreviated as mEq. Although the milliequivalent measure of a drug can be converted to a metric weight measure, there is little practical reason to do so in nursing.

Practice Notations

(answers on page 78)

Match the measurement system in the first column with the correct unit of measure in the second column.

1. SI metric system _____   **a.** IU

2. Milliequivalents _____   **b.** fluid ounce, pound, mile

3. Household system _____   **c.** liter, gram, meter

4. International Units _____   **d.** mEq

Write the correct notation for these quantities.

5. 3 fluid ounces _____

6. 4 pounds _____

7. 5 teaspoons _____

8. 2 cups _____

9. 6 inches _____

10. 12 milliequivalents _____

Identify these equivalent measures.

11. 1 gal = _____ L

12. 0.9 m = _____ yd

13. 2.5 cm = _____ in

14. 30 mL = _____ fl oz

15. 1 tsp = _____ mL

16. 1 c   = _____ mL

17. 15 mL = _____ Tbsp

Key Points

1. The SI metric system is the preferred system of measurement for prescribing and dispensing medications in the United States.

2. The basic units of the SI metric system include the meter (m), the kilogram (kg), and the liter (L).

3. The SI metric system is based on the powers of 10.

4. Abbreviations used to express medication dosages may be different than those used in the SI metric system due to increased risk of error when handwritten.

5. The household system of measurement should not be used in prescribing or administering medications.

6. The International Unit system of measurement reflects the biological activity of a drug compared to similar drugs with a known International Unit value.

7. A drug measured in milliequivalents reflects the ability of the medication to mix with another substance.

Chapter Post-Test

(answers in Unit 4)

Choose *True* or *False* for each statement.

1. The SI metric system is based on the power of 12.   True   False

2. The basic metric units are the inch (in) for length, the kilogram (kg) for weight, and the liter (L) for volume.   True   False

3. The apothecary system of measure should not be used to prescribe, compound, dispense, or administer medications.   True   False

4. The International Unit system of measurement assigns values to medications based on the biological activity of similar drugs.   True   False

5. Milliequivalent measures the ability of a substance to mix with another substance.   True   False

In each group of quantities, identify and circle the notation error.

6. 5 mg   6.1 gm   3 cm   8.32 kg

7. 76 kg   49 mcg   0.22 g   412 mgm

8. 297 g   9.26 L   6 mLs   13.3 mg

9. 23 mm   8 k   14 km   67 g

10. 0.09 mcgs   6.9 mL   31mg   918 m

11. 1 tsp   4 ou   3 Tbsp   2 pt

Write the correct notation for these quantities.

12. 42 milligrams _____

13. 3 cups _____

14. 700 micrograms _____

15. 35.4 millimeters _____

16. 12 liters _____

17. 7 teaspoons _____

18. 55 grams _____

19. 4 fluid ounces _____

Identify these equivalent measures.

20. 1 g = _____ mg

21. 1000 g = _____ kg

22. 1 kg = _____ lb

23. 1 tsp = _____ mL

24. 1000 mcg = _____ mg

25. 1 km = _____ m

26. 10 mm = _____ cm

27. 240 mL = _____ c

28. 1 in = _____ cm

29. 100 cm = _____ m

30. 1 lb = _____ g

31. 1 cm = _____ mm

32. 1 t = _____ kg

33. 1000 mg = _____ g

34. 1 ft = _____ cm

35. 30 mL = _____ fl oz

Answers to Practice Questions

Measures and Equivalents

1. b
2. 4.1 L
3. 2.5 km
4. 69.4 kg
5. 231 mcg
6. 532 g
7. 10 mL
8. 775 cm
9. 1 mg
10. 1 cm
11. 1000 g
12. 1 L
13. 1000 mL
14. 1000 m
15. 1 m

Notations

1. c
2. d
3. b
4. a
5. 3 fl oz
6. 4 lb
7. 5 tsp
8. 2 c
9. 6 in
10. 12 mEq
11. 3.8 L
12. 1 yd
13. 1 in
14. 1 fl oz
15. 5 mL
16. 240 mL
17. 1 Tbsp

Chapter 6
Conversions

Objectives

After completing this chapter, the learner will be able to—
1. Convert units of measure within the metric system, including simple and complex conversions.
2. Convert between metric and household systems of measure.

Conversions Within the Metric System

Converting between units in the metric system requires understanding the basic units of the metric system and their relationships. For example, a kilogram (kg) is 1000 times larger than a gram (g), which is 1000 times larger than a milligram (mg), which is 1000 times larger than a microgram (mcg). (See Figure 6-1.) Understanding the relationship between units helps set up equations and determine the accuracy of your answers.

Simple conversions require only one conversion factor because the units are directly related. In contrast, complex conversions require two or more conversion factors because the units are *not* directly related.

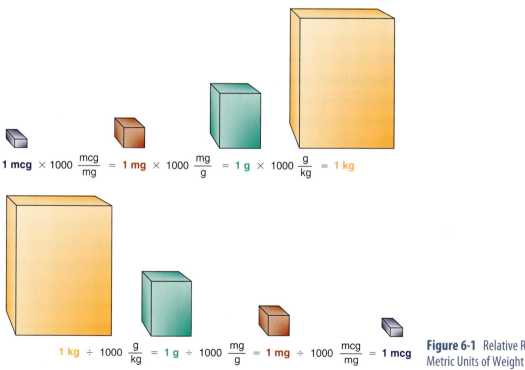

Figure 6-1 Relative Relationship Among Metric Units of Weight

Simple Metric Conversions

Simple conversions can be calculated by using dimensional analysis, which decreases the risk of making errors. An alternate method of converting metric units of measure is discussed in Box 6-1.

Example 1: 287 mcg = _____ mg

1. Establish the answer's unit of measure (mg), and place the equal sign to the right of mg.

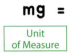

mg =

Unit of Measure

2. Normally, the next step would be to insert the given quantities. However, since we are converting from one unit of measure to another, the conversion factor must be inserted first.

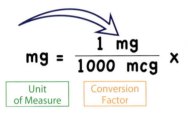

$$mg = \frac{1 \ mg}{1000 \ mcg} \ X$$

Unit of Measure Conversion Factor

3. Now insert the given quantity *287 mcg* and cancel units.

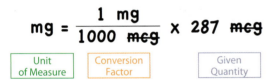

$$mg = \frac{1 \ mg}{1000 \ \cancel{mcg}} \times 287 \ \cancel{mcg}$$

Unit of Measure Conversion Factor Given Quantity

■ Box 6-1 Converting Metric Measures by Moving the Decimal Point

To convert closely related units of measure in the same system, move the decimal point.

Example 1: 349 mcg = _____ mg

In this example, a small unit (mcg) must be converted into a larger unit (mg). Because 1000 mcg are in 1 mg and 349 mcg is smaller than 1000 mcg, the final answer should be less than 1. Therefore, the decimal point must move to the *left* as many spaces as the number of zeros in the conversion factor. Sometimes, placing the decimal point at the end of a whole number helps identify the starting point.

$$.349. \ mcg = 0.349 \ mg$$

Example 2: 6.454 L = _____ mL

In this example, a large unit (L) must be converted into a smaller unit (mL). Because 1000 mL is equivalent to 1 L and the original quantity is greater than 6 L, the final answer should be at least 6000 mL. Therefore, the decimal point must move to the *right* by as many spaces as the number of zeros in the conversion factor.

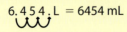

$$6.454. \ L = 6454 \ mL$$

4. Calculate the answer.

$$mg = \frac{1 \text{ mg}}{1000 \text{ mcg}} \times 287 \text{ mcg} = \frac{1 \text{ mg} \times 287}{1000} = 0.287 \text{ mg}$$

Unit of Measure	Conversion Factor		Given Quantity

5. Critically evaluate the answer. Since 1 mg is 1000 times larger than 1 mcg, it makes sense that 287 mcg will be only a fraction of 1 mg. Therefore, 287 mcg = 0.287 mg is a logical answer.

For Examples 2–5, refer to the directions in Example 1.

Example 2:   23 kg = _____ g

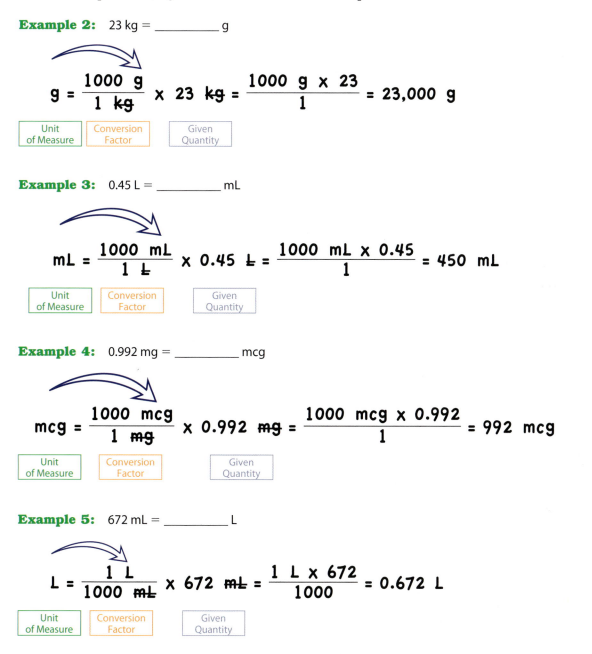

$$g = \frac{1000 \text{ g}}{1 \text{ kg}} \times 23 \text{ kg} = \frac{1000 \text{ g} \times 23}{1} = 23{,}000 \text{ g}$$

Unit of Measure	Conversion Factor	Given Quantity

Example 3:   0.45 L = _____ mL

$$mL = \frac{1000 \text{ mL}}{1 \text{ L}} \times 0.45 \text{ L} = \frac{1000 \text{ mL} \times 0.45}{1} = 450 \text{ mL}$$

Unit of Measure	Conversion Factor	Given Quantity

Example 4:   0.992 mg = _____ mcg

$$mcg = \frac{1000 \text{ mcg}}{1 \text{ mg}} \times 0.992 \text{ mg} = \frac{1000 \text{ mcg} \times 0.992}{1} = 992 \text{ mcg}$$

Unit of Measure	Conversion Factor	Given Quantity

Example 5:   672 mL = _____ L

$$L = \frac{1 \text{ L}}{1000 \text{ mL}} \times 672 \text{ mL} = \frac{1 \text{ L} \times 672}{1000} = 0.672 \text{ L}$$

Unit of Measure	Conversion Factor	Given Quantity

Practice Simple Metric to Metric Conversions

(answers on page 89)

Calculate these simple conversions. Do not round the answers.

1. 6.5 mg = _____ mcg

2. 5829 mcg = _____ mg

3. 93 mL = _____ L

4. 1.6 L = _____ mL

5. 2.3 kg = _____ g

6. 0.082 g = _____ mg

7. 1.9 L = _____ mL

8. 32 mg = _____ mcg

9. 0.3 kg = _____ g

10. 33 mg = _____ g

Complex Metric Conversions

Complex conversions require two or more conversion factors to solve the equation.

Example 1: 18,340 mcg = _____ g

   Two conversion factors are needed in this equation: one to convert g to mg and one to convert mg to mcg. Recall that 1 g = 1000 mg, and 1000 mcg = 1 mg.

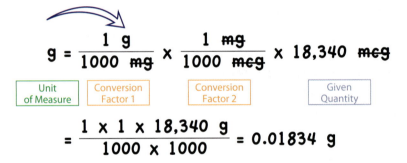

$$g = \frac{1\ g}{1000\ mg} \times \frac{1\ mg}{1000\ mcg} \times 18{,}340\ mcg$$

| Unit of Measure | Conversion Factor 1 | Conversion Factor 2 | Given Quantity |

$$= \frac{1 \times 1 \times 18{,}340\ g}{1000 \times 1000} = 0.01834\ g$$

For Examples 2–5, refer to the directions in Example 1.

Example 2: 3 kg = _____ mg

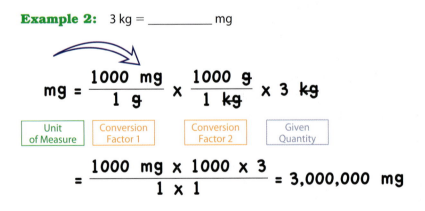

$$mg = \frac{1000\ mg}{1\ g} \times \frac{1000\ g}{1\ kg} \times 3\ kg$$

| Unit of Measure | Conversion Factor 1 | Conversion Factor 2 | Given Quantity |

$$= \frac{1000\ mg \times 1000 \times 3}{1 \times 1} = 3{,}000{,}000\ mg$$

Example 3:   2.5 kg = _____ mg

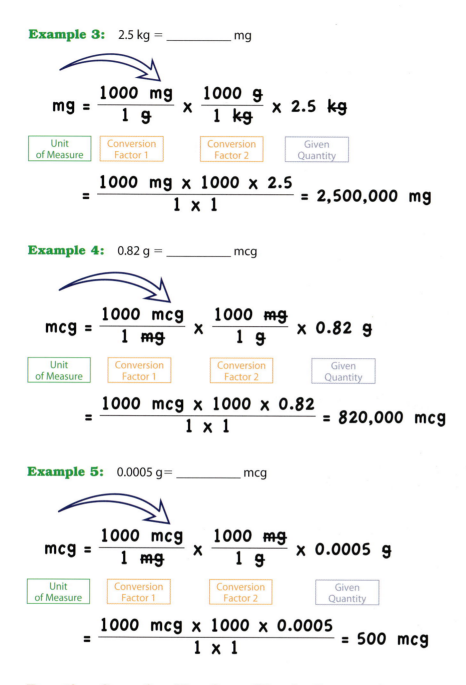

$$mg = \frac{1000\ mg}{1\ g} \times \frac{1000\ g}{1\ kg} \times 2.5\ kg$$

| Unit of Measure | Conversion Factor 1 | Conversion Factor 2 | Given Quantity |

$$= \frac{1000\ mg \times 1000 \times 2.5}{1 \times 1} = 2,500,000\ mg$$

Example 4:   0.82 g = _____ mcg

$$mcg = \frac{1000\ mcg}{1\ mg} \times \frac{1000\ mg}{1\ g} \times 0.82\ g$$

| Unit of Measure | Conversion Factor 1 | Conversion Factor 2 | Given Quantity |

$$= \frac{1000\ mcg \times 1000 \times 0.82}{1 \times 1} = 820,000\ mcg$$

Example 5:   0.0005 g = _____ mcg

$$mcg = \frac{1000\ mcg}{1\ mg} \times \frac{1000\ mg}{1\ g} \times 0.0005\ g$$

| Unit of Measure | Conversion Factor 1 | Conversion Factor 2 | Given Quantity |

$$= \frac{1000\ mcg \times 1000 \times 0.0005}{1 \times 1} = 500\ mcg$$

Practice Complex Metric to Metric Conversions

(answers on page 90)

Calculate these complex conversions. Do not round the answers.

1. 1367 mcg = _____ g

2. 4.52 g = _____ mcg

3. 1.08 kg = _____ mg

4. 45 g = _____ mcg

5. 603 mg = _____ kg

6. 0.007 g = _____ mcg

7. 0.176 kg = _____ mg

8. 0.0015 g = _____ mcg

9. 7670 mg = _____ kg

10. 25,000 mcg = _____ g

Conversions Between Household and Metric Measurements

The necessity to convert between household and metric units is becoming less common in administrating medication, but the skill is required in other nursing functions such as computing a patient's fluid volume oral intake and converting a patient's weight from pounds into kilograms.

Example 1:   3 fl oz = _____ mL

To convert 3 fl oz into mL, remember that 1 fl oz = 30 mL. Because the two measures are directly related to each other, only one conversion factor is needed in the equation.

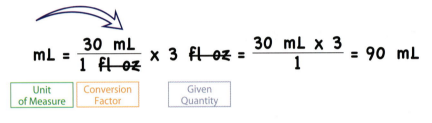

$$mL = \frac{30\ mL}{1\ fl\ oz} \times 3\ fl\ oz = \frac{30\ mL \times 3}{1} = 90\ mL$$

| Unit of Measure | Conversion Factor | Given Quantity |

Example 2:   0.81 L = _____ fl oz

In this example, there is no direct conversion from liters (L) into fluid ounces (fl oz). Therefore, liters (L) must be converted into milliliters (mL), then milliliters (mL) into fluid ounces (fl oz). As a result, this equation must have two conversion factors.

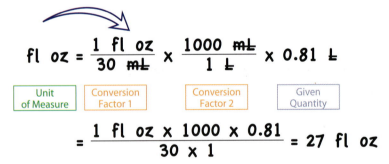

$$fl\ oz = \frac{1\ fl\ oz}{30\ mL} \times \frac{1000\ mL}{1\ L} \times 0.81\ L$$

| Unit of Measure | Conversion Factor 1 | Conversion Factor 2 | Given Quantity |

$$= \frac{1\ fl\ oz \times 1000 \times 0.81}{30 \times 1} = 27\ fl\ oz$$

For Examples 3– 5, refer to the directions in Examples 1 and 2.

Example 3:   8 lb = _____ kg (Round your answer to the nearest hundredth kg.)

Remember that 1 kilogram (kg) is equal to 2.2 pounds (lb).

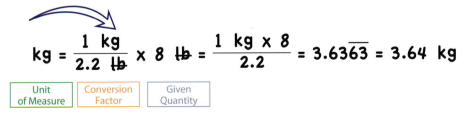

$$kg = \frac{1\ kg}{2.2\ lb} \times 8\ lb = \frac{1\ kg \times 8}{2.2} = 3.63\overline{63} = 3.64\ kg$$

| Unit of Measure | Conversion Factor | Given Quantity |

Example 4: 6 tsp = _____ mL

Remember that 5 milliliters (mL) is equal to 1 teaspoon (tsp).

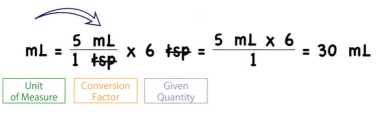

| Unit of Measure | Conversion Factor | Given Quantity |

Example 5: 2 c = _____ mL

This conversion can be calculated in one of two ways: as a simple conversion [1 cup (c) contains 240 milliliters (mL)] or as a complex conversion (30 mL = 1 fl oz).

Simple Conversion:

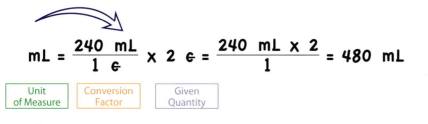

| Unit of Measure | Conversion Factor | Given Quantity |

Complex Conversion:

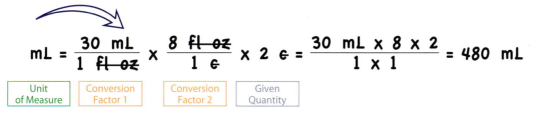

| Unit of Measure | Conversion Factor 1 | Conversion Factor 2 | Given Quantity |

Example 6: 7 lb, 2 oz = _____ kg (Round your answer to the nearest hundredth kg.)

There are two ways to solve this equation.

Method 1:

This conversion requires more than one step, since two different units must be converted (lb and oz).

1. Convert pounds (lb) into kilograms (kg).

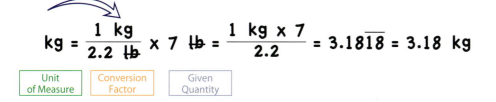

| Unit of Measure | Conversion Factor | Given Quantity |

2. Convert ounces (oz) into kilograms (kg).

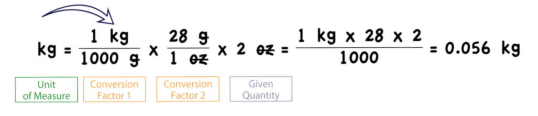

$$kg = \frac{1\ kg}{1000\ \cancel{g}} \times \frac{28\ \cancel{g}}{1\ \cancel{oz}} \times 2\ \cancel{oz} = \frac{1\ kg \times 28 \times 2}{1000} = 0.056\ kg$$

Unit of Measure	Conversion Factor 1	Conversion Factor 2	Given Quantity

3. Add the weights.

$$3.18\ kg + 0.06\ kg = 3.24\ kg$$

Method 2:
A shorter method of converting pounds and ounces into kilograms is to convert pounds into ounces, then ounces into kilograms.

1. Convert pounds into ounces [16 ounces (oz) = 1 pound (lb)].

$$oz = \left(\frac{16\ oz}{1\ \cancel{lb}} \times 7\ \cancel{lb} \right) + 2\ oz =$$

$$\left(\frac{16\ oz \times 7}{1} \right) + 2\ oz = 112\ oz + 2\ oz = 114\ oz$$

2. Convert ounces (oz) into kilograms (kg).

$$kg = \frac{1\ kg}{100\ \cancel{g}} \times \frac{28\ \cancel{g}}{1\ \cancel{oz}} \times 114\ \cancel{oz} = \frac{1\ kg \times 28 \times 114}{1000} = 3.192 = 3.19\ kg$$

Alert! Notice that the answer from the second calculation method is different from the first by 0.05 kg. This discrepancy occurs because metric equivalents of household measures are only approximations of the true weight (for example, 1 ounce equals *approximately* 28 grams). To be precise, 1 ounce is equivalent to 28.3495231 grams. In most cases, using approximate metric equivalencies is acceptable. If a more precise answer is needed, use the more precise (longer) equivalent measure in the conversion factor. See Box 6-2.

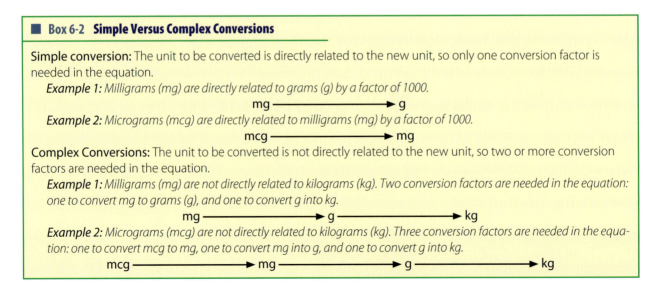

■ **Box 6-2 Simple Versus Complex Conversions**

Simple conversion: The unit to be converted is directly related to the new unit, so only one conversion factor is needed in the equation.
  Example 1: Milligrams (mg) are directly related to grams (g) by a factor of 1000.
  mg ⟶ g
  Example 2: Micrograms (mcg) are directly related to milligrams (mg) by a factor of 1000.
  mcg ⟶ mg
Complex Conversions: The unit to be converted is not directly related to the new unit, so two or more conversion factors are needed in the equation.
  Example 1: Milligrams (mg) are not directly related to kilograms (kg). Two conversion factors are needed in the equation: one to convert mg to grams (g), and one to convert g into kg.
  mg ⟶ g ⟶ kg
  Example 2: Micrograms (mcg) are not directly related to kilograms (kg). Three conversion factors are needed in the equation: one to convert mcg to mg, one to convert mg into g, and one to convert g into kg.
  mcg ⟶ mg ⟶ g ⟶ kg

Practice Conversions Between Household and Metric Measures

(answers on page 91)

Calculate these conversions. Round the answers to the nearest tenth.

1. 14 cm = _____ in

2. 3 tsp = _____ mL

3. 20 mL = _____ Tbsp

4. 7 fl oz = _____ mL

5. 60 cm = _____ ft

6. 12 kg = _____ lb

7. 8 oz = _____ g

8. 44 lb = _____ kg

9. 5 ft = _____ cm

10. 63 mL = _____ tsp

Key Points

1. Converting quantities from one unit of measure to another, whether within the same system or between different systems, requires an understanding of how the quantities relate to each other.
2. Simple conversions are those that require only one conversion factor in the equation because the units are directly related to each other.
3. Complex conversions are those that require two or more conversion factors in the equation because the units are not directly related to each other.

Chapter Post-Test

(answers in Unit 4)

Calculate these conversions. Do not round the answers.

1. 12 mm = _____ cm

2. 432 mcg = _____ mg

3. 9926 mL = _____ L

4. 627 cm = _____ m

5. 8264 mg = _____ g

6. 0.015 L = _____ mL

7. 0.73 kg = _____ g

8. 45,600 mcg = _____ g

9. 1.3 kg = _____ mg

10. 4.5 km = _____ cm

11. 7.9 g = _____ mg

12. 3.2 m = _____ mm

13. 0.00522 g = _____ mcg

14. 9850 mg = _____ kg

15. 67 mL = _____ L

Calculate these conversions. Round the answers to the nearest tenth.

16. 6 lb = _____ kg

17. 10 cm = _____ in

18. 6 fl oz = _____ mL

19. 1.5 c = _____ mL

20. 25 kg = _____ lb

21. 96 in = _____ cm

22. 38 lb = _____ g

23. 560 g = _____ oz

24. 77 mL = _____ fl oz

25. 30 mL = _____ tsp

26. 9 fl oz = _____ mL

27. 5 Tbsp = _____ mL

28. 165 cm = _____ in

29. 44 kg = _____ lb

30. 2 tsp = _____ mL

Answers to Practice Questions

Simple Metric to Metric Conversions

1. $\text{mcg} = \dfrac{1000 \text{ mcg}}{1 \text{ mg}} \times 6.5 \text{ mg} = \dfrac{1000 \text{ mcg} \times 6.5}{1} = 6500 \text{ mcg}$

2. $\text{mg} = \dfrac{1 \text{ mg}}{1000 \text{ mcg}} \times 5829 \text{ mcg} = \dfrac{1 \text{ mg} \times 5829}{1000} = 5.829 \text{ mg}$

3. $\text{L} = \dfrac{1 \text{ L}}{1000 \text{ mL}} \times 93 \text{ mL} = \dfrac{1 \text{ L} \times 93}{1000} = 0.093 \text{ L}$

4. $\text{mL} = \dfrac{1000 \text{ mL}}{1 \text{ L}} \times 1.6 \text{ L} = \dfrac{1000 \text{ mL} \times 1.6}{1} = 1600 \text{ mL}$

5. $\text{g} = \dfrac{1000 \text{ g}}{1 \text{ kg}} \times 2.3 \text{ kg} = \dfrac{1000 \text{ g} \times 2.3}{1} = 2300 \text{ g}$

6. $\text{mg} = \dfrac{1000 \text{ mg}}{1 \text{ g}} \times 0.082 \text{ g} = \dfrac{1000 \text{ mg} \times 0.082}{1} = 82 \text{ mg}$

7. $\text{mL} = \dfrac{1000 \text{ mL}}{1 \text{ L}} \times 1.9 \text{ L} = \dfrac{1000 \text{ mL} \times 1.9}{1} = 1900 \text{ mL}$

8. $\text{mcg} = \dfrac{1000 \text{ mcg}}{1 \text{ mg}} \times 32 \text{ mg} = \dfrac{1000 \text{ mcg} \times 32}{1} = 32{,}000 \text{ mcg}$

9. $\text{g} = \dfrac{1000 \text{ g}}{1 \text{ kg}} \times 0.3 \text{ kg} = \dfrac{1000 \text{ g} \times 0.3}{1} = 300 \text{ g}$

10. $\text{g} = \dfrac{1 \text{ g}}{1000 \text{ mg}} \times 33 \text{ mg} = \dfrac{1 \text{ g} \times 33}{1000} = 0.033 \text{ g}$

Complex Metric to Metric Conversions

1. $g = \dfrac{1g}{1000 \text{ mg}} \times \dfrac{1 \text{ mg}}{1000 \text{ mcg}} \times 1367 \text{ mcg} = \dfrac{1g \times 1 \times 1367}{1000 \times 1000} = 0.001367 \text{ g}$

2. $\text{mcg} = \dfrac{1000 \text{ mcg}}{1 \text{ mg}} \times \dfrac{1000 \text{ mg}}{1 \text{ g}} \times 4.52 \text{ g} = \dfrac{1000 \text{ mcg} \times 1000 \times 4.52}{1 \times 1} = 4{,}520{,}000 \text{ mcg}$

3. $\text{mg} = \dfrac{1000 \text{ mg}}{1 \text{ g}} \times \dfrac{1000 \text{ g}}{1 \text{ kg}} \times 1.08 \text{ kg} = \dfrac{1000 \text{ mg} \times 1000 \times 1.08}{1 \times 1} = 1{,}080{,}000 \text{ mg}$

4. $\text{mcg} = \dfrac{1000 \text{ mcg}}{1 \text{ mg}} \times \dfrac{1000 \text{ mg}}{1 \text{ g}} \times 45 \text{ g} = \dfrac{1000 \text{ mcg} \times 1000 \times 45}{1 \times 1} = 45{,}000{,}000 \text{ mcg}$

5. $\text{kg} = \dfrac{1 \text{ kg}}{1000 \text{ g}} \times \dfrac{1 \text{ g}}{1000 \text{ mg}} \times 603 \text{ mg} = \dfrac{1 \text{ kg} \times 1 \times 603}{1000 \times 1000} = 0.000603 \text{ kg}$

6. $\text{mcg} = \dfrac{1000 \text{ mcg}}{1 \text{ mg}} \times \dfrac{1000 \text{ mg}}{1 \text{ g}} \times 0.007 \text{ g} = \dfrac{1000 \text{ mcg} \times 1000 \times 0.007}{1 \times 1} = 7000 \text{ mcg}$

7. $\text{mg} = \dfrac{1000 \text{ mg}}{1 \text{ g}} \times \dfrac{1000 \text{ g}}{1 \text{ kg}} \times 0.176 \text{ kg} = \dfrac{1000 \text{ mg} \times 1000 \times 0.176}{1 \times 1} = 176{,}000 \text{ mg}$

8. $\text{mcg} = \dfrac{1000 \text{ mcg}}{1 \text{ mg}} \times \dfrac{1000 \text{ mg}}{1 \text{ g}} \times 0.0015 \text{ g} = \dfrac{1000 \text{ mcg} \times 1000 \times 0.0015}{1 \times 1} = 1500 \text{ mcg}$

9. $\text{kg} = \dfrac{1 \text{ kg}}{1000 \text{ g}} \times \dfrac{1 \text{ g}}{1000 \text{ mg}} \times 7670 \text{ mg} = \dfrac{1 \text{ kg} \times 1 \times 7670}{1000 \times 1000} = 0.00767 \text{ kg}$

10. $g = \dfrac{1 \text{ g}}{1000 \text{ mg}} \times \dfrac{1 \text{ mg}}{1000 \text{ mcg}} \times 25{,}000 \text{ mcg} = \dfrac{1 \text{ g} \times 1 \times 25{,}000}{1000 \times 1000} = 0.025 \text{ g}$

Conversions Between Household and Metric Measures

1. in = $\dfrac{1 \text{ in}}{2.5 \text{ cm}}$ x 14 cm = $\dfrac{1 \text{ in} \times 14}{2.5}$ = 5.6 in

2. mL = $\dfrac{5 \text{ mL}}{1 \text{ tsp}}$ x 3 tsp = $\dfrac{5 \text{ mL} \times 3}{1}$ = 15 mL

3. Tbsp = $\dfrac{1 \text{ Tbsp}}{15 \text{ mL}}$ x 20 mL = $\dfrac{1 \text{ Tbsp} \times 20}{15}$ = 1.3̄3 Tbsp = 1.3 Tbsp

4. mL = $\dfrac{30 \text{ mL}}{1 \text{ fl oz}}$ x 7 fl oz = $\dfrac{30 \text{ mL} \times 7}{1}$ = 210 mL

5. ft = $\dfrac{1 \text{ ft}}{30 \text{ cm}}$ x 60 cm = $\dfrac{1 \text{ ft} \times 60}{30}$ = 2 ft

6. lb = $\dfrac{2.2 \text{ lb}}{1 \text{ kg}}$ x 12 kg = $\dfrac{2.2 \text{ lb} \times 12}{1}$ = 26.4 lb

7. g = $\dfrac{28 \text{ g}}{1 \text{ oz}}$ x 8 oz = $\dfrac{28 \text{ g} \times 8}{1}$ = 224 g

8. kg = $\dfrac{1 \text{ kg}}{2.2 \text{ lb}}$ x 44 lb = $\dfrac{1 \text{ kg} \times 44}{2.2}$ = 20 kg

9. cm = $\dfrac{30 \text{ cm}}{1 \text{ ft}}$ x 5 ft = $\dfrac{30 \text{ cm} \times 5}{1}$ = 150 cm

10. tsp = $\dfrac{1 \text{ tsp}}{5 \text{ mL}}$ x 63 mL = $\dfrac{1 \text{ tsp} \times 63}{5}$ = 12.6 tsp

Chapter 7

Safety Considerations in Medication Administration

Objectives

After completing this chapter, the learner will be able to—
1. Define *medication error*.
2. Describe the functions of U.S. organizations that are involved with ensuring medication safety.
3. Differentiate between the various medication delivery systems.
4. Explain the six rights and three checks of medication administration.
5. Describe how point-of-care barcode technology improves the accuracy of medication administration.
6. Discuss the purpose of medication reconciliation.
7. Recognize acceptable and unacceptable abbreviations associated with medication orders.

Medication Errors

A medication error is any preventable event that may cause or lead to inappropriate medication use or patient harm while the medication is in the control of the healthcare professional, patient, or consumer. Such events may be related to professional practice, health care products, procedures, and systems, including prescribing; order communication; product labeling, packaging, and nomenclature; compounding; dispensing; distribution; administration; education; monitoring; and use. (National Coordinating Council for Medication Error Reporting and Prevention, 2018)

Each year in the United States, medication errors in healthcare facilities cause hundreds of thousands of patients to suffer illness or injury, and cost patients, hospitals, healthcare providers, and insurance companies billions of dollars. A 1999 study revealed that 7000 Americans die each year from medication errors (Kohn, Corrigan, & Donaldson, 2000). In 2001, the costs of drug-related problems were estimated to be $177.4 billion annually (Ernst & Grizzle, 2001). Another 2001 study revealed that human factors, such as performance or knowledge deficits, accounted for 65.2 percent of patient deaths from medication errors, followed by communication problems, which accounted for 15.8 percent of deaths (Phillips et al., 2001). A 2013 literature review revealed that the incidence of patient harm is even higher than these early estimates—up to 440,000 people die or experience injury from medical errors annually, including mistakes related to medications (James, 2013).

Organizations Involved in Safe Medication Practices

In the United States, many organizations monitor the strength, purity, and efficacy of medications, oversee the safety of the manufacturing and labeling processes, formulate policies and procedures to reduce medication errors, and conduct research into medication errors to prevent future harm.

U.S. Food and Drug Administration

The U.S. Food and Drug Administration (FDA) is a public health agency that oversees the safety of consumer products, such as medications, biologics, cosmetics, food, and medical devices. The organization's roots extend back to 1862 when a chemist was employed by the U.S. Department of Agriculture to investigate the adulteration of agricultural commodities. In 1906, after investigating complaints about food product contamination and misleading labeling of medicines, Congress passed the Pure Food and Drug Act and created today's FDA. Presently, the U.S. Department of Health and Human Services oversees the FDA, which is composed of nine divisions that regulate products consumed by the public. Two divisions within the FDA deal specifically with medications: the Center for Drug Evaluation and Research (CDER) and the Center for Biologic Evaluation and Research (CBER). See Boxes 7-1 and 7-2 and Figure 7-1.

■ Box 7-1 History of Significant Drug Legislation

1906: The Pure Food and Drugs Act (The Wiley Act)
The manufacture, sale, or transportation of misbranded food products and medications is prohibited. Drugs must meet standards of strength and purity. Meat products must be inspected by the government prior to sale.

1912: The Sherley Amendment
The labeling of medications with false therapeutic claims is banned.

1914: The Harrison Narcotic Act
The production, import, and distribution of narcotics become federally regulated. Physicians and pharmacists who dispense narcotics must improve their record-keeping.

1938: The Federal Food, Drug, and Cosmetic Act
Medical devices and cosmetics become federally regulated. Drugs must be labeled with directions for safe use. Manufacturers of drugs have to prove that their medications are safe prior to being released for sale to the public. False therapeutic claims cannot be made about drugs. Government inspectors are authorized to inspect manufacturing facilities.

1951: The Durham-Humphrey Amendment
This amendment establishes the difference between over-the-counter drugs and drugs needing a prescription from a physician.

1962: The Kefauver-Harris Drug Amendments
Drug manufacturers must prove that their medicines are safe and effective prior to sale.

1970: The Controlled Substance Act
The manufacture, import, distribution, possession, and use of certain substances, particularly narcotics, fall under regulatory control. Narcotics are categorized into "schedules" from I to V depending on whether the drugs have legitimate medicinal use and on their potential for causing abuse and addiction.

Continued

■ Box 7-1 History of Significant Drug Legislation—cont'd

1983: The Orphan Drug Act
This act creates financial incentives for pharmaceutical manufacturers to research and develop drugs needed to treat rare diseases.

2012: The Food and Drug Administration Safety and Innovation Act (FDASIA)
This act provides the FDA with the authority to collect user fees to fund reviews of innovator drugs, medical devices, generic drugs, and biological products; to promote innovation to allow faster access to safe and effective products; to increase stakeholder involvement in FDA processes; and to enhance the safety of the drug supply chain.

■ Box 7-2 Medication Tragedies

Radithor
Radithor was manufactured in New Jersey in the 1920s. This elixir, composed of distilled water and small quantities of radium, was marketed as a cure-all, and subjected those who drank it to radiation poisoning.

Elixir Sulfanilamide
A pharmaceutical company in Tennessee marketed the elixir sulfanilamide to treat streptococcal infections. In 1937, in response to public request for a liquid form of the drug, the company's chief chemist found that sulfanilamide dissolved well in diethylene glycol, a chemical relative to modern-day antifreeze. The drug was not tested before release to the public. More than 100 people in 15 states died from poisoning.

Thalidomide
Manufactured by a German company in the 1950s and early 1960s, thalidomide was marketed as a sleeping pill and an antiemetic drug for pregnant women. Ingestion of the drug by these women resulted in thousands of infants in Europe being born with severe birth defects involving the limbs.

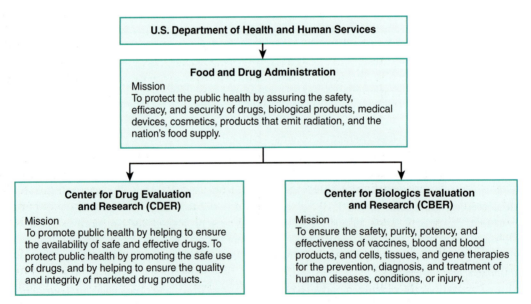

Figure 7-1 Organization of the FDA

U.S. Pharmacopeia

The U.S. Pharmacopeia (USP) was founded in 1820 to create a system of standards and quality control. The organization has also developed a national formulary, admitting only those drugs that meet the criteria of being the most established and the best understood. Today, the mission of the

U.S. Pharmacopeia is to ensure the quality, safety, and benefit of medicines, food ingredients, and dietary supplements. The USP sets the standards for quality, purity, strength, and consistency of those products.

Institute for Safe Medication Practices

The Institute for Safe Medication Practices (ISMP) is a nonprofit, independent watchdog organization devoted solely to safe medication use and error prevention. Created in 1975, the functions of the ISMP include the following:

- Collecting and analyzing medication-related errors and near misses
- Educating consumers and healthcare providers on safe medication practices
- Formulating error-prevention strategies
- Collaborating with other organizations concerned with patient safety
- Advocating for safe medication practices
- Conducting research into evidence-based safe medication practices

The ISMP publishes several newsletters designed to alert healthcare providers to current safety issues and error-avoidance strategies.

The National Coordinating Council for Medication Error Reporting and Prevention

Consumer and healthcare organizations formed the National Coordinating Council for Medication Error Reporting and Prevention (NCC MERP) in 1995 in recognition of the fact that medication errors occur for multiple reasons and that no single organization can adequately address the danger to patient safety. As a group, the NCC MERP has the authority and resources to tackle the complex nature of medication errors and develop appropriate solutions.

The Institute for Healthcare Improvement

In 1991, the Institute for Healthcare Improvement (IHI) was founded in an effort to improve healthcare throughout the world. The IHI's goals focus on improving worldwide health and healthcare. From 2006 to 2008, the IHI launched the "5 Million Lives Campaign," an educational initiative that focused on improving patient safety, concentrating on preventing patient harm from high-risk medications such as anticoagulants, sedatives, narcotics, and insulin. Now, in its third decade, IHI is focusing on the Triple Aim—improving population health and patient-centered care and containing healthcare costs.

The Joint Commission

The mission of The Joint Commission (formerly known as The Joint Commission on the Accreditation of Healthcare Organizations, or JCAHO) is to improve patient safety in healthcare facilities through accreditation and certification services that support performance improvement. The goal of The Joint Commission is to reduce the risk of adverse outcomes for patients receiving care in hospitals, laboratories, ambulatory care clinics, behavioral healthcare agencies, and long-term care facilities.

In January, 2003, The Joint Commission published the first of its National Patient Safety Goals (NPSGs). The purpose of these goals was to help organizations address specific areas of concern with patient safety, such as improving the accuracy of patient identification, improving communication between caregivers, standardizing medical abbreviations, and reducing errors in surgery. NPSGs are reviewed annually, and some are revised, eliminated, or added depending on information gathered from practitioners, consumers, and other interested parties. Each NPSG contains specific performance criteria that must be met by the healthcare facility to be in compliance with the goal. For example, the purpose of NPSG Goal One for hospitals is to identify patients correctly. (The Joint Commission, 2018). The performance criteria that must be met by the accredited hospital includes the use of two patient identifiers when administering medications or blood products, providing treatments, collecting specimens for testing, and labeling of specimens.

Nurse Practice Acts

Each state has Nurse Practice Acts, which are laws defining the scope of practice and responsibilities for nurses. Nurse Practice Acts are designed to protect the health, safety, and welfare of the public, including protection from unsafe nurses. Each state has a Board of Nursing that defines nursing education requirements and scope of practice, and establishes disciplinary procedures for nurses who break the law.

Healthcare Facilities

Every healthcare facility should have written policies and procedures that outline a nurse's scope of practice and responsibilities for medication administration and documentation. For example, some facilities may allow Licensed Practical/Vocational Nurses (LPN/LVN) to administer certain intravenous medications after additional education and practice has been established. Other facilities may allow LPN/LVNs to administer oral medications only. It is the nurse's responsibility to become familiar with the policies and procedures of the facility in which he or she practices.

Medication Delivery Systems

Medication delivery systems refer to the methods by which drugs are delivered to nursing units for administration to patients. Medications are typically supplied by the pharmacy in either unit doses or multiple doses.

Unit Dose Systems

Unit dose medications are packaged individually in sterile, clearly marked packages (Fig. 7-2). Most unit dose medications come in solids—such as tablets or capsules—or in liquids—such as prefilled containers or syringes. The advantages of unit dose medication systems are twofold: ease of administration for the nurse and increased safety for the patient. The unit dose system reduces the time necessary to prepare drugs for administration, lessens the risk of drug contamination through inappropriate handling techniques, and reduces the chance of mixing different medications in a common container. Unit dose medications should be transported to the bedside in their original packaging to further reduce the chance of errors.

Multiple Dose Systems

Multiple dose medication delivery systems package more than one dose in a container because such packaging is sometimes more cost-effective and practical than unit dose packaging (Fig. 7-3). The nurse who is withdrawing drugs from a multiple dose container, however, must ensure that the medication is within its expiration date and that it has been handled carefully to reduce the chance of contamination. If the medication is to be injected into tissues or veins (parenterally), the nurse must also read the drug label and package insert carefully to make sure that the manufacturer intended the container to have multiple doses. If the label states "Single Use Only," then multiple doses should not be drawn from the container (Fig. 7-4).

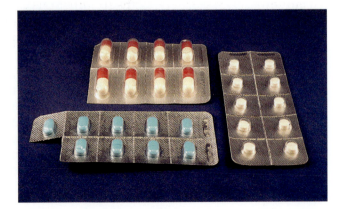

Figure 7-2 Unit Dose Medications

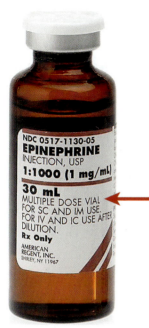

Figure 7-3 This vial provides multiple doses of the medication epinephrine.

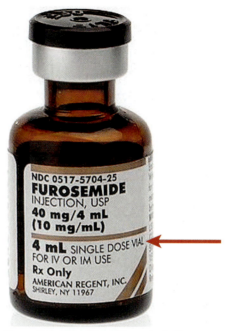

Figure 7-4 This vial provides a single dose of the medication furosemide.

Automated Medication Dispensing Systems

Automated medication dispensing (AMD) systems are computer-operated storage and dispensing devices for medications and healthcare-related supplies (Figs. 7-5 and 7-6). A typical AMD system consists of a medication storage cabinet, keyboard, monitor, and software. Medications are stored in locked drawers in the cabinet. Users must input a user identification code and password in order to access medications.

The benefits of AMD systems include:

- The ability to track medication and supply inventory in real time, which reduces costs and improves efficiency.
- Enhanced security of stored medications. Users must log onto the system in order to access and withdraw drugs. All transactions for every patient and every user are recorded, providing an audit trail in case of discrepancies.
- Enhanced access to patient medications. Some cabinets are mobile and may be moved from room to room.
- Improved patient safety. Software programs alert users to potential drug interactions and patient allergies. Many systems have barcode readers that compare the medication being dispensed with the patient's identification to assure that the right drug is being administered to the right patient at the right time.

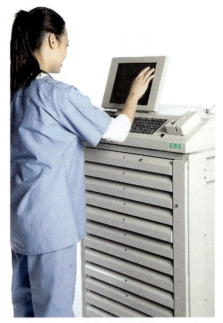

Figure 7-5 Omnicell Automated Dispensing System

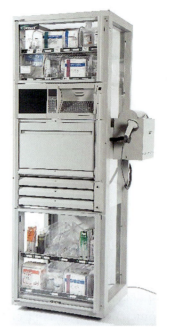

Figure 7-6 Omnicell Storage Cabinet

Practice Medication Errors

(answers on page 115)

Choose True or False for each statement.

1. Human factors, such as knowledge deficits, contribute to medication errors.   True   False

2. One of the missions of the Food and Drug Administration is to protect public health by ensuring the safety, efficacy, and security of drugs.   True   False

3. The National Patient Safety Goals were formulated to punish hospitals for medication errors.   True   False

4. The Center for Drug Evaluation and Research is a division of the Institute for Healthcare Improvement.   True   False

Select the best answer.

5. The nurse removes a tablet from a bottle of acetaminophen. This is an example of a(n):
   a. unit dose delivery system.
   b. multiple dose delivery system.
   c. automated delivery system.
   d. dual dose delivery system.

6. One disadvantage of a multiple dose delivery system is:
   a. increased risk of contaminating the contents of the container.
   b. reduction in time to administer the drug.
   c. increased risk of mixing more than one medication in one container.
   d. a and c.

7. The nurse is preparing to administer a single-dose medication to a patient. Which of these actions is correct?
   a. The nurse opens the unit dose package outside the patient's room.
   b. The nurse takes the medication from a bottle that the patient brought from home.
   c. The nurse opens the unit dose package at the patient's bedside.
   d. The nurse opens the unit dose package inside the patient's room.

Insert the correct answer.

8. Computer-operated storage and dispensing devises for medications are called _____ _____ systems.

9. The organization responsible for setting the standards for the quality, purity, strength, and consistency of medicines, food ingredients, and dietary supplements is the _____.

10. The organization that has the authority and resources to tackle the complex nature of medication errors and develop appropriate solutions is the _____.

Preventing Medication Errors: Six Rights and Three Checks

Preventing medication errors from reaching patients requires careful attention. Nurses should use the six rights of medication administration when preparing and administering medications. (See Box 7-3).

Nurses should also check medication labels against the medication administration record (MAR) at least three times before administering drugs. Unfortunately, following the six rights and the three checks does not always guarantee that drugs are given without error. Human factors such as interruptions, fatigue, or lack of knowledge, combined with weaknesses in a facility's medication administration system can also contribute to adverse outcomes for patients even if the six rights and three checks have been followed.

Right 1: The Right Patient

The Joint Commission requires nurses in healthcare facilities to use two patient-specific identifiers when administering medications. The term *identifier* refers to the person-specific information by which the patient can be identified. Acceptable items include the patient's name, date of birth, social security number, address, medical record number, and facility account number. To identify a patient correctly, the nurse might use one of the following methods: (1) Have the patient state his or her name and date of birth and compare the patient's response with the name and birth date on the MAR or (2) have the patient state his or her name and compare it with the patient's armband, then compare the patient's medical record number on the MAR with the medical record number on the patient's armband. Electronic forms of identification technology, such as barcode scanning, that include two or more patient identifiers are also acceptable. Room

---

■ **Box 7-3   The Six Rights and Three Checks of Medication Administration**

The Six Rights

Ensure that the six rights are being followed when preparing drugs for administration:

1. The Right Patient
2. The Right Drug
3. The Right Dose
4. The Right Route
5. The Right Time
6. The Right Documentation

The Three Checks

Check the medications with the medication administration record:

1. When collecting the medications
2. Prior to entering the patient's room
3. At the patient's bedside

numbers may not be used as a form of patient identification since patients may be moved to different rooms or units.

Healthcare facilities should have policies regarding acceptable forms of patient identifiers, and should address how to identify patients who are confused or nonverbal.

Patients should be encouraged to take an active role in their medical care. They should be educated about the medications they are taking, including benefits and risks, proper administration, side effect management, and necessary follow-up care, such as laboratory testing. They should be encouraged to ask questions about their medications—a free exchange of information between providers and patients can help reduce misunderstandings and medication errors.

Right 2: The Right Drug

Administering the wrong drug to a patient is one of the most common preventable drug errors. Factors that lead to giving the wrong medication include the following:

- Drug names that look alike or sound alike
- Drug labels that look similar or are misleading
- Poorly written prescriptions
- Errors in transcribing the medication to the MAR
- Lack of knowledge by the care provider about the medication being prescribed

A medication usually has three names: a generic name, a trade name, and a chemical name. For example, Tylenol is a trade name for the generic form of acetaminophen, which also has the chemical name of *N*-acetyl-*p*-aminophenol. Chemical names reflect the chemical composition of the drug and are not used in prescribing medications. However, drugs may be ordered by either the generic or the trade name. Because of the thousands of medications on the market, inevitably many names may look or sound similar.

The ISMP has published a list of easily confused drugs that look alike when written or sound alike when spoken (see the ISMP's List of Confused Drug Names at http://www.ismp.org). For example, two medications that may look alike in poor handwriting are Taxol and Paxil. Two medications that may sound alike when spoken are Foradil and Toradol. Many drugs also have extended-release forms, such as Depakote and Depakote ER. Depakote ER is administered once daily, whereas Depakote is typically administered twice daily. Confusing one form for the other could result in an overdose, which may cause a patient to experience serious health problems.

To reduce the chance of confusing drug names, The Joint Commission requires healthcare facilities to identify a list of at least 10 look-alike or sound-alike drugs used by the facility. The facility must take action to prevent errors involving the drugs on the list. The FDA, The Joint Commission, and the ISMP have also recommended the use of "tall man" letters to help differentiate certain look-alike drugs (Institute for Safe Medication Practices, 2016). Here are some examples:

acetoHEXAMIDE versus acetaZOLIMIDE

buPROPion versus busPIRone

clomiPHENE versus clomiPRAMINE

Using technology can also help lessen medication mistakes. For instance, many healthcare facilities use electronic prescriptions, or e-prescriptions, to reduce the errors generated by illegible handwritten prescriptions. Such software not only decreases the chances of misreading a prescription but provides easy access to patient information and checks automatically for drug allergies, appropriate dosages, and drug-drug interactions. In addition, most AMDs have software that includes drug reference information that is easily accessed by nursing staff. Drug information is also available for downloading from the Internet on tablets or smart phones.

Right 3: The Right Dose

Administering the wrong dose of a medication is one of the most common types of medication errors. Factors that contribute toward dosage errors include the following:

- Poor handwriting
- Inaccurate calculation of dosages that are based on body weight or body surface area
- Incorrect transcription of the dosage from the order onto the medication record
- Use of unapproved abbreviations (Fig. 7-7)
- Use of trailing zeros in the dosage prescription (Fig. 7-8)
- Availability of highly concentrated drug products (Fig. 7-9)

℞

20U Lantus insulin

Figure 7-7 Using the abbreviation *u* instead of writing out *units* makes this order for 20 units of Lantus look like 200 units.

℞

50 mg lisinopril

Figure 7-8 Using a trailing zero and the nearly invisible period between the 5 and the 0 makes this order for lisinopril 5 mg look like lisinopril 50 mg.

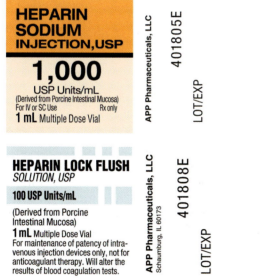
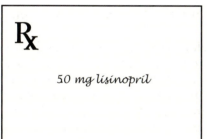

HEPARIN SODIUM INJECTION, USP
1,000 USP Units/mL
(Derived from Porcine Intestinal Mucosa)
For IV or SC Use   Rx only
1 mL Multiple Dose Vial

APP Pharmaceuticals, LLC
401805E
LOT/EXP
3 63323-540-01 2

HEPARIN LOCK FLUSH
SOLUTION, USP
100 USP Units/mL
(Derived from Porcine Intestinal Mucosa)
1 mL Multiple Dose Vial
For maintenance of patency of intravenous injection devices only, not for anticoagulant therapy. Will alter the results of blood coagulation tests.

APP Pharmaceuticals, LLC
Schaumburg, IL 60173
401808E
LOT/EXP
3 63323-545-01 7

Figure 7-9 Two Concentrations of Heparin

Ensuring that prescribed medication dosages are within the limits directed by the drug manufacturer is part of a nurse's responsibility. Healthcare providers who prescribe medications are human and sometimes make mistakes. Therefore, nurses should always question dosages outside the safe dose limit. They should also be familiar with their facility's policies regarding medications that need to be double-checked by two registered nurses or a registered nurse and a pharmacist. Certain medications, such as insulin and heparin, may cause severe adverse effects if the wrong dose is administered.

Right 4: The Right Route

Medications are prepared in liquid, solid, or powered form. They may be administered in a variety of ways, such as by mouth (orally), through injection into tissue or into veins (parenterally), or by direct contact with skin or mucous membranes (topically). The form of the drug and the route by which it is taken determines how quickly the medication is absorbed, distributed throughout the body, metabolized, and then excreted. For example, medications in liquid form are absorbed in the stomach faster than solids, and drugs given by injection are absorbed more rapidly than those given orally (Tables 7-1 and 7-2). Nurses should always check the drug label or package insert to determine the route(s) of administration to verify the route selected by the prescriber. See also Box 7-4.

Table 7-1	Drug Formulations
	Solids
Tablets	Tablets are hard, solid forms of medications that contain the active ingredient of the drug plus binders and fillers to give it bulk. They come in many colors and shapes and may be • scored to allow them to be broken into pieces for lower dosing. • enteric-coated to prevent them from being dissolved in the stomach. • chewable to aid in ease of administration. Not all tablets are chewable, however. • formulated to be slowly released into the body. Look for the suffixes "SR" (slow- or sustained-release), "XL" or "ER" (extended-release), "CR" (controlled-release), or "LA" (long-acting).
Capsules	Capsules contain medication that is enclosed within a soft gelatinous shell or a hard, two-piece casing.
Caplets	Caplets are coated, elongated tablets.
Lozenges	Lozenges are hard, sugar-based tablets that are not meant to be swallowed but to be allowed to dissolve slowly in the mouth to provide topical application of the medication to the oral cavity and throat.
Troches or pastilles	Like lozenges, troches and pastilles are meant to be dissolved in the mouth.
Suppositories	Suppositories contain medications that are mixed in a base of glycerin or cocoa butter and administered rectally or vaginally.
Transdermal patches	Transdermal patches are applied to the skin and contain medication that is slowly released and absorbed into the blood supply.
	Liquids
Syrups	Syrups are liquids that contain medication in a thick, sweetened, and flavored water base.
Elixirs	Elixirs are similar to syrups, but the medication is mixed in a base of water and alcohol.
Suspensions	Suspensions consist of undissolved particles of the medication suspended in an oil or water base. Suspensions must be shaken thoroughly before being administered as the drug particles tend to settle to the bottom of the bottle.
Solutions	Solutions contain medications in a sterile base of water or saline. These medications are usually meant to be administered by injection into tissues or veins.
Lotions	Lotions are similar to liquid suspensions but are thicker. They are used to apply medication to the skin.
	Semi-solids
Ointments	Ointments are thick petroleum- or lanolin-based substances that are applied for their topical effects.

Table 7-2   Routes of Medication Administration

Routes of Administration	Medication Formulation	Examples
Enteral		
Oral (by mouth)	Tablets, capsules, caplets, extended-release tablets or capsules, chewable tablets, liquids, elixirs, suspensions, syrups, lozenges, troches, pastilles	Acetaminophen tablets, diltiazem extended-release capsules, chewable aspirin tablets, amoxicillin/clavulanate suspension, clotrimazole lozenges
Rectal	Suppositories	Bisacodyl suppository
Via tube placed into the stomach or small intestine.	Liquids, tablets that can be crushed, capsules that can be opened	Refer to a "do not crush" list before crushing and administering medications through a feeding tube.
Parenteral		
Intravenous	Liquids, reconstituted powders	Furosemide for injection, morphine sulfate for injection
Intramuscular	Liquids, reconstituted powders	Cefazolin sodium powder for injection, penicillin G potassium powder for injection
Subcutaneous	Liquids	Heparin sodium for injection, insulin
Intradermal	Liquids	Purified protein derivative
Topical		
Direct application	Creams, ointments, lotions	Ketoconazole cream, nitroglycerin ointment
Transdermal patch	Patches impregnated with medication	Estrodial transdermal patch, fentanyl transdermal patch, nicotine transdermal patch
Other routes		
Inhaled	Droplets or fine powder	Albuterol, levoalbuterol, pentamidine
Sublingual (under the tongue) or buccal (in the cheek pocket)	Fast-dissolving tablets or lozenges, liquids, and sprays	Nitroglycerin sublingual spray
Vaginal	Suppositories	Dinosprostone, miconazole vaginal suppository
Intrathecal (epidural or spinal) via injection	Liquids	Ropivacaine 2% solution, morphine sulfate

---

■ Box 7-4   "Do Not Crush" Drugs

As a rule of thumb, do not crush medications that are:

• enteric coated or have other specialized coatings.
• extended-, sustained-, controlled-, or slow-release.
• effervescent (fizzy) tablets when placed in liquid.
• foul tasting in the patient's mouth.
• a cause of mucous membrane (mouth, esophagus, stomach, or small intestine) ulceration.
• meant to be given buccally or sublingually.

A complete list of "do not crush" medications is available at: http://www.ismp.org/tools/donotcrush.pdf.

Right 5: The Right Time

Prescribers may order medications to be administered on a routine basis (for example, once daily, three times per day, or at bedtime), on a STAT basis (immediately), as needed (PRN, or *pro re nata*), or as based on certain clinical criteria (for example, a particular lab result or vital sign reading). The institution's pharmacy, however, usually determines the actual timing of routine administration. In most instances, those medications must be given within 30 to 60 minutes of the scheduled time. For example, a drug that is ordered to be given every six hours may be scheduled for administration at 6:00 a.m., 12:00 p.m., 6:00 p.m. and 12:00 a.m. Therefore, a medication scheduled for 6:00 a.m. may be given between 5:30 a.m. and 6:30 a.m.

Certain medications, however, must be given at the same time each day to be effective or to maintain a therapeutic blood level of the drug. For example, the drug insulin lispro must be given 15 minutes before a meal in order to effectively control the rise in blood glucose level from the meal. The anti-HIV drug zidovudine must be given in evenly spaced intervals throughout the day and night to keep the blood level of the drug at a steady state. Some drugs must be given before meals and other drugs may be given with food.

At all times, nurses must exercise sound judgment in administering medications; sometimes that means withholding medications. For example, a patient whose blood pressure is extremely low should not take the routinely scheduled dose of antihypertensive medication, and the nurse should consult with the provider in a timely manner that the medication is being held, why it is being held, and if additional orders are needed.

Right 6: The Right Documentation

After giving a medication, the nurse should immediately document the occurrence on the MAR (paper or electronic). Documented information should include the name of the drug, the dose, the route, and the time of administration. The nurse giving the medication should sign or initial each medication given and document in the patient's progress notes if the drug was given on an as-needed (PRN) basis or if any special circumstances indicated a need for the drug. The entry should emphasize the assessment of the need, the intervention taken, and the patient's response to the medication.

Example 1: 04/10/18 Patient complaining of right knee incision pain of 8 on a scale of 0 to 10. Medicated
0030 with morphine sulfate, 2 mg intravenously. ....**N. Jones, RN**
04/10/18 Patient reports that right knee pain now 2 on a scale of 0 to 10. States being comfortable.
0130 No further needs identified. ....**N. Jones, RN**

Example 2: 04/10/18 Patient's blood pressure 210/108. Dr. Smith notified via telephone. Enalapril 1.25 mg given IV
0030 as ordered. ....**N. Jones, RN**
04/10/18 Patient's blood pressure 158/92. Denies headache, dizziness, or nausea.......**N. Jones, RN**
0130

The Three Checks

To reinforce the six rights of drug administration, the nurse should check medications at least three times prior to administering the drug to the patient. Remember that the three checks are reliable only if the medication has been correctly transcribed to the MAR! These are the three checks:

1. **Check** the time of administration, the name of the medication, and the dose against the MAR as medications are pulled from the drawer (medication cart or the AMD cabinet),
2. **Check** the medications with the MAR after all the medications have been obtained but prior to entering the patient's room.
3. **Check** the medications with the MAR at the patient's bedside after ensuring that the right patient is about to receive the medications.

Barcode Medication Administration and the Six Rights

Many facilities use point-of-care barcode medication administration technology to improve the accuracy of medication administration and reduce the number of drug-related errors. Variations exist depending on the system and facility policies, but barcode technology typically works this way:

1. A patient is admitted to the hospital. A barcoded identification bracelet is placed on the patient's wrist that links the patient to his or her unique electronic medical record.
2. The admitting provider orders medications for the patient. These orders are entered into the computer, then verified and approved by the pharmacy.
3. At the time of drug administration, the nurse logs onto the AMD system computer and selects the patient from a list. The screen will display the patient's ordered medications.
4. The nurse selects the medications to be administered. After the selection is complete, the machine will unlock the drawers where the medication is stored. The nurse retrieves the medications.
5. After the medications are obtained from the AMD, the nurse takes the drugs and barcode scanner to the patient's bedside. The nurse will scan the patient's identification bracelet barcode, then the barcodes on the medications that are being administered. The computer will compare the patient's current drug orders and compare it to each drug being scanned to ensure that they match. If the drug and the record do not match, an error message will appear on the screen. The nurse would then investigate the discrepancy.
6. The nurse documents the medication and associated nursing care in the patient's record.

Point-of-care barcode medication administration is not perfect. While it can prevent medication errors from occurring, it cannot prevent all types of errors, and the technology and support services associated with barcode systems tend to be expensive. See Figure 7-10.

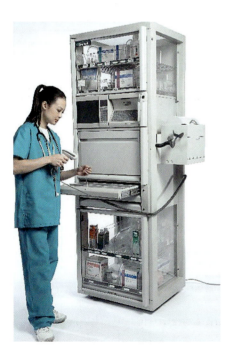

Figure 7-10 Automated Dispensing Medication System With Barcode Reader

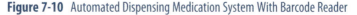

Medications Across the Continuum of Care: Medication Reconciliation

The Joint Commission's NPSG 03.06.01 states that healthcare facilities make a good faith effort to maintain and communicate accurate information about patient medications (The Joint Commission, 2018). The purpose of medication reconciliation is to identify and resolve discrepancies between current medications and those that patients should be taking. The process of medication reconciliation includes comparing prescribed medications with current medications to look for allergies, duplications, omissions, interactions, contraindications, and need to continue medications.

The nurse's responsibility in medication reconciliation is as follows (see Figs. 7-11 and 7-12):

- Upon admission to a healthcare facility, the admitting nurse collects a complete list of the patient's medications, including name, dose, route, frequency, duration, purpose, and last

---

MEDICATION RECONCILIATION FORM

Date: _____04/22/18_____   Allergies: ___*Penicillin, sulfa*___

Source of Information (patient, family, retail pharmacy, primary care provider, bottles/list): _____*Patient*_____

Home Medication (Include Herbal/OTC/ Vitamins/Supplements)	Dose/Route/Frequency	Last Dose	Continue on admission?	Continue on transfer or discharge?
Pantoprazole	*40 mg, by mouth, daily*	4/22/18 0900	(YES) NO	YES NO
Spironolactone	*10 mg, by mouth, daily*	4/22/18 0900	YES (NO)	YES NO
			YES NO	YES NO
			YES NO	YES NO
			YES NO	YES NO
			YES NO	YES NO

Medication history taken by: _____*Rose Haley, RN*_____ Date: ___4/22/18___ Time: ___1835___

Admission medication orders reconciled by: _____*Rose Haley, RN*_____ Date: ___4/22/18___ Time: ___2055___

Admission Medications Reviewed by: _____M. Jones, MD_____ Date: ___4/22/18___ Time: ___2055___

Discharge Medications Reviewed by: _____ Date: _____ Time: _____

WHITE COPY: CHART	PINK COPY: PATIENT	YELLOW COPY: PRIMARY CARE PROVIDER

Donald L. Harvey
DOB: 07/05/1941
MRN: 01700980984

Figure 7-11 Medication Reconciliation Form

| | Patient Profile | Allergies | Orders | Lab Results | **Medications** | Nursing Assessment | Provider Notes |

ALLERGIES: Penicillin, Sulfa, Eggs *(last validated 10/7/2018)*

Medications last reviewed with patient 10/5/2018 by Leslie Hall, RN

| Active Medications | Inactive Medications | Discharge Medications | **Medication Reconciliation** |

NR	Medication	Start Date	Prescribed by	Status	Action
☐	**Tylenol (acetaminophen)** **325 mg tablet** Take 2 tablets by mouth every 6 hours for headache. Do not take more than 12 tablets in 24 hours.	10/5/2018	Kirk, J. MD	Active	**Inactivate Renew Discontinue Hold Modify**
☐	**Prilosec (omeprazole)** **40 mg capsule** Take 1 tablet by mouth once daily before breakfast for 2 weeks.	10/5/2018	Kirk, J. MD	Active	**Inactivate Renew Discontinue Hold Modify**
☐	**Tenormin (atenolol)** **25 mg tablet** Take 1 tablet by mouth once daily.	3/28/2015	Merriweather, R. MD	Hold	**Inactivate Renew Discontinue Hold Modify**

Figure 7-12 Sample Electronic Medication Reconciliation Form

dose taken of each drug. All prescribed medications, over-the-counter medications, and any nutritional supplements that the patient is taking should be included in this list. The patient (and the family, if necessary) should be involved in this process.

- After the list has been created, the medications on the list are compared to the medications ordered for the patient by the provider(s) caring for the patient in the hospital. Any discrepancies between the listed drugs and ordered drugs must be explored and explanations documented in the patient's chart. The provider must be notified of any discrepancies.
- At the time of discharge from the hospital, the patient must receive a copy of the current list of reconciled medications.
- If the patient is transferred to another facility, the list must be communicated to the receiving provider.

Abbreviations Used in Medication Administration

Using abbreviations in prescribing, dispensing, and administering medications has been strongly discouraged in the past several years by The Joint Commission and the ISMP, which have both published guidelines for medical abbreviations. The ISMP has published a list of error-prone abbreviations, symbols, and dose designations that should not be used as they have been reported to contribute to medication errors. See the ISMP's List of Error-Prone Abbreviations, Symbols, and Dose Designations at http://www.ismp.org/Tools/errorproneabbreviations.pdf. See Tables 7-3 and 7-4.

Table 7-3	"Do Not Use" Abbreviations, Symbols, and Dose Designations		
Abbreviation, Symbol or Dose Designation	**Intended Meaning**	**Error Risk**	**Substitution**
μg	microgram	May be mistaken for "mg."	mcg
cc	cubic centimeter	May be mistaken for "u" in units.	mL
hs	hour of sleep (at bedtime)	May be mistaken for "half-strength."	at bedtime
q.d.	every day	The period may be mistaken for an "i" in "qid."	daily
q.o.d.	every other day	The "o" may be mistaken for the period in "q.d." or the "i" in "q.i.d."	every other day
SC, sq, or sub q	subcutaneous	The "s" may be mistaken for a 5, or the "q" mistaken for "every."	subcut *or* subcutaneously
U, u, or IU	Units	The "u" may be mistaken as the number "0" or "4" or the letters "cc." The "IU" may be mistaken for a "1."	units *or* international units
Trailing zeros (e.g., 3.0 g)	3 g	The decimal point before the zero may be missed, resulting in a tenfold increase in dose.	*Avoid trailing zeros after whole numbers.*
Leading decimal point (e.g., .5 mg)	0.5 mg	The decimal point before the number may be missed, resulting in a tenfold increase in dose.	*Place a zero in front of any numbers that are less than a whole number.*
Drug name abbreviations, such as $MgSO_4$, MS, MSO_4	$MgSO_4$ = magnesium sulfate	May be mistaken for "morphine sulfate."	*Use the complete drug name.*
	MS = morphine sulfate	May be mistaken for "magnesium sulfate."	
	MSO_4 = morphine sulfate	May be mistaken for "magnesium sulfate."	
Ʒ	dram	May be mistaken for "3."	*Use the metric system.*
♏	minim	May be mistaken for "mL."	*Use the metric system.*
> and <	greater than and less than	May be mistaken for each other.	greater than *and* less than
@	at	May be mistaken for "2".	at
^{0} (e.g., every 2^0)	hour(s)	May be mistaken for "0."	hr, h, *or* hour

Table 7-4	**Acceptable Abbreviations, Symbols, and Dose Designations**				
Abbreviation	Meaning	Abbreviation	Meaning	Abbreviation	Meaning
ac	Before meals	PEG	Percutaneous endoscopic gastrostomy	ER	extended-release
pc	After meals	NG	Nasogastric	SR	sustained-release
ad lib	As desired	PR	Per rectum	CR	controlled-release
IV	Intravenous	PO	Per os (by mouth)	g	gram
subcut	Subcutaneous	supp	Suppository	mg	milligram
IM	Intramuscular	NPO	Nothing by mouth	kg	kilogram
ID	Intradermal	b.i.d.	Twice daily	mcg	microgram
SL	Sublingual	t.i.d.	Three times daily	tsp	teaspoon
STAT	Immediately	q	Every	NKA	no known allergies
PRN *or* prn	As needed	q2hr	Every 2 hours	NKDA	no known drug allergies
IVP	Intravenous push	q4h	Every 4 hours		
IVPB	Intravenous piggyback	gtt	Drop		

Practice Six Rights and Three Checks

(answers on page 115)

Select the best answer.

1. Factors that may lead to giving the wrong medication to a patient include:
   a. look-alike medication names.
   b. sound-alike medication names.
   c. errors in transcribing the medication to the medication administration record.
   d. all of the above.

2. Which patient identifier would not be acceptable?
   a. the patient's social security number
   b. the patient's date of birth
   c. the patient's medical record number
   d. the patient's room number

3. Which drug route refers to a drug that is applied directly to the skin?
   a. intramuscular
   b. subcutaneous
   c. topical
   d. intravenous

4. Which right is not one of the six rights of medication administration?
   a. right patient
   b. right place
   c. right dose
   d. right route

5. Which dosage is written incorrectly?
   a. 0.2 mg
   b. 2.0 mg
   c. 2.02 mg
   d. 0.02 mg

6. A nurse makes the decision to withhold a medication for a patient. Which action should the nurse take next?
   a. Notify the patient's next of kin.
   b. Notify the nursing supervisor.
   c. Notify the pharmacy.
   d. Notify the patient's provider.

7. Which statement is incorrect regarding the nurse's role in medication reconciliation?
   a. Upon admission to the hospital, the nurse must gather and verify the patient's list of medications taken at home.
   b. The nurse must notify the provider about any discrepancies noted between the medications ordered for the patient while in the hospital and those that are on the patient's list from home.
   c. The nurse must give the patient a complete list of medications upon discharge from the hospital.
   d. The nurse is not involved in the process of medication reconciliation; that is the provider's responsibility.

Place the steps in the correct order.

8. The nurse should check medications at least three times before giving them to a patient.
   a. _____ Check the medication at the patient's bedside.
   b. _____ Check the medication as it is being gathered from its storage location.
   c. _____ Check the medication prior to entering the patient's room.

Read Case Study 7–1 and answer the questions.

Case Study 7–1

Ira Rosenburg, 76 years old, is admitted to the medical floor of the hospital. He has pneumonia, a history of mild dementia, type 2 diabetes mellitus, and Parkinson's disease. Mr. Rosenburg's wife, who is at the bedside, hands you (the RN) a list of the medications that Mr. Rosenburg takes at home. Mrs. Rosenburg states that Mr. Rosenburg also takes a multivitamin every morning and occasionally takes acetaminophen tablets for headaches. For a list of Mr. Rosenburg's medications see Figure 7-13.

1. *Review the medication reconciliation form shown in Figure 7-14. What other information do you need from Mr. or Mrs. Rosenburg to complete the form? (Assume that the date is current.)*
2. *What medications will you list on the medication reconciliation form?*
3. *After obtaining the missing information from Mrs. Rosenburg and filling out the form, what is your next step?*
4. *Mr. Rosenburg has been discharged from the hospital. You are preparing his discharge papers. What are your responsibilities in making sure that Mr. Rosenburg has a complete list of his current medications?*

Ira Rosenburg's Daily Medications

- *Lisinopril 10 mg, by mouth, daily*
- *Metformin 1000 mg, by mouth, every morning with breakfast*
- *Metformin 1000 mg, by mouth, every evening with dinner*
- *Levodopa/Carbidopa 25/100 mg, by mouth, four times per day*
- *Donepezil 5 mg, by mouth, daily*

Figure 7-13 Ira Rosenburg's Daily Medications

MEDICATION RECONCILIATION FORM

Date: _____   Allergies: _____

Source of Information (patient, family, retail pharmacy, primary care provider, bottles/list): _____

Home Medication (Include Herbal/OTC/ Vitamins/Supplements)	Dose/Route/Frequency	Last Dose	Continue on admission?		Continue on transfer or discharge?	
			YES	NO	YES	NO
			YES	NO	YES	NO
			YES	NO	YES	NO
			YES	NO	YES	NO
			YES	NO	YES	NO
			YES	NO	YES	NO

Medication history taken by: _____   Date: _____ Time: _____

Admission medication orders reconciled by: _____   Date: _____ Time: _____

Admission Medications Reviewed by: _____   Date: _____ Time: _____

Discharge Medications Reviewed by: _____   Date: _____ Time: _____

WHITE COPY:	PINK COPY:	YELLOW COPY:
CHART	PATIENT	PRIMARY CARE PROVIDER

Ira M. Rosenburg
MR # A93710745
Acct: 7391759
DOB: 07/05/1933

Dr. John Crockett

Figure 7-14 Medication Reconciliation Form for Ira Rosenburg

Key Points

1. Medication errors are preventable events that may lead to patient harm. Causes of medication errors are related to failures during production, distribution, administration, or use.

2. Numerous organizations are involved in protecting the public against medication errors:

   a. The Food and Drug Administration (FDA) is responsible for overseeing the safety, efficacy, and security of medications manufactured and sold in the United States.

   b. The Institute for Safe Medication Practices (ISMP) is dedicated to safe medication use and the prevention of errors.

   c. The National Coordinating Council for Medication Error Reporting and Prevention (NCC MERP) researches the causes of medication errors and develops prevention strategies.

   d. The Institute for Healthcare Improvement (IHI) focuses on improving patient safety and preventing injury from high-risk medications.

   e. The Joint Commission requires accredited facilities to comply with safety-related activities, such as those outlined in the National Patient Safety Goals.

   f. State Nurse Practice Acts are laws enacted to protect the public from harm related to nursing practice.

   g. Healthcare institutions formulate policies and procedures that guide nurses in carrying out procedures in a safe manner.

3. Medication delivery systems include unit dose systems, multiple dose systems, and automated medication dispensing systems.

   a. Unit dose medications are dispensed one dose at a time in prepackaged containers or syringes that are easy to use.

   b. Multiple dose medications are supplied in bulk containers. The disadvantage to multiple dose medications includes the risk of contamination; however, it is not practical to package all medications in unit dose form.

   c. Automated medication dispensing systems provide additional security for medications along with the advantages of easier control over inventory, better tracking, and faster access to medications for nurses.

4. The six rights of medication administration are the right patient, the right drug, the right dose, the right route, the right time, and the right documentation.

5. Medications should be checked by the nurse at least three times prior to a patient's taking the drug. The provider's original order should be compared to the medication administration record to verify accuracy of the transcription.

6. Point-of-care barcode technology can improve the accuracy of the medication administration process, but it is expensive and cannot reduce all types of errors.

7. The process of gathering, verifying, and communicating a patient's drug information is called medication reconciliation and is necessary to prevent the inadvertent omission of a needed drug.

8. Abbreviations should be used appropriately in prescribing and documenting medication administration.

References

1. Ernst, F. R., & Grizzle, A. J. (2001). Drug-related morbidity and mortality: Updating the cost-of-illness model. *Journal of the American Pharmaceutical Association, 41*(2), 192–199.

2. Institute for Healthcare Improvement. (2016). Reconcile medications at all transition points. Retrieved from http://www.ihi.org/resources/Pages/Changes/ReconcileMedicationsatAllTransitionPoints.aspx

3. Institute for Safe Medication Practices. (2016). FDA and ISMP lists of look-alike drug name sets with recommended tall man letters. Retrieved from https://www.ismp.org/tools/tallmanletters.pdf

4. James, J. T. (2013). A new, evidence-based estimate of patient harms associated with hospital care. *Journal of Patient Safety, 9*(3), 122–128.

5. Kohn, L. T., Corrigan, J. M., and Donaldson, M. S. (Eds.). (2000). *To err is human: Building a safer health system.* Washington, DC: National Academy Press.

6. National Coordinating Council for Medication Error Reporting and Prevention. (2018). *What is a medication error?* Retrieved from http://www.nccmerp.org/about-medication-errors

7. Phillips, J., Beam, S., Brinker, A., Holquist, C., Honig, P., Lee, L.Y., et al. (2001). Retrospective analysis of mortalities associated with medication errors. *American Journal of Health-System Pharmacists, 58*(19), 1824–1829.

8. The Joint Commission. (2018). Accreditation Program: Hospital. Chapter: National Patient Safety Goals. *National Patient Safety Goals Manual.* Retrieved from http://www.jointcommission.org

Chapter Post-Test

(answers in Unit 4)

Multiple Choice

Select the best answer.

1. According to the 2001 study by Phillips et al., what was the most common cause of medication errors?
   a. human factors
   b. system factors
   c. communication factors
   d. manufacturing factors

2. Which organization develops and publishes the National Patient Safety Goals?
   a. The Institute for Healthcare Improvement
   b. The Joint Commission
   c. The U.S. Pharmacopeia
   d. The Food and Drug Administration

3. The purpose of a state's Nurse Practice Act is to:
   a. protect the nurse from unsafe patients.
   b. safeguard the practice of nursing from lawmakers.
   c. protect the public from unsafe nurses.
   d. punish nurses who make errors.

4. Which patient identifier is inappropriate?
   a. patient's name
   b. patient's address
   c. patient's date of birth
   d. patient's room number

5. A nurse is teaching a patient about medications. Which of the following statements by the nurse demonstrates that the nurse needs additional education regarding medication administration?
   a. "This medication may cause nausea and drowsiness. These side effects can be managed by eating crackers with the medication and taking the medication at night."
   b. "I can't answer any questions about your medications. That's your physician's job."
   c. "This medication must be taken on an empty stomach to be fully absorbed. It is best to take it before breakfast."
   d. "You will need to have blood drawn every 2 weeks to monitor the blood level of the medication."

6. Which of the following is not one of the three names that a medication might have?
   a. generic name
   b. trade name
   c. chemical name
   d. therapeutic name

7. Which dosage is written incorrectly?
   a. 18 mcg
   b. 1.8 mcg
   c. 180.0 mcg
   d. 0.18 mcg

8. A nurse is preparing to give a medication to a patient. In reviewing the dosage information for the medication, the nurse notes that the dose prescribed by the provider is outside the manufacturer's recommended safe dosage range. Which of the following actions is appropriate?
   a. Give the medication as prescribed by the provider.
   b. Call the provider to question the accuracy of the order.
   c. Ignore the order.
   d. Have another nurse give the medication as ordered.

9. A medication is ordered to be given parenterally. The medication will be:
   a. injected into tissues or a vein.
   b. applied directly to the skin.
   c. given by mouth.
   d. inserted into a body cavity.

10. A drug that is ordered to be administered t.i.d. should be given:
    a. once per day.
    b. twice per day.
    c. three times per day.
    d. four times per day.

11. The law that organized narcotic drugs into separate categories based on medical need and potential for addiction is:
    a. the Pure Food and Drug Act.
    b. the Durham-Humphrey Amendment.
    c. the Orphan Drug Act.
    d. the Controlled Substance Act.

12. The second check of a medication should be conducted:
    a. at the patient's bedside.
    b. as the medication is being pulled from the storage cabinet.
    c. after the medication has been obtained, but prior to entering the room.
    d. after the patient has taken the medication.

13. Which abbreviation should not be used in charting dosages?
    a. subcut
    b. unit
    c. q.d.
    d. mcg

14. Which statement regarding medication reconciliation is false?
    a. The purpose of medication reconciliation is to improve communication between providers.
    b. Medication reconciliation serves to reduce the number of medications a patient is receiving.
    c. Nurses are responsible for verifying the patient's medications with the patient and family.
    d. When a patient is discharged from the hospital, the nurse ensures that the patient has a copy of his or her current list of medications.

15. Which of the following statements most accurately describes the function of a lozenge?
    a. to apply medication topically to the oral cavity
    b. to apply medication throughout the body
    c. to apply medication directly into a vein
    d. to apply medication deep into a muscle

True or False

16. Adhering to the six rights and three checks of medication administration ensures that the nurse will not make a mistake when giving medications to patients.   True   False

17. The purpose of "tall man" letters is to differentiate sound-alike drugs from one another.   True   False

18. The abbreviation "NPO" means "nothing by mouth."   True   False

19. The nurse should document administration of a medication on the medication administration record before it is given.   True   False

Matching

Match column A with the correct meaning in column B.

Column A	Column B
20. _____ pc	a. intravenous
21. _____ ad lib	b. microgram
22. _____ gtt	c. subcutaneously
23. _____ mg	d. as desired
24. _____ ac	e. immediately
25. _____ b.i.d.	f. every
26. _____ mcg	g. milligram
27. _____ subcut	h. intramuscular
28. _____ NKDA	i. after meals
29. _____ IM	j. per rectum
30. _____ IV	k. before meals
31. _____ tsp	l. kilogram
32. _____ q	m. teaspoon
33. _____ kg	n. drop
34. _____ STAT	o. no known drug allergies
35. _____ PR	p. gram
36. _____ g	q. twice per day

Answers to Practice Questions

Medication Errors

1. True
2. True
3. False
4. False
5. b
6. d
7. c
8. automated medication dispensing system
9. U.S. Pharmacopeia
10. National Coordinating Council for Medication Error Reporting and Prevention (NCC MERP)

Six Rights and Three Checks

1. d
2. d
3. c
4. b
5. b
6. d
7. d
8. a. 3, b. 1, c. 2

■ Answers to Case Study 7–1

1. The missing information includes Mr. Rosenburg's allergies, and the date and time that Mr. Rosenburg took the last dose of each of his medications.
2. The medications that will be listed on the form are as follows:
   - lisinopril
   - metformin (morning dose)
   - metformin (evening dose)
   - levodopa/carbidopa
   - multivitamin
   - acetaminophen
   - donepezil

   The multivitamin and acetaminophen must be added to the list of Mr. Rosenburg's medication even though they are over-the-counter medications, and the acetaminophen is taken only occasionally. It is important that providers have a complete list of all medications.
3. After completing the medication reconciliation form, it is important to verify the list with the patient and/or the family. The provider should be notified of any differences between the medications listed on the medication reconciliation form and those ordered by the provider. The provider will either order the missing medications or discontinue them.
4. Before discharging Mr. Rosenburg from the hospital, the nurse must make sure all current medications have been listed on the discharge form. The nurse does this by comparing the medications listed on the medication reconciliation form with the medications listed on the discharge form. Any discrepancies must be resolved with the provider.

Chapter 8
Prescriptions and Medication Orders

Glossary

DEA: Drug Enforcement Agency
Prescriptive authority: The legal authority to write prescriptions.
Telephone orders: Provider orders that are received over the telephone.
Transcribe (transcription): To transfer information from one source to another.
Verbal orders: Provider orders that are received in person or over the telephone.

Objectives

After completing this chapter, the learner will be able to—
1. Compare and contrast prescriptions and medication orders.
2. Differentiate between the types of medication orders.
3. Describe safe practices as they relate to medication orders.
4. Identify the components of the medication administration record (MAR).

Prescriptions and Medication Orders

Prescriptions are written by licensed healthcare providers and contain instructions to a pharmacist about compounding, dispensing, and administering a patient's medication (Fig. 8-1). Medication orders, as compared to prescriptions, are generated inside an organization such as a hospital or long-term care facility and are valid only inside that facility.

Prescriptions

The word *prescription* comes from the Latin word *praescriptio*, which means *preface* or *to write before*. Prescriptions are required for medications that require provider supervision, such as antibiotics, anticoagulants, or drugs that have a potential to cause abuse or addiction. A prescription is composed of four main parts (Fig. 8-1):

1. **Superscription.** The superscription consists of the traditional symbol for prescription R_x, which means *take thou* or *recipe*.
2. **Inscription.** The inscription is the body of the prescription and contains the name of the medication, the dosage strength, and the dose form (for example, capsules, tablets, or elixir).
3. **Subscription.** The subscription gives directions to the pharmacist.
4. **Signatura.** The signatura, or signa, gives instructions to the patient. It tells the patient the number of units to take per dose, the route of administration, the frequency of dosing, the purpose of the prescription, and any special warnings or instructions.

Dr. M. Merriweather
1421 Lancaster Ave., Ste 100
Seattle, WA
(206) 555-1111
DEA # A-93810-09

Date 2/22/2018

Patient Name Mary Lambert   DOB 12/15/1957
Address 9678 Sunshine Dr., Harvest, CA 90041
Phone 555-4231

R_X: penicillin V, 500 mg #30

Sig.:   1 capsule, by mouth, tid × 10 days

May refill: _____0_____ times

M. Merriweather, MD
Dispense as written   May substitute

Figure 8-1 Sample Prescription

A prescription also includes the following information (see Fig. 8-1):

- The date the prescription was written
- Information about the patient (name, address, date of birth)
- Information about the prescriber (name, address, phone number, qualification or degree held, DEA registration number). See Box 8-1.
- Signature lines
- Number of refills allowed

Medication Orders

Medication orders may be handwritten by the prescriber or entered into a computer. Medication orders are valid only for the nursing unit where the patient is currently located. For example, if a patient is admitted to the intensive care unit, then transferred to a medical floor, a new set of orders for the medical floor must be written by the provider.

■ **Box 8-1 Who Can Write Prescriptions and Medication Orders?**

Only providers who have the legal authority to prescribe medications can write prescriptions and medication orders. Such providers include physicians and surgeons (including both doctors of medicine [MDs] and doctors of osteopathy [DOs]), podiatrists, physician assistants, nurse practitioners, dentists, and naturopaths.

Some states may limit the ability of certain providers to prescribe potentially dangerous or addictive medications such as chemotherapy agents and narcotics. Prescribing narcotic drugs to patients requires that the provider be registered with the federal Drug Enforcement Administration (DEA) and the appropriate state agency. Nurses need to know whether a provider is limited in his or her prescriptive authority before administering ordered medication. Check with the facility's pharmacists or nursing supervisors if there is any question about a prescriber's qualifications or limitations.

Date	Physicians Orders
10/01/18	Mefoxitin (cefoxitin) 2 g intravenously every 6 hours for 4 doses.
1000	Reglan (metoclopramide) 10 mg intravenously every 12 hours.
	Lovenox (enoxaparin) 40 mg subcut daily.
	——————————————————— *Mary Jones, MD*
	Noted C. Lopez, HUC, 10/01/18 1010
	Noted B. Smith, RN, 10/01/18 1015
10/01/18	Dilaudid (hydromorphone) 0.4 mg intravenously every 2 hours as needed for right hip pain.
1500	Zofran (ondansetron) 4 mg intravenously every 6 hours as needed for nausea or vomiting.
	——————————— *T.O. Mary Jones, MD/Read Back/B. Smith, RN*
	Noted B. Smith, RN, 10/01/18 1505

Sidebar: Sarah Dillon / MR 00382991 / Account A9184028 / Dr. Mary Jones, MD / DOB: 04/16/1975

Figure 8-2 Sample Medication Order

Components of a Handwritten Medication Order

Medication orders are written on the provider's order sheet in the patient's chart (Fig. 8-2). Provider medication orders must contain these components:

- **Patient identifying information.** The patient's full name must be written on the order. Other information on the order sheet includes the patient's date of birth, medical record number, account number, and/or admitting physician.
- **Date and time that the order was written.** Most facilities utilize the 24-hour clock (also known as "military time") when entering information into a patient's medical record.
- **Name of the medication.** Either the trade name or the generic name of the drug may be used, although the generic name is preferred to reduce confusion.
- **The medication's dosage.** Example: 500 mg, 20 mEq, 100 units, 30 mL.
- **The route of administration.** Example: orally, subcutaneously, intramuscularly, intravenously, per rectum.
- **The frequency and/or time of administration.** Example: daily, three times daily, every 6 hr, at bedtime, with meals. Most facilities use the 24-hour clock to record time of administration. See Appendix C, Changing Conventional Time to Military Time.
- **The prescriber's name and credentials.** Example: Susan Whitmore, DO.
- **Name of the person transcribing the order.** The health unit secretary (HUC) is the person responsible for copying the handwritten order to the medication administration record (MAR). After the order has been transcribed, the HUC "notes" the order with a signature, date, and time. The transcribed order must be double-checked and cosigned by a nurse or pharmacist before the medication is administered to the patient.

The prescriber's orders are sent to the pharmacy to be filled. The disadvantage of handwritten orders is the time delay from the time the order was written until it is filled by the pharmacy, verified by the nurse, and finally administered to the patient.

Components of an Electronic Medication Order

Providers may directly enter medication orders into the patient's electronic medical record via computer. This is known as computerized prescriber order entry, or CPOE for short. The advantage of CPOE is that prescribers have access to information regarding patient identification, allergies, dosage recommendations, anticipated adverse reactions, drug interactions, and necessary laboratory tests. Because orders are typed instead of handwritten, the occurrence of illegible orders is reduced and patient safety is enhanced. Physicians, pharmacists, and nurses can review orders immediately, allowing for faster processing of orders.

Special Types of Medication Orders

Some medication orders must be handled differently from routine, ongoing medication orders. These types of orders include one-time-only orders, STAT orders, standing orders, and PRN orders.

One-Time-Only Orders

A provider may wish to order a medication to be given only once. Medications for nausea or pain may be ordered as a one-time-only dose, with the intent to limit the quantity received by the patient. See Figure 8-3.

STAT Orders

The term *STAT* comes from the Latin word *statim*, which means immediately or without delay. STAT orders must be carried out right away as they take priority over routine orders. Most STAT orders are for a single, one-time-only dose of medication. See Figure 8-4.

Standing Orders

Standing orders are pre-written, standardized instructions for patients whose medical care is similar. Standing orders are individualized to the patient based on the patient's medical status and must be approved and signed by the patient's provider. See Figure 8-5.

PRN Orders

Medications are sometimes ordered on an *as-needed* basis. These orders are called *PRN* (*pro re nata*) orders. Common PRN orders include medications needed to treat pain, anxiety, or nausea. PRN orders should be written with the medication name, dosage, frequency, and medical indication for the drug with *PRN* or *as needed* clearly indicated. Most facilities also require the nurse to write a progress note in the patient's chart that addresses the patient's problem, the nurse's assessment, the action taken, and the re-evaluation of the problem after the intervention. See Figure 8-6.

Zofran (ondansetron) 4 mg, intravenously, once only for nausea.

——————————————————— J. Thomas, MD

Figure 8-3 Example of a One-Time Order

Diphenhydramine (Benadryl) 25 mg, intravenously STAT for anaphylaxis.

——————————————— M. McMillan, MD

Figure 8-4 Example of a STAT Order

STANDING ORDERS
Chest Pain/Unstable Angina/Rule Out Acute Myocardial Infarction

DATE:	TIME WRITTEN:	ALLERGIES:	PATIENT:

PHYSICIAN: Complete the blank or check the box. Unmarked orders will NOT be implemented.

Admit to:	☐ Dr. _____	
	☐ Observation ☐ ICU/CCU ☐ Intermediate care	
	☐ Other: _____	
Diagnosis:	☐ Chest pain ☐ Unstable angina ☐ Acute myocardial infarction	
	☐ Other: _____	
Vital Signs:	☐ Per unit routine ☐ Every 4 hours ☐ Every 2 hours ☐ Other: _____	
Diet:	☐ Clear liquids ☐ 2 g sodium, low cholesterol ☐ No caffeine	
	☐ Calorie restricted: _____ ☐ Other: _____	
Activity:	☐ Strict bedrest ☐ Bedrest with bedside commode ☐ Bathroom privileges	
	☐ Other	
Diagnostics:	☐ CBC ☐ CMP ☐ PT ☐ aPTT ☐ INR ☐ Fasting lipid profile in a.m.	
(STAT)	☐ Troponin on admission, and at ☐ _____ , and ☐ _____	
	☐ Urinalysis	
	☐ Chest X-Ray	
	☐ EKG in a.m. and STAT for any complaints of chest pain	
Treatments:	☐ Oxygen via _____ at _____ LPM	
	☐ Pulse oximetry every _____ hours.	
IV:	☐ Saline lock. Flush every 12 hours.	
	☐ Start IV fluid of _____ at _____ mL/hr	
Anticoagulation:	☐ _____	
Medications:	☐ Aspirin (enteric coated) 325 mg orally STAT, and daily. ☐ Patient has aspirin allergy - aspirin contraindicated.	
	☐ Plavix (clopidogrel) 100 mg orally for first dose, then 75 mg once daily.	
	☐ Beta blocker: _____	
	☐ Nitroglycerin (nitrostat) 0.3 mg sublingual every 5 minutes × 3 doses PRN chest pain	
	☐	
	☐	
	☐	
Other meds:	☐	
	☐	
	☐	
☐ Telephone Order Read Back to Prescriber and Verified		

Nurse's Signature:	Physician's Signature:
Date: Time:	Date: Time:

Figure 8-5 Sample Standing Orders

Morphine sulfate 1 mg, intravenously, every 2 hours, as needed for right leg pain greater than 6 on a scale of 1 to 10. ————— *K. Lutz, MD*

Nurse's note in the patient's chart:

| 04/11/18 0510 | Patient complaining of right leg pain of 9 out of 10 on a scale of 1 to 10. Right leg in cast to knee. Circulation, sensation, and movement intact. Capillary refill 2 sec. Toes are pink. Medicated with morphine sulfate 1 mg, intravenously. ————— *T. Fallon, RN* |
| 04/11/18 0600 | Patient states pain in right leg now 3 out of 10. Denies need for further pain relief. ————— *T. Fallon, RN* |

Figure 8-6 Example of a PRN Order and Nurse's Note

Safety Considerations in Ordering and Transcribing Medications

Receiving Verbal Orders

Verbal orders are those given by a provider in a face-to-face situation or over the telephone. Verbal orders carry an inherent danger of error and should be used only in urgent situations. See Table 8-1 and Figures 8-7 and 8-8.

Illegible and Incomplete Orders

Handwritten medication orders must be legible and complete. The order should be printed—not written in cursive—and should contain all necessary components. Illegible and incomplete medication orders can easily lead to errors: wrong medication, wrong dosage, wrong time, and wrong route. Only approved abbreviations should be used when writing medication orders, and even then, abbreviations should be used sparingly. If an order is illegible or incomplete, the nurse or pharmacist must call the provider to clarify the order.

Table 8-1	The Do's and Don'ts of Taking Verbal and Telephone Orders
Do:	**Don't:**
Ensure that the order is complete before ending the conversation with the provider.	Write a verbal or telephone order if you did not hear it yourself.
Spell out unfamiliar drug names. Include both the generic and the trades names of the drug to reduce the risk of error.	Try to guess what the provider is ordering if you are not sure.
Read back the order in its entirety. Include documentation in the order that signifies the order has been "read-back" to the provider.	End the conversation until you are absolutely sure that you understand the provider's order.
Write the order directly onto the provider's order sheet.	Write orders on paper towels or scrap paper. Rewriting the order to the provider's order sheet increases the chances of error.
Indicate that the order was received verbally by writing the abbreviation *V.O.* next to the provider's name. Telephone orders should be indicated by the abbreviation *T.O.*	Get distracted while taking an order. If possible, talk to the provider in a quiet area to minimize interruptions.
Limit verbal orders to urgent situations only.	Accept a verbal order if you are not in a position to take one, for example, in the middle of patient care when you are unable to write it down.
Follow your facility's policy regarding verbal orders.	Accept a verbal order for chemotherapy.

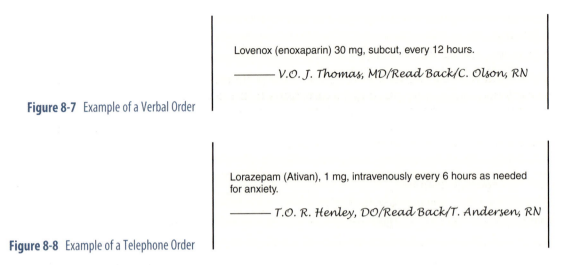

Figure 8-7 Example of a Verbal Order

Figure 8-8 Example of a Telephone Order

Look-Alike/Sound-Alike Medications

Because some medication names may look alike or sound alike, the purpose for the medication should be included in the medication order if the potential for confusion exists. This minimizes the possibility that the patient will receive the wrong medication. See Box 8-2.

Outdated Systems of Measurement

The metric system of measurement for dispensing and administering medications is preferred to the apothecary or household systems of measurement. Most medications are manufactured using the metric system, and having to convert alternative measurements to the metric system increases the risk of errors. Orders written in household or apothecary systems should be clarified with the provider.

Knowledge of the Medication Being Ordered

Nurses are obligated to have knowledge of the medication they are administering to their patients. They need to know the usual indications for the drug being ordered, the contraindications or precautions to giving the medication, the usual dosage, the route(s) of administration, common or life-threatening adverse reactions, potential interactions with other drugs or foods, the appropriate patient or family teaching, and any necessary laboratory follow-up.

Nurses must research new or unfamiliar medications before administering a drug to a patient. To find drug information, nurses can access nursing drug handbooks, medication package inserts, online medication guides such as Micromedex or Lexicomp, and pharmacy staff. The Internet may be used as a source of information about medications, but caution must be used to ensure that the source of information is credible and reliable.

■ **Box 8-2 Example of Look-Alike/Sound-Alike Medications**

A provider orders:

"Celebrex 100 mg by mouth twice daily."

Celebrex, a nonsteroidal anti-inflammatory agent, may be confused for Cerebyx, which is prescribed for seizures. The two drugs may be mistaken for each other if the provider has poor handwriting or speaks with an accent. Confusion over a look-alike or sound-alike drug may be reduced if the provider includes the indication for the medication.

"Celebrex (celecoxib) 100 mg by mouth twice daily for osteoarthritis."

Practice Prescription and Medication Order Questions

(answers on page 130)

Choose True or False for each statement.

1. Registered nurses can prescribe medications for patients.   True   False
2. The *inscription* on a prescription gives directions to the pharmacist.   True   False
3. Nurses must never take verbal orders from physicians.   True   False
4. The medication order in Figure 8-9 is written correctly.   True   False
5. The medication order in Figure 8-10 is written correctly.   True   False

Date	Physicians' Orders	
10/01/18	Prozac (fluoxetine) 20 mg by mouth daily.	Sarah Dillon
1000	———————————————————— Mary Jones, MD	MR 00382991 / Account A9184028 / Dr. Mary Jones, MD / DOB: 04/16/1975

Figure 8-9 Practice Prescription and Medication Orders

Date	Physicians' Orders	
05/23/18	Namenda 5 mg bid.	Matthew Simpson
2220	———————————————————— S. Mendez	MR 937295991 / Account S93750402 / Dr. S. Mendez, DO / DOB: 12/19/1947

Figure 8-10 Practice Prescription and Medication Orders

The Medication Administration Record

The medication administration record (MAR) is used to document medications administered to a patient. After a provider writes a medication order, it is transcribed to the MAR by either the unit secretary or a nurse. The nurse then double-checks that the order was transcribed to the MAR accurately and co-signs the original order. A copy of the order is sent to the pharmacy where it is processed and filled.

> **Note:** The transcription process does not occur in facilities that use CPOE. However, the nurse is still responsible to make sure the MAR is accurate.

Each facility has its own MAR design, but most contain the following information:

- **Patient information.** Name, date of birth, unique identifying numbers (medical record number and/or account number), attending physician, and room number.
- **Patient's allergies to medications.**
- **Current date.** Most MARs in the hospital setting are used for a 24-hour period. Long-term care facilities may use the same MAR for an entire month.
- **Time that medication is due to be administered.** Most facilities use the 24-hour clock (military time).
- **Specific medication information.** Medication name (generic or trade, or both names), dosage, route, and frequency of administration.
- **Identification of person administering medications.** Signature and initials.
- **Other pertinent information.** The MAR may include special instructions, such as when to hold the medications, how to mix the medications, or specific food or drug interactions.

Documenting Administered Medications

The MAR is a legal document and part of the patient's medical record. The following information should be documented on the MAR after administering the medication to the patient (Figs. 8-11 and 8-12):

- Date and time of administration
- Route of administration (include injection site for medications given intramuscularly or subcutaneously)
- Initials and/or signature (nurse administering the medication)

Medication Administration Record
General Hospital

Date: April 13, 2018

Room #	Patient Name	Date of Birth	Age	Sex	Height	Weight	Allergies
ICU-1	Johnson, John K.	02-12-73	45	M	5' 8"	170.5 kg	**Sulfa, Penicillin**

Medical Record Number		Account Number	Physician
A3985028881		100827959	Dr. M. Jones

Date	Medication	2300-0729			0730-1529			1530-2259		
			Route	Init		Route	Init		Route	Init
4/12/18	Mefoxitin (cefoxitin) 2 g intravenously every 6 hours *HS*	2400 0600	IV IV	CJ CJ	1200	IV	MR	1800	IV	MR
4/12/18	Nexium (esomeprazole) 20 mg intravenously daily. Reconstitute with 5 mL sterile normal saline. *HS*	0600	IV	CJ						
4/12/18	Levothyroxine 125 mcg by mouth daily in the morning before breakfast *HS*	0600	PO	CJ						
4/12/18	Lovenox (enoxaparin) 40 mg subcut twice daily *HS*				0900	Sub-cut	MR	2100	Sub-cut	HS
4/12/18	Dilaudid (hydromorphone) 0.4 mg intravenously every 2 hours as needed for breakthrough left knee pain *HS*	0215 0530	IV IV	CJ CJ	1040	IV	MR	1950	IV	HS

Initial	Signature	Initial	Signature
CJ	C. Johnson, RN		
MR	Mary Richardson, RN		
HS	H. Swanson, RN		

Figure 8-11 Sample Medication Administration Record

PATIENT: SMITH, JANICE   MRN: 9067489012
DOB: 12/12/1960   PROVIDER: ALEX JONES, MD

| Patient Profile | Allergies | Orders | Lab Results | Medications | Nursing Assessment | Provider Notes |

ALLERGIES: Aspirin (last validated 10/3/2018)

Medications last reviewed with patient 10/3/2018 by L. Hall, RN

| Active Medications | Inactive Medications | Discharge Medications | Medication Reconciliation |

Medication	Rx	Start Date	Instruction	Last Dose Administered	Next Dose Due
Medication: acetaminophen (Tylenol) **Strength/Form:** 325 mg per tablet	650 mg by mouth every 6 hours as needed for headache.	10/3/2018	Do not take more than 12 tablets in 24 hours.	10/04/2018 at 2215 by L. Hall	*PRN MED
Medication: omeprazole (Prilosec) **Strength/Form:** 40 mg per capsule	40 mg by mouth once daily before breakfast for 2 weeks.	10/3/2018	Take 1 hour before breakfast.	10/05/2018 at 0605 by J. Peters	10/06/2018 0600
Medication: atenolol (Tenormin) **Strength/Form:** 25 mg tablet	25 mg by mouth once daily.	10/5/2018	Hold for systolic BP less than 110 mm Hg.	10/05/2018 at 0910 by L. Hall	10/06/2018 0900

Figure 8-12 Sample Electronic Medication Administration Record

Do not initial the MAR before the medication is administered. If the medication was not administered at the prescribed time (perhaps because the patient was vomiting or having a CT scan), then the nurse should follow the institution's policy for documenting held medications. Most facilities also require a note in the patient's chart about the reason for holding the medication.

Practice Medical Administration Record Questions

(answers on pages 130–131)

Read Case Studies 8-1 and 8-2 and answer the questions.

Case Study 8–1

You are the nurse caring for Margaret M. Bell. She has been admitted to the hospital for pneumonia. Dr. Mary Jones writes medication orders for Ms. Bell. See Figure 8-13.

1. *Transcribe the orders above onto the MAR. See Figure 8-14.*
2. *You administer the pantoprazole and enoxaparin to Ms. Bell at 1600 on August 15, 2018. Document the time and route of administration, your initials, and signature on the MAR. See Figure 8-13.*

Date	Physicians' Orders	
08/15/18	Rocephin (ceftriaxone) 1 g intravenously every 12 hours.	Margaret M. Bell MR 00382991 Account A9184028 Dr. Mary Jones, MD DOB: 10/3/1954
1030	Protonix (pantoprazole) 40 mg by mouth daily.	
	Lovenox (enoxaparin) 30 mg subcut every 12 hours.	
	———————————————— Mary Jones, MD	

Figure 8-13 Case Study 1: Physicians' Orders

Medication Administration Record
General Hospital

Date: August 15, 2018

Room #	Patient Name	Date of Birth	Age	Sex	Height	Weight	Allergies
256-1	Margaret M. Bell	10/03/1954	63	F	162.5 cm	73.63 kg	NKA

Medical Record Number	Account Number	Physician
00382991	A9184028	Dr. M. Jones

Date	Medication	2300-0729	Route	Init	0730-1529	Route	Init	1530-2259	Route	Init

Initial	Signature	Initial	Signature

Figure 8-14 Case Study 1: MAR

Case Study 8–2

You are the nurse caring for Samuel Barker, who was admitted to the medical floor for treatment of cellulitis and mild congestive heart failure. Mr. Barker's physician writes medicine orders for Mr. Barker. See Figure 8-15.

1. Transcribe Dr. Smith's orders onto the MAR in Figure 8-16.
2. You administer Mr. Barker's Unasyn at 1200 and 1800 on November 21, 2018. Document the time and route of administration, your initials, and signature on the MAR in Figure 8-16.

Date	Physicians' Orders	
11/21/18	Potassium chloride 20 mEq by mouth daily.	Samuel L. Barker MR 00382991 Account A9184028 Dr. Martin Smith, MD DOB: 02/22/1982
0530	Lasix (furosemide) 40 mg intravenously daily.	
	Ampicillin/sulbactam (Unasyn) 2 g intravenously every 6 hours.	
	———————————————————————— *Martin Smith, MD*	

Figure 8-15 Case Study 2: Physicians' Orders

Medication Administration Record
General Hospital

Date: November 21, 2018

Room #	Patient Name	Date of Birth	Age	Sex	Height	Weight	Allergies
240	Samuel L. Barker	02/22/1982	36	M	6' 2"	195 lb	**Sulfa**

Medical Record Number	Account Number	Physician
00382991	A9184028	Martin Smith, MD

Date	Medication	2300-0729		0730-1529		1530-2259	
		Route	Init	Route	Init	Route	Init

Initial	Signature	Initial	Signature

Figure 8-16 Case Study 2: MAR

Key Points

1. Prescriptions are written orders for medications requiring supervision by a healthcare provider who has prescriptive authority. Prescriptions consist of four main parts: the superscription, the inscription, the subscription, and the signature.

2. Medication orders are typically generated inside a healthcare agency such as a hospital or long-term care facility. Medication orders must contain this information: the patient's identifying information; the date and time the order was written or electronically generated; the medication's name, the dosage, route of administration, and frequency; the prescriber's name and credentials; and the transcriptionist's name.

3. Medication orders may be obtained verbally or by telephone, or may be handwritten or electronically generated. Routine verbal and telephone orders are discouraged as they increase the risk of medication errors.

4. Medication orders are of different types: STAT medication orders should be implemented immediately. Standing orders are prewritten, standardized instructions. PRN orders are for medications administered as needed.

5. Medication error risks can be reduced by following certain safety precautions: reading back verbal and telephone orders, clarifying illegible or incomplete handwritten orders, spelling back the name of the medication, using the metric system for dispensing and administering medications, and having complete knowledge of the medication being administered.

6. The medication administration record (MAR) is used to document the administration of medications. Although facilities may have MARs that look different, most MARs contain the same information: patient information, patient allergies, information about medications, special instructions, and room for documenting drug administration.

Chapter Post-Test

(answers in Unit 4)

Multiple Choice

Choose the best answer.

1. The *signatura* on a prescription:
   a. provides instructions for the patient.
   b. provides instructions for the pharmacist.
   c. is the signature of the provider who prescribed the medication.
   d. consists of the body of the prescription.

2. Medication orders must provide which of the following information?
   a. name of the medication
   b. name of the provider ordering the medication
   c. name of the patient
   d. all of the above.

3. A STAT medication order must be carried out:
   a. within 15 minutes.
   b. after routine medications have been given.
   c. immediately.
   d. as soon as the nurse can get to it.

4. When receiving a telephone order from a provider, the nurse must:
   a. have another nurse verify the order with the provider.
   b. read back the order to the provider.
   c. have the pharmacist co-sign the order.
   d. ask the provider to come in to write the order because nurses cannot take telephone orders.

5. The most appropriate action for the nurse to take if a handwritten medication order is illegible or incomplete is to:
   a. make a guess as to what the medication order says.
   b. ignore the order.
   c. wait for the provider to come back to the facility so it can be rewritten.
   d. call the provider to clarify the order.

6. Medications that are ordered PRN should be administered:
   a. as needed.
   b. immediately.
   c. every 12 hours.
   d. as soon as possible.

7. Medications should be ordered and administered using which of the following measurement systems?
   a. apothecary
   b. household
   c. metric
   d. international units

True or False

8. The medication administration record (MAR) is a legal document.   True.   False

9. The nurse should initial the MAR before the medication is administered to the patient.   True.   False

Multiple Choice

Select all that apply.

10. Which of the following information should the nurse know before administering a medication to a patient?
    a. common or life-threatening adverse reactions
    b. the usual dosage
    c. route(s) of administration
    d. potential interactions with other medications
    e. the cost of the medication

Answers to Practice Questions

Prescription and Medication Orders

1. False

2. False

3. False

4. True

5. False

Medical Administration Record Questions

■ *Answers to Case Study 8–1*

See Figure 8-17.

Medication Administration Record
General Hospital

Date: August 15, 2018

Room #	Patient Name	Date of Birth	Age	Sex	Height	Weight	Allergies
256-1	Margaret M. Bell	10/03/1954	63	F	162.5 cm	73.63 kg	NKA

Medical Record Number		Account Number		Physician	
00382991		A9184028		Dr. M. Jones	

Date	Medication	2300-0729			0730-1529			1530-2259		
			Route	Init		Route	Init		Route	Init
08/15/18	Rocephin (ceftriaxone) 1 g intravenously every 12 hours. SB									
08/15/18	Protonix (pantoprazole) 40 mg by mouth daily. SB							1600	PO	SB
08/15/18	Lovenox (enoxaparin) 30 mg subcut every 12 hours. SB							1600	Sub-cut	SB

Initial	Signature	Initial	Signature
SB	Sharon Bradley, RN		

Figure 8-17 Case Study 1: Completed MAR

■ *Answers to Case Study 8–2*

See Figure 8-18.

Medication Administration Record
General Hospital

Date: November 21, 2018

Room #	Patient Name	Date of Birth	Age	Sex	Height	Weight	Allergies
240	Samuel L. Barker	02/22/1982	36	M	6' 2"	195 lb	Sulfa

Medical Record Number		Account Number		Physician	
00382991		A9184028		Martin Smith, MD	

Date	Medication	2300-0729		0730-1529		1530-2259	
		Route	Init	Route	Init	Route	Init
11/21/18	Potassium chloride 20 mEq by mouth daily. *KL*						
11/21/18	Lasix (furosemide) 40 mg intravenously daily. *KL*						
11/21/18	Ampicillin/sulbactam (Unasyn) 2 g intravenously every 6 hours. *KL*			1200 IV	KL	1800 IV	KL

Initial	Signature	Initial	Signature
KL	Kenneth Lambert, RN		

Figure 8-18 Case Study 2: Completed MAR

Chapter 9

Reading Medication Labels and Syringes

☙ Glossary

Enteral: By way of the gastrointestinal tract.
Form: The physical form in which a medication is manufactured and dispensed (e.g., solid tablet or a liquid elixir).
Hypodermic: Inserted under or into the skin.
Intradermal injection: An injection into the skin layer.
Intramuscular injection: An injection into the muscle.
Intravenous injection: An injection directly into the vein.
Meniscus: The curved surface of a liquid in a container.
Parenteral: By way of a route other than through the gastrointestinal tract (for example, by injection into tissue or into a vein).
Proprietary: Owned by an individual or company under a patent or trademark.
Subcutaneous injection: An injection into the tissue under the skin, but above the muscle.
Reconstitution: The process of bringing a powder to normal strength by adding a liquid.

Objectives

After completing this chapter, the learner will be able to—

1. Identify the components of a medication label.
2. Describe the information found on a package insert.
3. Discuss the different types of solid and liquid forms of medications.
4. Calculate oral dosages of medications.
5. Select the correct dosage on an oral dosing cup or syringe.
6. Identify the parts of a hypodermic syringe.
7. Calculate parenteral doses of medications.
8. Select the correct dosage on various types of hypodermic syringes.

Medication Labels

Medication labels and package inserts contain a wealth of information about a medication, such as the chemical composition of the drug, prescribing guidelines, and known adverse drug reactions. The nurse must be able to read and interpret this information in order to fulfill the six rights of safe medication administration.

Identifying the Components of a Medication Label

Medication labels include the name(s) of the medication, the National Drug Code number, the form of the medication, route of administration, dosage strength, total volume, lot number, and expiration date. They may also include information such as usual dosage or storage instructions.

132

Name of the Medication

Medications typically have three names:

1. The **chemical name** of a drug describes its chemical properties. For example, the chemical name for acetaminophen is *N-acetyl-para-aminophenol*. The chemical name is usually not printed on the drug label, but should be included in the package insert.
2. The **generic name** is the name of the medication as registered with the United States Pharmacopeia National Formulary (USP-NF). The generic name is identified by the abbreviation *USP* after the drug name on a drug label. Acetaminophen is a generic name.
3. The **trade name** (also called the **brand name**) is the name that the manufacturer applies to the drug. This name is proprietary and can be used only by the company that owns the trademark. A trademarked name will be signified by the symbol ®, which means the name is registered with the United States Patent and Trademark Office. The most common trade name for acetaminophen in the United States is Tylenol.

National Drug Code Number

The National Drug Code (NDC) number is a three-segment, 10-digit number used for all prescription drugs and insulin products made for commercial distribution. The NDC number identifies the labeler of the drug, which is the firm that manufactures or distributes the drug; the product code, which identifies the specific strength, dosage, form, and formulation of the drug; and the package size of the drug, which identifies the size and type of package. For example, the drug with the NDC number 55154-4225-5 belongs to the drug with the trade name Protonix (generic name pantoprazole), specifically the intravenous form of Protonix in the 40 mg/vial marketed by Cardinal Health.

The NDC number is also contained within the barcode on the medication package. Barcode scanning technology helps to reduce errors by matching the correct medication with the correct patient at the time the drug is to be administered.

Form of the Medication

Medications come in many forms: aerosols, capsules, creams, elixirs, emulsions, enemas, granules, injections, powders, solutions, suspensions, tablets, and troches, just to name a few. Drug labels must list the form of the medication.

Route of Administration

Medication labels must list the route(s) of administration. The label may also warn the user about ways the drug should *not* be administered if it is a high-risk drug. For example, some medications may be designed to be administered through an intramuscular injection, but must not be given intravenously.

Dosage Strength

The dosage strength of a drug is the amount of active ingredient per dosage unit. The amount of the active ingredient will be listed in g, mg, mcg, units, or milliequivalents (mEq). The dosage unit is the form of the medication—the most common are mL (for liquids) and tablets or capsules (for solids). For example, a bottle of tablets may have a dosage strength of 325 mg per tablet. An intravenous medication may contain 50 mg per 1 mL. A liquid oral medication may contain 80 mEq per 5 mL.

Some medications have two or more active ingredients that may be present in varying amounts. For example, the drug Sinemet, prescribed to treat the symptoms of Parkinson's disease, contains the drugs carbidopa and levodopa. A prescriber can order one of three strengths of Sinemet: 25-100, 10-100, or 25-250. The first number in the sequence indicates the amount of carbidopa in the tablet; the second number indicates the amount of levodopa.

Volume/Number

Drug labels also indicate the total number of dosage units (that is, number of tablets or total volume of solution) in the container.

> **Alert!** Take care not to confuse the total volume of medication in the container with the dosage strength! For example: A bottle of medication contains 300 capsules (total volume in the container) with a dosage strength of 250 mg per capsule.

Lot Number and Expiration Date

The lot number is an identification number that is assigned to a particular quantity of medication made by a manufacturer. If a medication is found to be contaminated, the lot number provides a trail by which the drug maker can examine the manufacturing process for errors.

The expiration date is the date by which the manufacturer guarantees that the medication will be chemically stable and its potency and safety maintained. Medications that have passed this date have expired and should be returned to the facility's pharmacy for disposal.

Other Label Information

Storage instructions: Some drugs must be stored in carefully controlled environments to maintain their potency and efficacy.

Directions for mixing or reconstituting: Medications in powdered form must be mixed with water or some other diluents before administration.

Warnings: Warnings on labels may include information about potentially harmful side effects, use during pregnancy and lactation, or other points deemed important by the manufacturer.

Manufacturer's name: The name of the manufacturer must be printed on the drug label.

Usual dosage: Some labels may provide usual dosage instructions. If not, this information can be found in the package insert. The usual dosage may be not the same as the dosage prescribed by the provider. See Figure 9-1.

Black box warning: Serious or life-threatening effects.

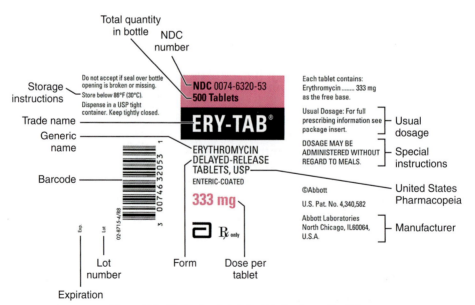

Figure 9-1 Medication Label: Oral Medication—Ery-Tab

Package Insert

The package insert is a document that is included in the medication's surrounding box or wrapper. The insert contains information about the medication in far more detail than the sticker label. This document contains highlights of prescribing information, which provides a short, concise summary of the information found within the document. The contents section contains the full prescribing information, including the following:

- Indications and usage
- Dosage and administration
- Dosage forms and strengths
- Contraindications (known hazards)
- Warnings and precautions (including black box warnings)
- Adverse reactions (clinical studies and post-marketing experiences)
- Drug and food interactions
- Use in specific populations (use in pregnancy/lactation, use with pediatric and geriatric patients, and use in patients with kidney or liver problems)
- How to treat an overdose
- Description of the drug
- Clinical pharmacology (mechanisms of action, pharmacokinetics, and pharmacodynamics)
- Nonclinical toxicology (ability of the drug to cause cancer or impair fertility)
- Clinical studies findings
- How the drug is supplied
- Storage and handling instructions
- Patient counseling information (teaching points)

The package insert is an invaluable resource for the provider and the nurse. Unfortunately, the insert is not always readily available on nursing units. However, most drug guidebooks contain a concise summary of the information needed to safely administer medications. Additional information about drugs can also be found on the Internet by accessing Web-based drug guides or by accessing the drug manufacturer's Web site. Some automated dispensing systems contain drug reference software that can be accessed while the nurse is withdrawing medications from the cabinet.

Practice Identifying the Components of a Medication Label

(answers on page 162)

Answer these questions for the medication label shown in Figure 9-2.

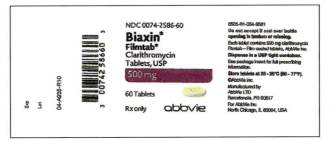

Figure 9-2 Medication Label: Biaxin

1. What is the trade name of this drug? _____

2. What is the generic name (USP) of this drug? _____

3. What is the dosage strength of this drug? _____

4. What form does this drug come in? _____

5. At what temperature range should this drug be stored? _____

Answer these questions for the medication label shown in Figure 9-3.

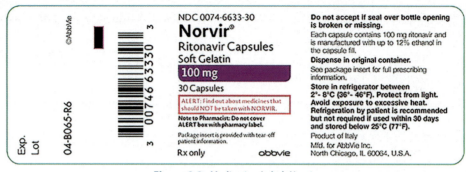

Figure 9-3 Medication Label: Norvir

6. What is the trade name of this drug? _____

7. What is the generic name (USP) of this drug? _____

8. What is the dosage strength of this drug? _____

9. What "alert" is posted on the label for this drug? _____

10. How many capsules are in this bottle? _____

Answer these questions for the package insert pictured in Figure 9-4.

**SIMULATED MEDICATION INSERT
FOR EDUCATIONAL PURPOSES ONLY**

PHENTL – fentanyl injection
XYZ Pharmaceuticals

HIGHLIGHTS OF PRESCRIBING INFORMATION
These highlights do not include all the information needed to use
PHENTL FOR INJECTION safely and effectively. See full
prescribing information for PHENTL FOR INJECTION.
PHENTL FOR INJECTION (fentanyl) for intravenous use
Initial U.S. Approval: 2018

**WARNING: ADDICTION, RESPIRATORY DEPRESSION &
MISUSE**
See full prescribing information for complete boxed warning.
- **Fentanyl injection exposes patients to addiction, abuse
and misuse, which may lead to overdose and death.
Assess individual for risk of abuse or misuse prior to
prescribing.**
- **Fentanyl Injection may lead to severe respiratory
depression. Monitor patients closely after administration.**
- **Concurrent use with benzodiazepines may increase risk
of respiratory depression. Limit dosage.**

-------------------------RECENT MAJOR CHANGES-------------------------
Warning and precautions, addiction, abuse, and misuse; severe
respiratory depression   4/2017

-------------------------INDICATIONS AND USAGE-------------------------
Fentanyl for injection is an opioid agonist indicated for:
- Short duration analgesia during anesthesia, premedication,
post-operative period.
- For the induction of anesthesia and to maintain anesthesia.

---------------------DOSAGE AND ADMINISTRATION---------------------
Fentanyl for Injection should be administered only by healthcare
providers who are trained in the use of intravenous anesthetics and
management of the respiratory effects of opioids.

Have an opioid antagonist, resuscitation and intubation equipment, and
oxygen readily available.

Dosage should be individualized based on age, body weight, physical
status, use of other medication, anesthesia to be used, and surgical
procedure.

Initial dosage in adults is 50 to 100 mcg (0.05 to 0.1 mg).

Initial dosage in children 2 to 12 years of age is 2 to 3 mcg/kg.

--------------------DOSAGE FORMS AND STRENGTHS--------------------
Solution for injection (sterile): 2 mL, 5 mL, and 10 mL ampules

-----------------------------CONTRAINDICATIONS-----------------------------
- Allergic reaction to fentanyl.

-----------------------WARNINGS AND PRECAUTIONS-----------------------
Cardiovascular depression: Monitor during initiation and titration of
dosage.

Serotonin syndrome: Life-threatening condition may result from
administering serotonin-containing drugs. Discontinue fentanyl if
serotonin syndrome is suspected.

Patients with increased intracranial pressure or head njuries: Monitor
for sedation and respiratory depression.

-------------------------------ADVERSE REACTIONS-------------------------------
Most common serious adverse reactions were respiratory depression,
apnea, muscle rigidity, and bradycardia.

**To report SUSPECTED ADVERSE REACTIONS, contact XYZ
Pharmaceutical at 800-555-1212 or FDA at 1-800-FDA-1088 or
www.fda.gov/medwatch.**

-----------------------------DRUG INTERACTIONS-----------------------------
Concurrent use of CNS depressants: May cause hypotension. Monitor
for potentiation of CNS depressant effects.
Mixed agonist/antagonist and partial agonist opioid analgesics: Avoid
use with fentanyl Injection because they may reduce analgesic effect
or precipitate withdrawal symptoms.

------------------------USE IN SPECIFIC POPULATIONS----------------------
Pregnancy: May cause harm to fetus.
Lactation: Monitor infants exposed to fentanyl Injection through breast
milk for increased sedation and respiratory depression.
Geriatric patients: Initiate at lowest possible dose. Monitor for CNS and
respiratory depression.

**See 17 for PATIENT COUNSELING INFORMATION and
FDA-approved patient labeling OR and Medication Guide.**

Revised: 11/2017

FULL PRESCRIBING INFORMATION: CONTENTS*

WARNING: TITLE OF WARNING
1 INDICATIONS AND USAGE
2 DOSAGE AND ADMINISTRATION
3 DOSAGE FORMS AND STRENGTHS
4 CONTRAINDICATIONS
5 WARNINGS AND PRECAUTIONS
6 ADVERSE REACTIONS
  6.1 Clinical Trials Experience
  6.2 Immunogenicity
  6.2 Postmarketing Experience
7 DRUG INTERACTIONS
8 USE IN SPECIFIC POPULATIONS
  8.1 Pregnancy
  8.2 Lactation
  8.3 Females and Males of Reproductive Potential
  8.4 Pediatric Use
  8.5 Geriatric Use
  8.6 Subpopulation

9 DRUG ABUSE AND DEPENDENCE
  9.1 Controlled Substance
  9.2 Abuse
  9.3 Dependence
10 OVERDOSAGE
11 DESCRIPTION
12 CLINICAL PHARMACOLOGY
  12.1 Mechanism of Action
  12.2 Pharmacodynamics
  12.3 Pharmacokinetics
  12.4 Microbiology
  12.5 Pharmacogenomics
13 NONCLINICAL TOXICOLOGY

Figure 9-4 Sample Package Insert

11. What are the indications for use of this drug? _____

12. What is the usual initial dosage for adults? _____

13. List the contraindication to receiving this drug._____

14. List one adverse reaction to this medication. _____

15. Besides oxygen and intubation equipment, what else would the nurse want to have available to treat an overdose? _____

Oral Medications

Drugs given orally (also called *enterally*) can be administered in solid or liquid form.

Solid Medications

Solid forms of medications include tablets, capsules, and granules.

Tablets

Tablets are medications that are mixed with a powder-based binder and molded into a particular shape. They may contain coloring and flavoring agents and may be coated or uncoated. Some tablets are scored to allow the tablet to be divided in half for administering smaller doses. Tablets come in many different forms:

Chewable: Flavored tablets meant to be chewed and easily swallowed.
Coated: The coating protects the tablet from being dissolved in the stomach or masks an unpleasant taste.
Effervescent: Releases carbon dioxide gas when dissolved in liquid.
Modified release:
  • Delayed-release tablets release the active ingredient at a time after administration.
  • Extended-release tablets release the active ingredient over an extended amount of time, allowing for less frequent dosing.
Multilayer: Contains multiple layers of ingredients.
Orally disintegrating: Dissolves rapidly in the mouth.
Soluble: Dissolves in liquid.
Troche: Flavored disks that are placed in the mouth and meant to dissolve slowly.
Lozenge: Contain active ingredients combined with a sweetened, flavored base. They are meant to dissolve slowly in the mouth.

Capsules

Capsules are solid forms of medications that are contained within hard or soft shells. They may be immediate-acting or of the delayed- or extended-release variety. Hard capsules usually contain powdered or granular form of medications and can be easily opened to empty their contents.

Soft capsules have thicker shells than hard capsules and are usually made in one piece. Soft capsules usually contain liquid medication. They must be punctured to discharge the medication.

Alert! Before opening or emptying a capsule, check the manufacturer's package insert to make sure it does not change the action of the drug. Some capsules should not be opened.

Granules

Granules are small particles containing the active ingredient. They are typically meant to be dissolved in liquid before dispensing. They may be designed to be delayed- or extended-release.

Liquid Medications

Liquid medications contain one or more active ingredients that are dissolved in a suitable fluid. Liquid drugs come in several categories:

Solutions: Clear fluids free from precipitates (solid particles).
Suspensions: Solutions that contain undissolved, solid particles. Suspensions must be mixed before administering to ensure even distribution of the particles.

Emulsions: Liquids that are suspended in another liquid in droplet form. Emulsions tend to separate upon standing and must be thoroughly mixed before administering.

Elixirs: Clear solutions that have been flavored or sweetened.

Syrups: Contain high amounts of sugar. They are sweet and generally thicker than solutions or elixirs.

Measuring Oral Medications

Most tablets and capsules are meant to be swallowed in their whole form. However, if a patient is unable to swallow, it may be necessary to crush tablets or open capsules. However, before crushing tablets or opening capsules, check a drug guide or other reliable source to make sure the intended activity of the drug will not change.

Liquid medications must be carefully measured using a calibrated measuring device, such as a dosing cup, oral syringe, dropper, or a cylindrical spoon. The oral syringe, dropper, or cylindrical spoon is used for small doses of liquid medications. If the medication comes with its own delivery device, the device should be used as it has been calibrated to deliver the correct amount of medication.

Dosing Cups

A plastic dosing cup is suitable for liquid medications that do not require precise dosing. The cup holds up to 30 mL of liquid and is calibrated in 5-mL markings. To use the cup, place it on a level surface. With the cup at eye level, pour the liquid into the cup until the bottom of the meniscus is level with the desired dose marking (Fig. 9-5). Some medication cups also contain calibrations for fluid ounces and the obsolete apothecary measure of drams, so nurses must take care not to confuse the dosage markings when pouring medications.

Oral Syringes

Oral syringes (Fig. 9-6) have several unique characteristics, depending on the manufacturer, that distinguish them from hypodermic syringes. The most important feature of an oral syringe is that the tip does *not* fit adapters and devices made for hypodermic syringes, such as intravenous tubing ports or needles. This prevents medications meant for oral administration from being administered intravenously or injected into tissues, which can cause injury or death. Some oral syringes have offset tips or orange-colored barrels and calibration markings on the side. They may also include

30 cc	30 mL
25 cc	
20 cc	
15 cc	15 mL
10 cc	
5 cc	5 mL

Figure 9-5 Dosing Cup

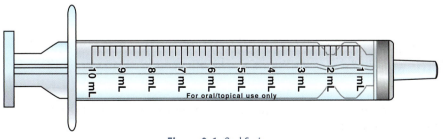

Figure 9-6 Oral Syringe

household measures (such as teaspoon), as well as metric measures. These differences are designed to alert staff that the syringe is for oral use only.

> **Alert!** Oral syringes are for measuring and administering oral medications only. Do not use an oral syringe for medications intended for injection. Conversely, do not use hypodermic syringes to administer oral medications.

Droppers

A dropper (Fig. 9-7) is for administering small amounts of medications, typically up to 5 mL. The size dropper selected should be appropriate to the amount of medication to be given. Even so, obtaining exact measurements can be difficult, depending on the pressure on the dropper's bulb.

Cylindrical Spoons

Since the cylindrical spoon (Fig. 9-8) is calibrated in 1-mL increments, it is good for administering liquid drugs that do not require precise measurements. The spoon is typically used for giving medications in the home environment rather than hospitals.

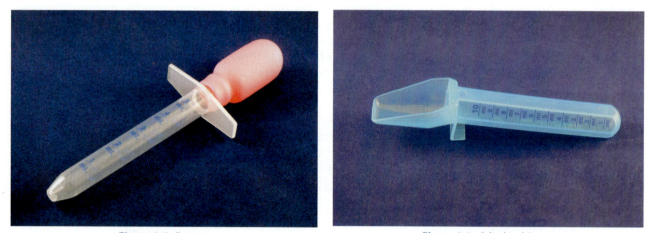

Figure 9-7 Dropper   **Figure 9-8** Cylindrical Spoon

Calculating Oral Dosages

In general, tablets are given whole or in halves if the tablet is scored. Tablets that are not pre-scored should not be divided.

Example 1: A provider orders levothyroxine 125 mcg, by mouth, daily. The pharmacy provides levothyroxine in tablets containing 250 mcg. Calculate the number of tablets to give. Round to the nearest half tablet.

1. Set up the equation using the principles of dimensional analysis. The unknown units of measure is the number of tablets to be administered. The first set of given quantities is the dosage strength of the tablets (250 mg/tablet).

$$\text{tablets} = \frac{1 \text{ tablet}}{250 \text{ mcg}}$$

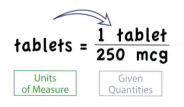

2. Enter the next given quantity. In this example, it is the dosage ordered by the provider (125 mcg).

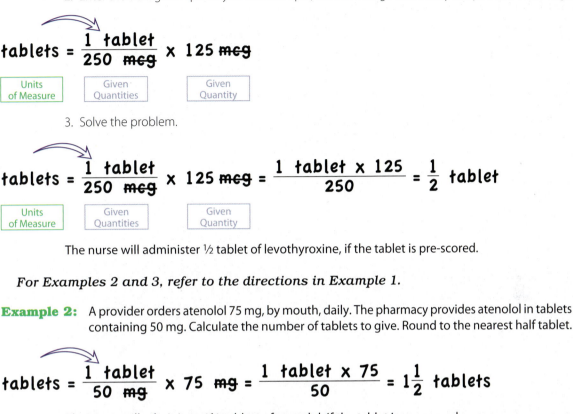

3. Solve the problem.

$$\text{tablets} = \frac{1 \text{ tablet}}{250 \text{ mcg}} \times 125 \text{ mcg} = \frac{1 \text{ tablet} \times 125}{250} = \frac{1}{2} \text{ tablet}$$

The nurse will administer ½ tablet of levothyroxine, if the tablet is pre-scored.

For Examples 2 and 3, refer to the directions in Example 1.

Example 2: A provider orders atenolol 75 mg, by mouth, daily. The pharmacy provides atenolol in tablets containing 50 mg. Calculate the number of tablets to give. Round to the nearest half tablet.

$$\text{tablets} = \frac{1 \text{ tablet}}{50 \text{ mg}} \times 75 \text{ mg} = \frac{1 \text{ tablet} \times 75}{50} = 1\frac{1}{2} \text{ tablets}$$

The nurse will administer 1½ tablets of atenolol, if the tablet is pre-scored.

Example 3: A provider orders digoxin 250 mcg, by mouth, daily. The pharmacy provides digoxin in tablets containing 0.25 mg. Calculate the number of tablets to give. Round to the nearest half tablet.

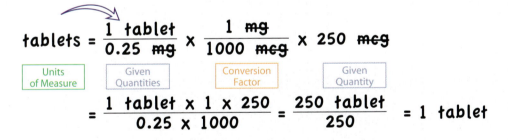

$$= \frac{1 \text{ tablet} \times 1 \times 250}{0.25 \times 1000} = \frac{250 \text{ tablet}}{250} = 1 \text{ tablet}$$

Note: In this example, a conversion factor is needed to convert mg into mcg.

The nurse will administer 1 tablet of digoxin to the patient.

Example 4: A provider orders amoxicillin suspension 500 mg, by mouth, every 8 hours. The pharmacy supplies amoxicillin suspension in bottles containing 250 mg in 5 mL. Calculate the amount of medication to administer. Round to the nearest whole mL.

1. Set up the equation using dimensional analysis and insert the first set of given quantities—the dosage strength of the medication (250 mg amoxicillin in 5 mL liquid).

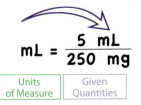

2. Insert the next given quantity—the dosage of amoxicillin ordered by the provider—and solve the equation.

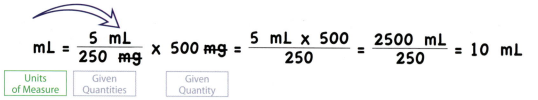

$$\underset{\substack{\text{Units}\\\text{of Measure}}}{mL} = \frac{5\ mL}{250\ \underset{\substack{\text{Given}\\\text{Quantities}}}{mg}} \times 500\ \underset{\substack{\text{Given}\\\text{Quantity}}}{mg} = \frac{5\ mL \times 500}{250} = \frac{2500\ mL}{250} = 10\ mL$$

The nurse should administer 10 mL of amoxicillin, using an oral syringe. See Figure 9-9 for the correct amount of medication to draw up.

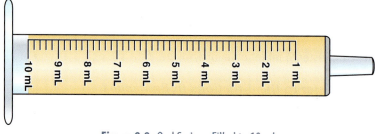

Figure 9-9 Oral Syringe Filled to 10 mL

For Example 5, refer to the directions in Example 4.

Example 5: A provider orders potassium chloride oral liquid 80 mEq, by mouth, twice daily. The pharmacy supplies potassium chloride oral liquid in bottles containing 40 mEq in 15 mL. Calculate the amount of medication to administer. Round to the nearest whole mL.

$$\underset{\substack{\text{Units}\\\text{of Measure}}}{mL} = \frac{15\ mL}{40\ \underset{\substack{\text{Given}\\\text{Quantities}}}{mEq}} \times 80\ \underset{\substack{\text{Given}\\\text{Quantity}}}{mEq} = \frac{15\ mL \times 80}{40} = \frac{1200\ mL}{40} = 30\ mL$$

The nurse should administer 30 mL of potassium chloride oral liquid in a dosing cup. See Figure 9-10 for the correct amount of medication.

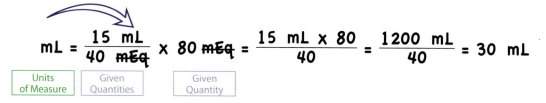
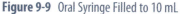

Figure 9-10 Dosing Cup Filled to 30 mL

Practice Calculating Oral Dosages

(answers on page 163)

Using the medication labels in the figures accompanying the question, calculate the amount of medication to be administered for the ordered dosages. Round tablets to the nearest half tablet and liquid amounts to the nearest whole mL unless otherwise specified.

1. The provider orders erythromycin (Ery-Tab) 333 mg, by mouth, every 8 hours. See Figure 9-11. Calculate the number of tablets to administer.

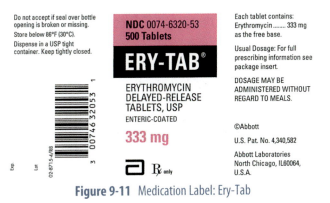

Figure 9-11 Medication Label: Ery-Tab

2. The provider orders lopinavir/ritonavir (Kaletra) oral solution 400/100 mg, by mouth, twice daily. See Figure 9-12.

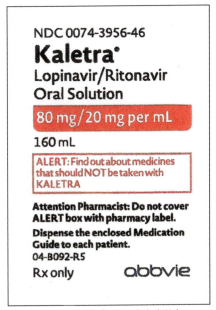

Figure 9-12 Medication Label: Kaletra

Calculate the amount of oral solution to administer. Indicate the dosage on the oral syringe in Figure 9-13.

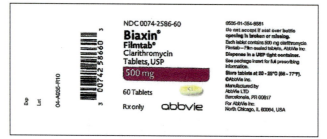

Figure 9-13 Indicate correct dosage.

3. The provider orders clarithromycin (Biaxin) 1000 mg, by mouth, every 12 hours for 14 days. See Figure 9-14. Calculate the number of tablets to administer.

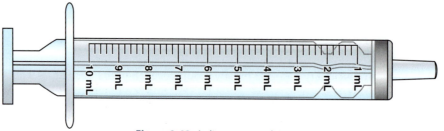

Figure 9-14 Medication Label: Biaxin

4. The provider orders ciprofloxacin (Cipro) 750 mg, by mouth, every 12 hours. See Figure 9-15. Calculate the number of tablets to administer.

For Educational Purposes Only

CIPROFLOXACIN HCL

250 mg

100 tablets
For prescription use only.

Usual Dosage:
See package insert.
Each tablet contains
ciprofloxacin hydrochloride
equivalent to 250 mg
ciprofloxacin.

Recommended storage:
Store below 84 degrees F

Figure 9-15 Medication Label: Ciprofloxacin

5. The provider orders ritonavir (Norvir) 300 mg, by mouth, twice daily. Calculate the number of capsules to administer. See Figure 9-16.

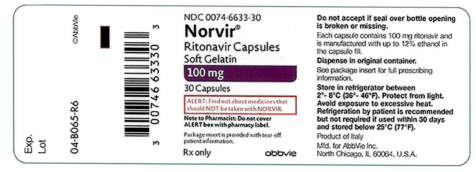

Figure 9-16 Medication Label: Norvir

6. The provider orders cefdinir (Omnicef) 225 mg, by mouth, daily. Calculate the amount of oral solution to administer. See Figure 9-17.

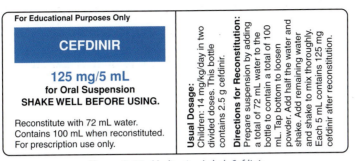

For Educational Purposes Only

CEFDINIR

125 mg/5 mL
for Oral Suspension
SHAKE WELL BEFORE USING.

Reconstitute with 72 mL water.
Contains 100 mL when reconstituted.
For prescription use only.

Usual Dosage: Children: 14 mg/kg/day in two divided doses. This bottle contains 2.5 g cefdinir.

Directions for Reconstitution: Prepare suspension by adding a total of 72 mL water to the bottle to contain a total of 100 mL. Tap bottom to loosen powder. Add half the water and shake. Add remaining water and shake to mix thoroughly. Each 5 mL contains 125 mg cefdinir after reconstitution.

Figure 9-17 Medication Label: Cefdinir

Indicate the dosage on the oral syringe in Figure 9-18.

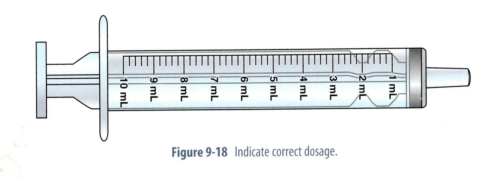

Figure 9-18 Indicate correct dosage.

Calculate the amount of medication to be administered for the dosages ordered in the following questions.

7. The provider orders guaifenesin (Mucinex) 200 mg, by mouth, every 4 hours. The pharmacy provides guaifenesin in a syrup containing 100 mg in 5 mL. Indicate the dosage on the dosing cup in Figure 9-19.

30 cc —— 30 mL

25 cc ——

20 cc ——

15 cc —— 15 mL

10 cc ——

5 cc —— 5 mL

Figure 9-19 Indicate correct dosage.

8. The provider orders digoxin pediatric elixir 60 mcg, by mouth, twice daily. The bottle of elixir contains 0.05 mg per 1 mL. Indicate the dosage on the oral syringe in Figure 9-20.

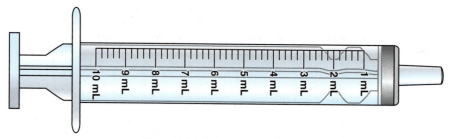

Figure 9-20 Indicate correct dosage.

9. The provider orders morphine sulfate 15 mg every 12 hours. The pharmacy provides liquid morphine sulfate in a solution containing 10 mg in 10 mL. Indicate the dosage on the dosing cup in Figure 9-21.

Figure 9-21 Indicate correct dosage.

10. The provider orders dimenhydrinate (Dramamine) 25 mg, by mouth, every 4 hours, as needed for nausea. The pharmacy provides dimenhydrinate in an oral solution containing 12.5 mg in 4 mL. Indicate the dosage on the oral syringe in Figure 9-22.

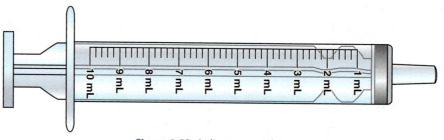
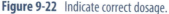

Figure 9-22 Indicate correct dosage.

Injected Medications

Medications given by injection into veins or into tissues are said to be given by the parenteral route. Drugs can be injected into the skin (intradermal, abbreviated ID), into the subcutaneous tissue under the skin (subcutaneous, or subcut), into muscles (intramuscular, or IM), directly into a vein (intravenous, or IV), or into other body cavities or parts (e.g., into the epidural space or intrathecal space in the spine). Nurses typically perform only intradermal, subcutaneous, intramuscular, and intravenous injections. To reduce the risk of medication errors, nurses should become familiar with the different types of syringes used by their facilities and the markings on those syringes.

Parts of a Hypodermic Syringe

Syringes have three basic parts: the needle (which may or may not be included with the syringe in the packaging), the barrel, and the plunger. Needles range in size from very short (1/4 inch) and fine (31 gauge) to long (4 inches) and large in diameter (14 gauge). Most needles have safety features, such as safety shields, that protect the nurse from accidental needlesticks.

The syringe barrel contains a printed dosing scale, with a tip on one end and a flange on the other. The tip of the syringe is either a slip or luer-lock tip. Needles attached to a slip tip can be easily removed (or slipped) from the syringe by pulling the two pieces apart. In contrast, luer-lock tips are threaded to allow needles and other devices to be connected securely to the syringe. The barrel's flange provides counterpressure for the plunger when injecting medication. See Figure 9-23.

The plunger slides within the interior of the syringe. One end of the plunger is usually made of a black rubber-like material and has two rings that make contact with the interior walls of the barrel. The ring closest to the medication is where the dose is read. The flange at the other end of the barrel allows the nurse to manipulate the plunger without touching the part of the plunger that must remain sterile when drawing up a medication.

Syringe Types and Sizes

Hypodermic syringes come in varying sizes: 1 mL, 3 mL, 5 or 6 mL, 10 or 12 mL, 20 or 30 mL, and 60 mL. The very small 1-mL syringe (Fig. 9-24) is also known as a tuberculin syringe as it is used to administer the tuberculosis (TB) skin test. It is calibrated in increments of 0.01 mL between the short lines, and 0.1 mL between the dark, longer lines. The medium-size lines in between the longer markings indicate 0.05 mL. Besides being used for the TB skin test, the 1-mL syringe is useful for administering very small, precise amounts of medication.

> **Alert!** Take care reading the TB syringe, especially if the syringe contains a scale for *minims*—a measure used in the apothecary system. Use the correct metric scale and count markings carefully when drawing up medications.

Insulin syringes are measured in calibrated units instead of mL and are designed to be used only with insulin. Insulin syringes come in varying sizes, from 30 units to 100 units and typically come with the needle permanently attached to the syringe.

The 3-mL, 5- or 6-mL, and 10-mL syringes are most commonly used for intramuscular injections or to draw up large amounts of medications for intravenous infusion. The short markings between the long lines indicate 0.1-mL increments. The long lines on the 3-mL syringe shown in Figure 9-25 indicate increments of 0.5 and 1 mL.

The long markings on the 5-mL syringe shown in Figure 9-26 and 10-mL syringe shown in Figure 9-27 are calibrated in increments of 1 mL, with the shorter lines indicating increments of

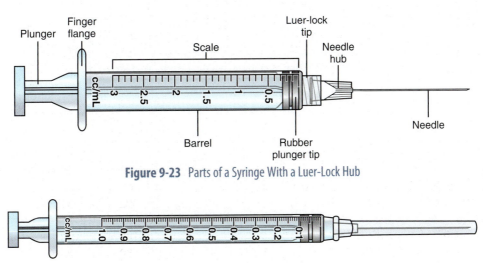

Figure 9-23 Parts of a Syringe With a Luer-Lock Hub

Figure 9-24 1-mL Syringe

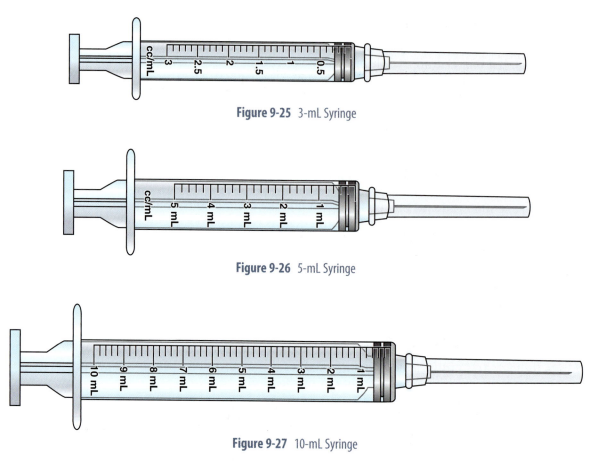

Figure 9-25 3-mL Syringe

Figure 9-26 5-mL Syringe

Figure 9-27 10-mL Syringe

0.2 mL. These syringes should not be used to draw medications that require precise doses (less than 0.2 mL).

Larger syringes, such as the 20- or 30-mL and 60-mL, are typically marked in increments of 1 mL. These syringes are rarely used in day-to-day medication administration because of their large capacity. Some large syringes may include a scale for ounces. Be sure to use the correct metric scale when drawing up medications.

Measuring Medications in a Hypodermic Syringe

Measuring medications in a syringe requires familiarity with the calibration markings on the selected syringe. The specific skills needed to draw medications using a hypodermic syringe (such as maintaining sterility and handling syringes in a safe manner) are beyond the scope of this textbook. Instead, this book's focus is on calculating parenteral dosages and drawing accurate amounts.

Example 1: 1-mL syringe filled to 0.83 mL.

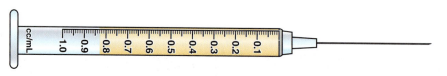

Figure 9-28 1-mL Syringe Filled to 0.83 mL

Example 2: 3-mL syringe filled to 1.4 mL.

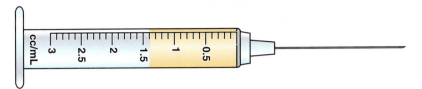

Figure 9-29 3-mL Syringe Filled to 1.4 mL

Example 3: 5-mL syringe filled to 3.8 mL.

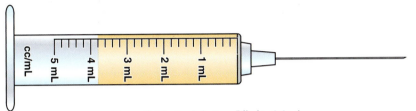

Figure 9-30 5-mL Syringe Filled to 3.8 mL

Example 4: 10-mL syringe filled to 7.2 mL.

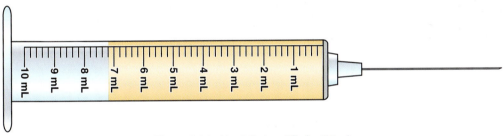

Figure 9-31 10-mL Syringe Filled to 7.2 mL

Practice Measuring Medications in a Hypodermic Syringe

(answers on page 165)

Indicate the quantities on the hypodermic syringes.

1. 0.6 mL

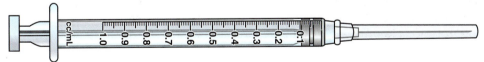

Figure 9-32 Indicate correct dosage.

2. 0.89 mL

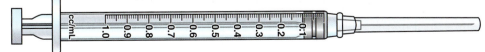

Figure 9-33 Indicate correct dosage.

3. 0.04 mL

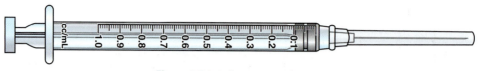

Figure 9-34 Indicate correct dosage.

4. 2.3 mL

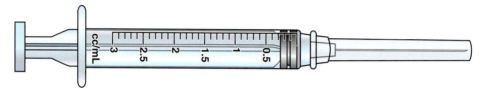

Figure 9-35 Indicate correct dosage.

5. 1.4 mL

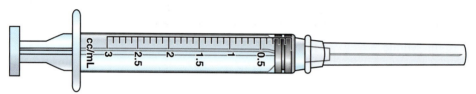

Figure 9-36 Indicate correct dosage.

6. 1 mL

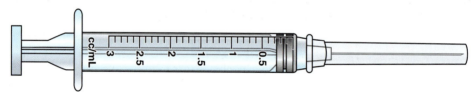

Figure 9-37 Indicate correct dosage.

7. 3.6 mL

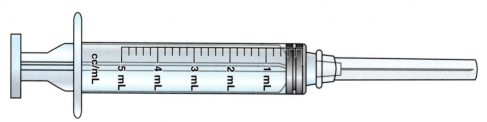

Figure 9-38 Indicate correct dosage.

8. 1.2 mL

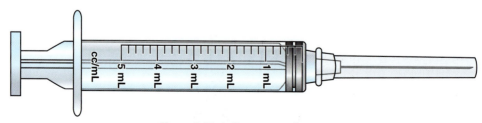

Figure 9-39 Indicate correct dosage.

9. 4.4 mL

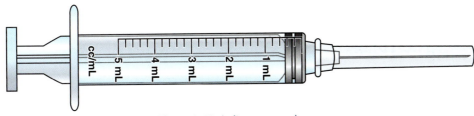

Figure 9-40 Indicate correct dosage.

10. 8.6 mL

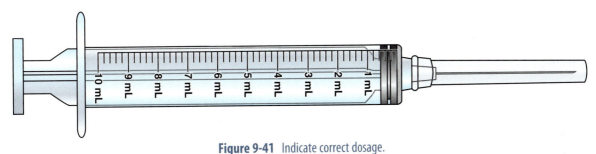

Figure 9-41 Indicate correct dosage.

Calculating Parenteral Dosages

Calculating dosages for medications given parenterally follows the same process as calculating dosages for oral liquid medications. The only difference is that the medication is drawn up with a syringe designed for parenteral use, not measured in a dosing cup.

Note: Medications that are to be injected intradermally, subcutaneously, or intramuscularly are given in relatively small quantities because of the limited capacity of these tissues to accept fluids. Intradermal injections usually do not exceed 0.1 mL. Subcutaneous injections are limited to 1 mL, and intramuscular injections do not exceed 4 to 5 mL for adults. Refer to a drug reference guide or package insert for restrictions and children's dosages. If you calculate an answer for a particular injection site that is greater than the guideline allows, recheck your math!

Example 1: A provider orders hydralazine 10 mg, IV, every 6 hours. Calculate the amount of hydralazine to draw up in the syringe, using the label in Figure 9-42. Round to the nearest tenth mL.

1. Set up the equation using dimensional analysis, and insert the first set of given quantities from the medication label (20 mg/mL).

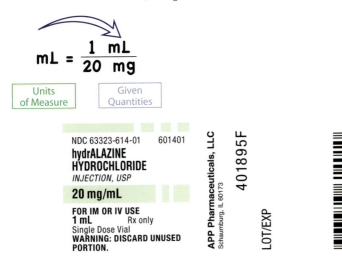

$$mL = \frac{1 \ mL}{20 \ mg}$$

Units of Measure   Given Quantities

NDC 63323-614-01   601401

hydrALAZINE
HYDROCHLORIDE
INJECTION, USP

20 mg/mL

FOR IM OR IV USE
1 mL   Rx only
Single Dose Vial
WARNING: DISCARD UNUSED PORTION.

APP Pharmaceuticals, LLC
Schaumburg, IL 60173

401895F

LOT/EXP

63323-614-01

Figure 9-42 Medication Label: Hydralazine

2. Insert the second given quantity. In this example, it is the dosage ordered by the provider.

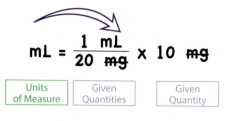

$$mL = \frac{1\ mL}{20\ \cancel{mg}} \times 10\ \cancel{mg}$$

| Units of Measure | Given Quantities | Given Quantity |

3. Solve the equation.

$$mL = \frac{1\ mL}{20\ \cancel{mg}} \times 10\ \cancel{mg} = \frac{1\ mL \times 10}{20} = \frac{10\ mL}{20} = 0.5\ mL$$

| Units of Measure | Given Quantities | Given Quantity |

The nurse should administer 0.5 mL of hydralazine. A 1-mL syringe is the best choice for administering the medication since that size provides the greatest accuracy.

Example 2: A provider orders epoetin alfa 1000 units subcut, three times weekly. The pharmacy supplies epoetin alfa in vials containing 3000 units in 1 mL. Calculate the amount of epoetin alfa to draw up. Round to the nearest hundredth mL.

1. Set up the equation, and insert the first set of given quantities (3000 units/mL).

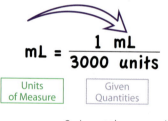

$$mL = \frac{1\ mL}{3000\ units}$$

| Units of Measure | Given Quantities |

2. Insert the second given quantity—the number of units ordered (1000 units).

$$mL = \frac{1\ mL}{3000\ \cancel{units}} \times 1000\ \cancel{units}$$

| Units of Measure | Given Quantities | Given Quantity |

3. Solve the equation.

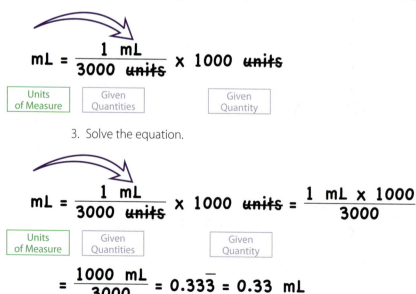

$$mL = \frac{1\ mL}{3000\ \cancel{units}} \times 1000\ \cancel{units} = \frac{1\ mL \times 1000}{3000}$$

| Units of Measure | Given Quantities | Given Quantity |

$$= \frac{1000\ mL}{3000} = 0.33\overline{3} = 0.33\ mL$$

The nurse will administer 0.33 mL of epoetin alfa. A 1-mL syringe is the best choice for administering the medication since that size provides the greatest accuracy.

For Examples 3–5, refer to the directions in Examples 1 and 2.

Example 3: A provider orders morphine sulfate 10 mg, IM, every 4 to 6 hours, as needed for pain. The pharmacy supplies morphine in vials containing 10 mg in 1 mL. Calculate the amount of morphine to draw up. Round the answer to the nearest tenth mL.

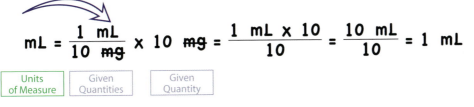

$$mL = \frac{1 \ mL}{10 \ mg} \times 10 \ mg = \frac{1 \ mL \times 10}{10} = \frac{10 \ mL}{10} = 1 \ mL$$

Units of Measure	Given Quantities	Given Quantity

The nurse should administer 1 mL of morphine sulfate. The 1-mL or 3-mL syringe is the best choice for drawing up the medication.

Example 4: A provider orders furosemide 40 mg, IV, daily. Calculate the amount of furosemide to draw up in the syringe, using the label in Figure 9-43. Round the answer to the nearest tenth mL.

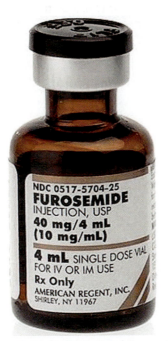

Figure 9-43 Medication Label: Furosemide

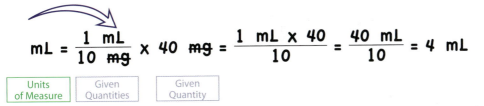

$$mL = \frac{1 \ mL}{10 \ mg} \times 40 \ mg = \frac{1 \ mL \times 40}{10} = \frac{40 \ mL}{10} = 4 \ mL$$

Units of Measure	Given Quantities	Given Quantity

The nurse should administer 4 mL of furosemide. The 5-mL syringe is the best choice for drawing up the medication.

Example 5: A provider orders betamethasone 4 mg, IM now. The pharmacy supplies betamethasone in vials containing 6 mg in 1 mL. Calculate the amount of betamethasone to draw up in the syringe. Round the answer to the nearest tenth mL.

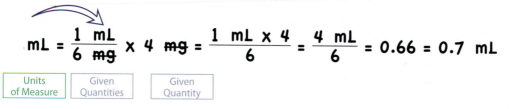

$$mL = \frac{1\ mL}{6\ mg} \times 4\ mg = \frac{1\ mL \times 4}{6} = \frac{4\ mL}{6} = 0.66 = 0.7\ mL$$

Units of Measure — Given Quantities — Given Quantity

The nurse should administer 0.7 mL of betamethasone. A 1-mL or 3-mL syringe may be used to draw up the medication; however, many 1-mL syringes have a needle that is an inappropriate size for an IM injection. The 3-mL syringe would be the best choice.

Practice Calculating Parenteral Dosages

(answers on page 167)

Using the medication labels shown in the figures, calculate the amount of medication (mL) to be drawn up in the syringe for these parenteral orders. Round the answers to the nearest tenth mL.

1. The provider orders epinephrine 1:1000 strength, 0.25 mg, IV stat (Fig. 9-44).

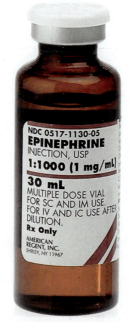

NDC 0517-1130-05
EPINEPHRINE
INJECTION, USP
1:1000 (1 mg/mL)
30 mL
MULTIPLE DOSE VIAL
FOR SC AND IM USE.
FOR IV AND IC USE AFTER
DILUTION.
Rx Only
AMERICAN
REGENT, INC.
SHIRLEY, NY 11967

Figure 9-44 Medication Label: Epinephrine

2. The provider orders magnesium sulfate 1 g, IM now (Fig. 9-45).

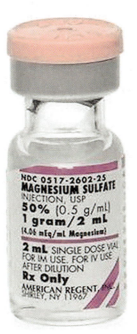

Figure 9-45 Medication Label: Magnesium Sulfate

3. The provider orders heparin 3000 units, subcut, daily (Fig. 9-46).

For Educational Purposes Only

STERILE

HEPARIN SODIUM
Injection, USP

5,000 USP Units/mL
Derived from Porcine Intestinal Mucosa
For IV or Subcut Use
10 mL
Multiple Dose Vial

Each mL contains 5,000 USP Units heparin sodium; 20 mg benzyl alcohol; 6 mg sodium chloride

Usual Dosage:
See insert.
Use only if solution is clear.
Store at 20–25 degrees C (68 to 72 degrees F).

Figure 9-46 Medication Label: Heparin Sodium (5000 units/mL)

Calculate the amount of medication to be drawn up in the syringe (mL) for these parenteral orders. Round the answer to the nearest tenth mL.

4. The provider orders lorazepam (Ativan) 2 mg, IM, prior to surgery. The pharmacy provides lorazepam in vials containing 4 mg in 1 mL.

5. The provider orders naloxone (Narcan) 0.4 mg, IM, STAT. The pharmacy provides naloxone in vials containing 0.4 mg in 1 mL.

6. The provider orders hydromorphone (Dilaudid) 1.5 mg, subcut every 4 hours, as needed for pain. The pharmacy provides hydromorphone in vials containing 2 mg per 1 mL.

7. The provider orders flumazenil (Romazicon) 0.2 mg, IV, STAT. The pharmacy provides flumazenil in vials containing 0.1 mg per 1 mL.

8. The provider orders methyldopa (Aldomet) 300 mg, IV, three times daily. The pharmacy provides methyldopa in vials containing 250 mg per 5 mL.

9. The provider orders fentanyl 75 mcg, IM, prior to surgery. The pharmacy provides fentanyl in vials containing 0.05 mg per 1 mL.

10. The provider orders ampicillin 1 g, IM, every 6 hours. The pharmacy provides ampicillin in vials containing 2 g per 5 mL after reconstitution.

Key Points

1. Drug labels and package inserts provide key information for prescribing, preparing, and administering medications.
2. Medications have three names: the chemical name, the trade (or brand) name, and the generic name.
3. Drug labels must contain the NDC number, the form of the medication, the route of administration, the dosage strength, the amount of dosage units in the container, the manufacturer's name, the lot number, and the expiration date.
4. Oral medications come in solid or liquid forms. Solid forms include tablets, capsules, and granules. Liquid forms include solutions, elixirs, syrups, suspensions, and emulsions.
5. Liquid oral medications should be administered using the device that allows for the most accurate measurement.
6. Parenteral medications (those given intradermally, subcutaneously, intramuscularly, or intravenously) are typically drawn up using the hypodermic syringe that allows for the most accurate measurement.
7. When using a syringe for drawing up medications, the correct scale must be used.

Chapter Post-Test   *(answers in Unit 4)*

True or False

1. The generic name of a drug is registered with the U.S. Patent and Trademark Office.   True   False

2. The National Drug Code number can be used to identify the labeler of the medication.   True   False

3. The dosage strength of a drug is the amount of active ingredient per dosage unit.   True   False

4. Medications may be used up to 24 hours after the expiration date on the label.   True   False

5. The package insert should contain full prescribing information for the drug.   True   False

Fill in the Blank

Refer to the medication label shown in Figure 9-47 to answer questions 6–10.

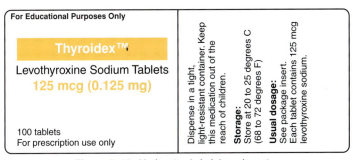

Figure 9-47 Medication Label: Levothyroxine

6. What is the trade name of this drug? _____

7. What is the generic name of this drug? _____

8. What form does this drug come in? _____

9. What is the dosage strength of this drug? _____

10. What is the recommended storage temperature of this drug? _____

Refer to the medication label shown in Figure 9-48 to answer questions 11–15.

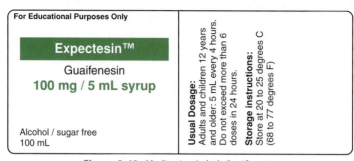

Figure 9-48 Medication Label: Guaifenesin

11. What is the trade name of this drug? _____

12. What is the generic name of this drug? _____

13. What is the dosage strength of this drug? _____

14. What form does this drug come in? _____

15. What is the total volume of drug contained in the bottle? _____

Refer to the medication label shown in Figure 9-49 to answer questions 16-20.

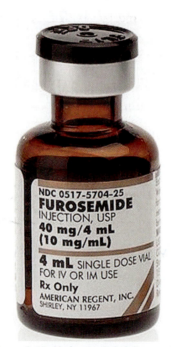

Figure 9-49 Medication Label: Furosemide

16. What is the generic name (USP) for this drug? _____

17. What is the dosage strength of this drug? _____

18. By which routes may this drug be administered? _____

19. What is the total volume of the vial? _____

20. Is this a single dose or multiple dose vial? _____

Calculate Dosages

Calculate the amount of medication to be administered for the oral medication dosages ordered. Round tablets to the nearest half tablet and liquids to the nearest tenth mL.

21. The provider orders acetaminophen (Tylenol) 220 mg, by mouth, every 4 hours, as needed for fever. The pharmacy provides acetaminophen in a suspension containing 160 mg in 5 mL.

22. The provider orders loperamide (Imodium) 2 mg, by mouth, after every loose stool. The pharmacy provides loperamide in a liquid containing 1 mg in 5 mL.

23. The provider orders dantrolene 50 mg, by mouth, twice daily. The pharmacy provides dantrolene in capsules containing 25 mg.

24. The provider orders metoclopramide (Reglan) 15 mg, by mouth, before meals. The pharmacy provides metoclopramide in tablets containing 5 mg.

25. The provider orders paroxetine (Paxil) 25 mg, by mouth, daily. The pharmacy provides paroxetine in tablets containing 10 mg.

26. The provider orders promethazine 6.25 mg, by mouth, three times daily. The pharmacy provides promethazine in a syrup containing 10 mg in 5 mL.

27. The provider orders oxycodone 7.5 mg, by mouth, every 4 hours, as needed for pain. The pharmacy supplies oxycodone in an oral solution containing 5 mg in 5 mL.

28. The provider orders hydroxyzine 75 mg, by mouth, every 6 hours, as needed for anxiety. The pharmacy supplies hydroxyzine in an oral suspension containing 25 mg/5mL.

29. The provider orders darifenacin (VesiGard) 7.5 mg, by mouth, daily. The pharmacy supplies darifenacin in tablets containing 15 mg.

30. The provider orders lamivudine (Lamivir) 150 mg, by mouth, every 12 hours. The pharmacy supplies lamivudine in an oral solution containing 10 mg in 1 mL.

Indicate the given quantities on the hypodermic syringes.

31. 0.11 mL (Fig. 9-50)

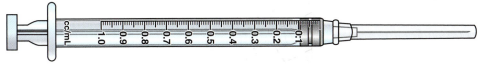

Figure 9-50 Indicate correct dosage.

32. 0.08 mL (Fig. 9-51)

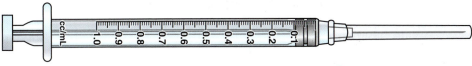

Figure 9-51 Indicate correct dosage.

33. 1.8 mL (Fig. 9-52)

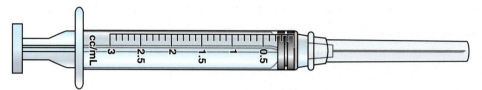

Figure 9-52 Indicate correct dosage.

34. 0.4 mL (Fig. 9-53)

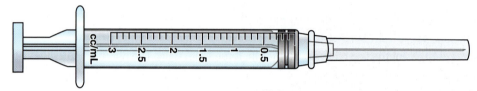

Figure 9-53 Indicate correct dosage.

35. 2.8 mL (Fig. 9-54)

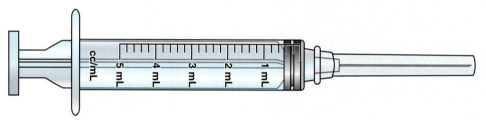

Figure 9-54 Indicate correct dosage.

36. 4.6 mL (Fig. 9-55)

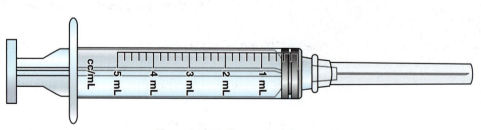

Figure 9-55 Indicate correct dosage.

Syringe Calculations

Using the medication labels shown in the figures, calculate the amount of medication (mL) to be drawn up in the syringe for these parenteral orders. Round the answers to the nearest tenth mL.

37. The provider orders hydralazine 30 mg, IV, STAT (Fig. 9-56).

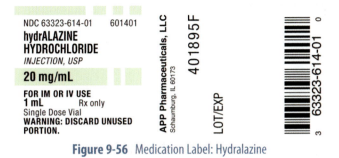

Figure 9-56 Medication Label: Hydralazine

38. The provider orders heparin 2500 units, subcut, daily (Fig. 9-57).

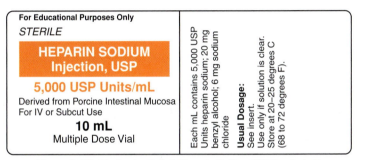

Figure 9-57 Medication Label: Heparin Sodium (5000 units/mL)

Calculate the amount of medication to be administered (mL) per dose for these parenteral orders. Round the answers to the nearest tenth mL.

39. The provider orders adenosine (Adenocard) 2 mg, IV, STAT. The pharmacy provides adenosine in vials containing 3 mg in 1 mL.

40. The provider orders procainamide (Pronestyl) 100 mg, IV, every 5 minutes up to 5 doses. The pharmacy provides procainamide in vials containing 100 mg in 1 mL.

41. The provider orders calcium gluconate 1.7 mEq, IV now. The pharmacy provides calcium gluconate in vials containing 0.45 mEq per 1 mL.

42. The provider orders ketorolac (Toradol) 60 mg, IM, every 6 hours. The pharmacy provides ketorolac in vials containing 30 mg per 1 mL.

43. The provider orders haloperidol (Haldol) 2 mg, IV, every 8 hours, as needed for agitation. The pharmacy provides haloperidol in vials containing 5 mg per 1 mL.

44. The provider orders meperidine (Demerol) 50 mg, subcut, every 4 hours, as needed for pain. The pharmacy provides meperidine in vials containing 100 mg per 1 mL.

45. The provider orders heparin sodium 7000 units, subcut, once daily. The pharmacy provides heparin sodium in vials containing 10,000 units per 1 mL.

Answers to Practice Questions

Identifying the Components of a Medication Label

1. Biaxin
2. clarithromycin
3. 500 mg per tablet
4. tablets (film-coated)
5. 20° to 25°C (68° to 77°F)
6. Norvir
7. ritonavir
8. 100 mg per capsule
9. Find out about which medications should not be taken with Norvir.
10. 30 capsules
11. Short duration analgesia; induction of anesthesia
12. 50–100 mcg (0.05–0.1 mg)
13. Allergic reaction to fentanyl
14. Respiratory depression
15. Opioid antagonist

Calculating Oral Dosages

1. $\text{tablets} = \dfrac{1 \text{ tablet}}{\cancel{333 \text{ mg}}} \times \cancel{333 \text{ mg}} = 1 \text{ tablet}$

2. Tip: You can calculate the amount of solution to administer using either the lopinavir or the ritonavir component in the solution since the drug is ordered in the same ratio as it is provided.)

$\text{mL} = \dfrac{1 \text{ mL}}{80 \text{ mg}} \times 400 \text{ mg} = \dfrac{1 \text{ mL} \times 400}{80} = \dfrac{400 \text{ mL}}{80} = 5 \text{ mL}$

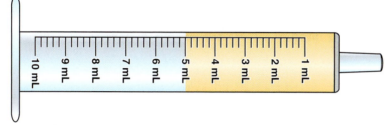

Figure 9-58 Oral Syringe Filled to 5 mL

3. $\text{tablets} = \dfrac{1 \text{ tablet}}{500 \text{ mg}} \times 1000 \text{ mg} = \dfrac{1 \text{ tablet} \times 1000}{500} = \dfrac{1000 \text{ tablets}}{500} = 2 \text{ tablets}$

4. $\text{tablets} = \dfrac{1 \text{ tablet}}{250 \text{ mg}} \times 750 \text{ mg} = \dfrac{1 \text{ tablet} \times 750}{250} = \dfrac{750 \text{ tablets}}{250} = 3 \text{ tablets}$

5. $\text{capsules} = \dfrac{1 \text{ capsule}}{100 \text{ mg}} \times 300 \text{ mg} = \dfrac{1 \text{ capsule} \times 300}{100} = \dfrac{300 \text{ capsules}}{100} = 3 \text{ capsules}$

6. $\text{mL} = \dfrac{5 \text{ mL}}{125 \text{ mg}} \times 225 \text{ mg} = \dfrac{5 \text{ mL} \times 225}{125} = \dfrac{1125 \text{ mL}}{125} = 9 \text{ mL}$

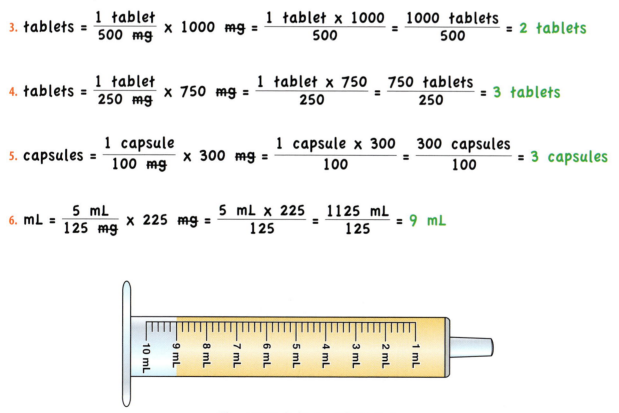

Figure 9-59 Oral Syringe Filled to 9 mL

Answers to Practice Questions

7. $mL = \dfrac{5\ mL}{100\ mg} \times 200\ mg = \dfrac{5\ mL \times 200}{100} = \dfrac{1000\ mL}{100} = 10\ mL$

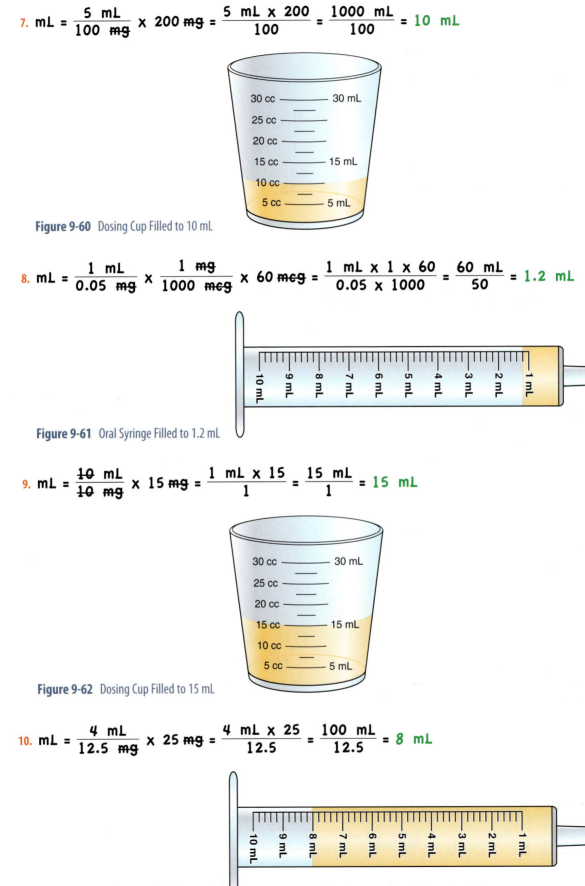

Figure 9-60 Dosing Cup Filled to 10 mL

8. $mL = \dfrac{1\ mL}{0.05\ mg} \times \dfrac{1\ mg}{1000\ mcg} \times 60\ mcg = \dfrac{1\ mL \times 1 \times 60}{0.05 \times 1000} = \dfrac{60\ mL}{50} = 1.2\ mL$

Figure 9-61 Oral Syringe Filled to 1.2 mL

9. $mL = \dfrac{10\ mL}{10\ mg} \times 15\ mg = \dfrac{1\ mL \times 15}{1} = \dfrac{15\ mL}{1} = 15\ mL$

Figure 9-62 Dosing Cup Filled to 15 mL

10. $mL = \dfrac{4\ mL}{12.5\ mg} \times 25\ mg = \dfrac{4\ mL \times 25}{12.5} = \dfrac{100\ mL}{12.5} = 8\ mL$

Figure 9-63 Oral Syringe Filled to 8 mL

Measuring Medications in a Hypodermic Syringe

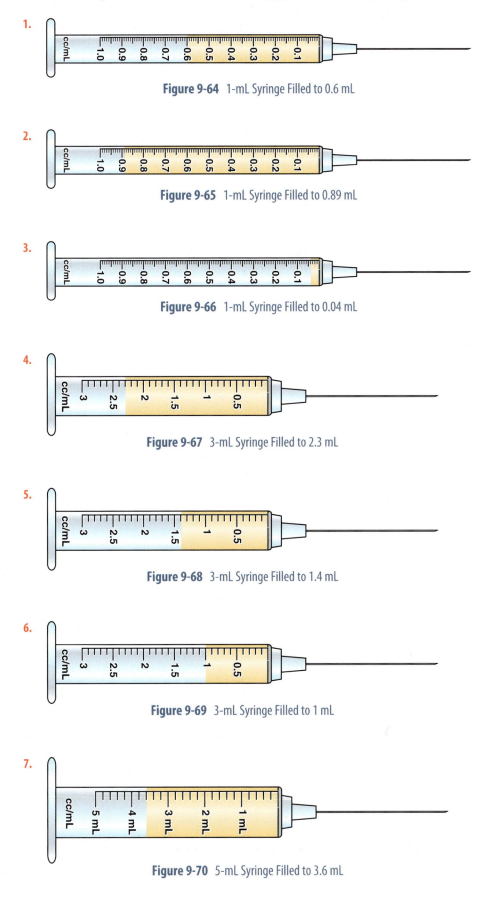

1.

Figure 9-64 1-mL Syringe Filled to 0.6 mL

2.

Figure 9-65 1-mL Syringe Filled to 0.89 mL

3.

Figure 9-66 1-mL Syringe Filled to 0.04 mL

4.

Figure 9-67 3-mL Syringe Filled to 2.3 mL

5.

Figure 9-68 3-mL Syringe Filled to 1.4 mL

6.

Figure 9-69 3-mL Syringe Filled to 1 mL

7.

Figure 9-70 5-mL Syringe Filled to 3.6 mL

8.

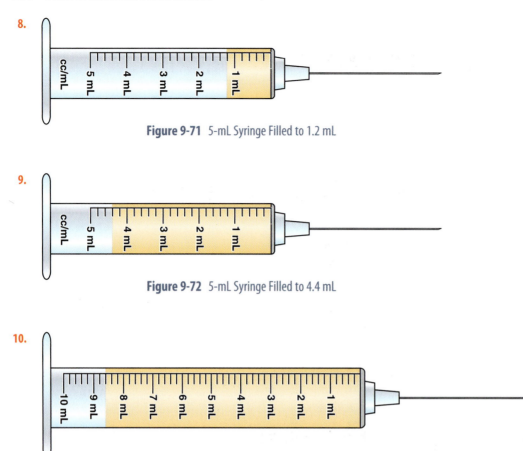

Figure 9-71 5-mL Syringe Filled to 1.2 mL

9.

Figure 9-72 5-mL Syringe Filled to 4.4 mL

10.

Figure 9-73 10-mL Syringe Filled to 8.6 mL

Calculating Parenteral Dosages

1. $mL = \dfrac{1\ mL}{1\ \cancel{mg}} \times 0.25\ \cancel{mg} = \dfrac{1\ mL \times 0.25}{1} = \dfrac{0.25\ mL}{1} = 0.25 = 0.3\ mL$

2. $mL = \dfrac{2\ mL}{1\ \cancel{g}} \times \cancel{1\ g} = 2\ mL$

3. $mL = \dfrac{1\ mL}{5000\ \cancel{units}} \times 3000\ \cancel{units} = \dfrac{1\ mL \times 3000}{5000} = \dfrac{3000\ mL}{5000} = 0.6\ mL$

4. $mL = \dfrac{1\ mL}{4\ \cancel{mg}} \times 2\ \cancel{mg} = \dfrac{1\ mL \times 2}{4} = \dfrac{2\ mL}{4} = 0.5\ mL$

5. $mL = \dfrac{1\ mL}{0.4\ \cancel{mg}} \times 0.4\ \cancel{mg} = \dfrac{1\ mL \times 0.4}{0.4} = \dfrac{0.4\ mL}{0.4} = 1\ mL$

6. $mL = \dfrac{1\ mL}{2\ \cancel{mg}} \times 1.5\ \cancel{mg} = \dfrac{1\ mL \times 1.5}{2} = \dfrac{1.5\ mL}{2} = 0.75\ mL = 0.8\ mL$

7. $mL = \dfrac{1\ mL}{0.1\ \cancel{mg}} \times 0.2\ \cancel{mg} = \dfrac{1\ mL \times 0.2}{0.1} = \dfrac{0.2\ mL}{0.1} = 2\ mL$

8. $mL = \dfrac{5\ mL}{250\ \cancel{mg}} \times 300\ \cancel{mg} = \dfrac{5\ mL \times 300}{250} = \dfrac{1500\ mL}{250} = 6\ mL$

9. $mL = \dfrac{1\ mL}{0.05\ \cancel{mg}} \times \dfrac{1\ \cancel{mg}}{1000\ \cancel{mcg}} \times 75\ \cancel{mcg} = \dfrac{1\ mL \times 1 \times 75}{0.05 \times 1000} = \dfrac{75\ mL}{50} = 1.5\ mL$

10. $mL = \dfrac{5\ mL}{2\ \cancel{g}} \times 1\ \cancel{g} = \dfrac{5\ mL \times 1}{2} = \dfrac{5\ mL}{2} = 2.5\ mL$

Chapter 10
Reconstituting Parenteral Medications From a Powder

Glossary

Bacteriostatic: Capable of inhibiting the reproduction of bacteria.

Diluent: A substance, usually a liquid, used to dilute another substance.

Lyophilized: Freeze-dried; the process of quickly freezing then drying a liquid substance in a vacuum; used to preserve a perishable material.

Reconstitute: The return of an altered substance to its original state, such as changing a powdered substance back into a liquid through the addition of water.

Objectives

After completing this chapter, the learner will be able to—
1. Describe the basic principles of reconstituting powdered medications.
2. Describe the process of reconstituting powdered medications.
3. List the ways that mistakes can be made during the reconstitution of medications.
4. Differentiate between single- and multiple-dose medication vials.
5. Analyze drug labels for single- and multiple-strength medications.
6. Calculate dosages based on drug strength after reconstitution.

Reconstituting Powdered Medications: Basic Principles

To extend the shelf life of unstable liquid medications, manufacturers package, store, and ship such drugs in a lyophilized form. These medications—labeled as "powder for injection," "powder for constitution," "powder for reconstitution," or "dry powder injection"—must be reconstituted prior to injection into a vein or tissue.

The fluid used to reconstitute a medication is called the **diluent**. Common diluents include 5% dextrose solution (D_5W), 0.9% sodium chloride solution (normal saline, or "NS"), bacteriostatic water, or sterile water for injection. Sometimes the drug manufacturer supplies the diluent with the medication, especially if the diluent is an uncommon solution, such as 0.8% normal saline. Do not use any other diluent than the one(s) directed by the manufacturer.

Reconstituting Powdered Medications

To reconstitute powdered medications, follow these steps:

1. Remove the caps from the medication and diluent vials and clean the vial tops as instructed by facility policy.
2. Determine the amount of diluent to be injected into the vial of powdered medication. This information is available on the medication label or package insert.

3. Using the appropriate size syringe, draw air up into the syringe in the same amount as the diluent determined in step 2.
4. Insert the needle (or vial access device if using a needleless system) into the vial of diluent and inject the air. Do not remove the needle from the vial.
5. Turn the vial upside down and withdraw the required amount of diluent into the syringe.
6. Withdraw the needle or vial access device from the vial.
7. Insert the needle or vial access device into the vial of the powdered medication.
8. Inject the diluent slowly into the vial.
9. Mix the medication as instructed by the drug label or package insert.
10. Withdraw the required amount of medication into the syringe and remove the needle from the vial. See Box 10-1.

> **Note:** The volume of the diluent added to reconstitute a medication is not always equal to the reconstituted volume. For example, 0.8 mL of sterile water for injection may be added to a vial of a drug to make a constituted volume of 1 mL. The powder itself has volume, even after it has been dissolved in the diluent.

Care must be taken to avoid errors when reconstituting medications. For example, needle-stick injuries may occur as vials are entered, or medications may be contaminated if the vial is not cleaned properly. Selecting the wrong diluents may inactivate a drug or cause it to react unpredictably, rendering it ineffective. In addition, inaccurate doses may be administered if the wrong concentration of medication is mixed.

■ Box 10-1 Principles of Safe Reconstitution

1. Take care to dissolve all the powder and be certain the fluid is completely clear, with no visible residue in the vial, before administering the drug to the patient.
2. To avoid small particles from getting into the patient's tissues or bloodstream, use a filter needle to withdraw the medication from the vial or, if the medication is being administered intravenously, add an inline filter to the IV tubing.
3. Avoid vigorously shaking the vial, an action that may cause some medications to foam. Foaming can inactivate some proteins in the medication and may delay administration while the foam dissipates. Follow the manufacturer's directions for mixing on the label or package insert.
4. Write the following information on the medication vial without obscuring other vital label information:
   • your initials
   • date
   • time of reconstitution
   • expiration date and time
   • amount of diluent added and the final concentration of the medication (this is critical if the vial will be used multiple times)
5. Do not reconstitute medications too early—some medications become ineffective a short time after reconstitution.
6. Store reconstituted medications according to the manufacturer's directions.
7. Discard unused medications according to facility policy.

Practice Reconstituting Medications

(answers on page 178)

Multiple choice. Select all answers that apply.

1. A "lyophilized" medication has been:
   a. sterilized to inhibit bacterial growth.
   b. reconstituted with sterile water.
   c. frozen in a liquid state.
   d. frozen then dried into a powder form.

2. Medications are produced, packaged, and shipped in a powdered form:
   a. to extend the shelf life of the drug.
   b. because they are unstable in their liquid form.
   c. to reduce manufacturing costs.
   d. to reduce the risk of contamination.

3. Which of the following items should be written on a vial of reconstituted medication?
   a. initials of the person mixing the medication
   b. the date
   c. the time the medication was mixed
   d. the time the medication was administered to the patient

4. An inline filter should be used when administering a reconstituted medication intravenously to:
   a. avoid air bubbles from being infused into the patient's bloodstream.
   b. prevent undissolved particles of medication from entering the patient's bloodstream.
   c. prevent the medication from foaming after mixing.
   d. prevent inactivation of the medication from damaged proteins.

Fill in the blanks.

5. List three errors or accidents that can occur while reconstituting drugs.
   a. _____
   b. _____
   c. _____

Reconstituting Single- and Multiple-Dose Medications

Closely examine package labels and inserts for medications that require reconstitution. Some reconstituted medications may be single-dose only (that is, they can be used just once, even if more than one dose is available after reconstitution). Reconstituted single-dose medications should be discarded after use. Other medications may be labeled multiple-dose (that is, two or more doses may be obtained from a single vial after mixing). For multiple-dose drugs, follow the instructions for proper storage to ensure that the drug will not expire prematurely. See Figures 10-1 and 10-2.

20 mg/mL (after reconstitution)

FOR IM OR IV USE
1 mL   Rx only
Single Dose Vial
WARNING: DISCARD UNUSED PORTION.

Figure 10-1 Single-Dose Vial

10 mg/mL (after reconstitution)

20 mL   Rx Only
Multiple Dose Vial

Figure 10-2 Multiple-Dose Vial

Reconstituting Single- and Multiple-Strength Medications

Some medications can be reconstituted in different strengths, or concentrations, by varying the amount of diluents added. Manufacturers of those multiple-strength drugs provide mixing directions for the various strengths. The flexibility of a multiple-strength drug is needed for patients, such as those with kidney or heart failure, who must restrict fluids. After preparing a multiple-strength medication, write the amount of diluent added and the medication's final concentration on the vial.

Example 1:   Examine the label for vancomycin in Figure 10-3.

1. What is the total amount of medication in this vial? _____
2. What is the usual adult dosage? _____
3. What diluent should be used to dilute this medication and how much should be used? _____
   _____
4. What are the storage instructions for vancomycin after it has been reconstituted?
   _____
5. What information do you still need to know that is *not* on the drug label?
   _____

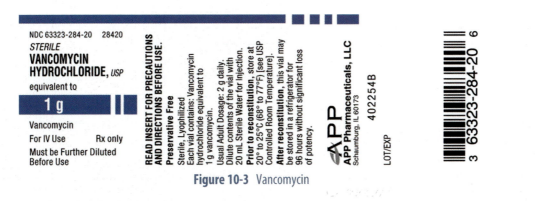

Figure 10-3 Vancomycin

Example 2:   Refer to the label facsimile for ampicillin in Figure 10-4.

1. What is the total amount of ampicillin in the vial? _____ mg
2. What are the two routes of administration? _____ and _____
3. What is the usual dosage? _____
4. What diluent should be used to dilute the medication? _____
5. How much diluent should be used to reconstitute the drug if is to be administered by IM injection?
   _____
6. What is the final concentration of the medication (mg/mL) after dilution for an IM injection? _____
   _____
7. A provider orders ampicillin 500 mg, IM, every 6 hours. If the drug is mixed according to label directions, how many mL of ampicillin should the nurse draw up in the syringe for each dose? _____
   _____

For Educational Purposes Only

STERILE

AMPICILLIN SODIUM for Injection

For IM, IV Injection

Each vial contains:
Ampicillin Sodium 1 gram

Store in a cool, dry place

Single Use Only

Usual Dosage: Weight 40 kg or more; 250 to 500 mg every 6 hours. **Directions for Reconstitution:** **IM Use:** 3.5 mL Sterile Water for Injection, for a final concentration of 250 mg/mL. **IV Use:** 7.4 mL Sterile Water for Injection. May further dilute with 50 mL NS, D5W or LR.

Figure 10-4 Simulated Ampicillin Label

Example 3: Refer to the label facsimile for ceftriaxone in Figure 10-5.

1. What is the total amount of ceftriaxone in the vial? _250mg_ _____ mg
2. What diluent is used to dilute the medication? _Sterile water or 0.9% sodium_
3. How much diluent should be used to reconstitute the drug initially if it is to be administered by IV injection?
   _100mg/ml 2.4_
4. What is the concentration of the medication (mg/mL) after the initial dilution for an IV injection?
   _500r100 ml_
5. How much diluent may be added to further dilute the ceftriaxone for IV administration? _____
6. After reconstitution, what are the storage instructions for this medication? _____

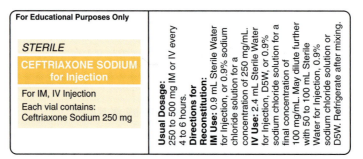

Figure 10-5 Simulated Ceftriaxone Label

Example 4: A provider orders penicillin G, 500,000 units, IV, every 6 hours. The pharmacy supplies the powdered penicillin G in a vial containing 1,000,000 units. The vial may be reconstituted to form solutions of varying concentrations as shown in Table 10-1.

1. To make a solution containing 50,000 units/mL, how much diluent should be added to the vial?
   _10ml_
2. To make a solution containing 250,000 units/mL, how much diluent should be added to the vial?
   _4ml_
3. If the nurse makes a solution containing 100,000 units/mL, how many mL should the nurse draw up in the syringe, based on the provider's order? _10ml_

Table 10-1	Penicillin G
Desired Concentration	**Amount of Diluent**
50,000 units/mL	20 mL
100,000 units/mL	10 mL
250,000 units/mL	4 mL
500,000 units/mL	1.8 mL

Example 5: A provider orders ampicillin 500 mg, IM, every 8 hours. The pharmacy supplies the powdered ampicillin in a vial containing 1 g. The vial may be reconstituted to form solutions of varying concentrations as shown in Table 10-2.

1. To make a solution containing 125 mg/mL, how much diluent should be added to the vial? _____4.8 ml_____

2. To make a solution containing 250 mg/mL, how much diluent should be added to the vial? _____3.6_____

3. To make a solution containing 500 mg/mL, how much diluent should be added to the vial? _____2.3_____

4. If the nurse makes a solution containing 250 mg/mL, how many mL should the nurse draw up in the syringe, based on the provider's order? _____

Table 10-2	Ampicillin
Desired Concentration	**Amount of Diluent**
125 mg/mL	4.8 mL
250 mg/mL	3.6 mL
500 mg/mL	2.3 mL
1 g/mL	1.2 mL

Practice Reconstituting Single- and Multiple-Dose Medications

(answers on page 178)

Refer to the label facsimile for ceftazidime shown in Figure 10-6.

1. What is the total amount of ceftazidime in the vial? _____ mg

2. What is the usual dosage of ceftazidime? _____

3. What diluent should be used to dilute the medication? _____

4. How much diluent should be used to reconstitute the drug? _____

5. What is the final concentration of the medication (mg/mL) after dilution? _____200mg/1ml_____

6. If the provider orders ceftazidime 1 g, IV, every 12 hours, how many mL of reconstituted medication will the nurse draw up in the syringe (without further dilution)?

For Educational Purposes Only

STERILE

CEFTAZIDIME SODIUM for Injection

For IV Use Only
Each vial contains:
Ceftazidime Sodium 2 grams
Store between 59° and 86°F.
Single Use Only

Usual Dosage: 1 g every 8 to 12 hours. Directions for Reconstitution: IV Use Only: Add 10 mL Sterile Water for Injection for a concentration of 200 mg per 1 mL. Shake vial well until solution is clear. After reconstitution, the solution is stable for one week under refrigeration (40°F).

Figure 10-6 Simulated Ceftazidime Label

A provider orders penicillin G, 1,000,000 units, IV, every 4 hours. The pharmacy supplies the powdered penicillin G in a vial containing 5,000,000 units. The vials may be reconstituted to form solutions of varying concentrations as shown in Table 10-1.

7. To make a solution with 100,000 units/mL, how much diluent should be added to the vial? _____

_____
10 ml

8. To make a solution with 500,000 units/mL, how much diluent should be added to the vial? _____

_____
1.8 ml

9. If the nurse makes a solution containing 500,000 units/mL, how many mL should be drawn up, based on the provider's order? _____

Refer to the label facsimile for clindamycin in Figure 10-7 to answer questions 10 through 15.

10. What is the total amount of clindamycin in the vial? _____ mg

11. What is the usual dosage of clindamycin? _____

12. What diluent should be used to dilute the medication? _____

13. How much diluent should be used to reconstitute the drug? _____

14. What is the final concentration of the medication (mg/mL) after dilution? _____100mg/ml_____

_____

15. If the provider orders clindamycin 400 mg, IM, every 8 hours, how many mL of reconstituted medication will the nurse draw up in the syringe? _____

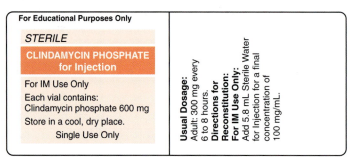

Figure 10-7 Simulated Clindamycin Label

Key Points

1. Powdered medications must be reconstituted with a diluent prior to injection into tissues or veins.

2. Opportunities for errors during reconstitution include needlesticks, contamination of vials, using the wrong diluent, or administering inaccurate doses.

3. Single-dose medications may be used only once after reconstitution. Multiple-dose vials may be used more than once provided the expiration date of the reconstituted medication has not passed.

4. Some powdered medications can be reconstituted with varying amounts of diluent. For such medications, the nurse must write the amount of diluent used and the final concentration of the contents on the vial.

Example 1 Answers

1. This vial contains 1 g of lyophilized vancomycin. Note that it is for IV use only, and must be diluted before using.
2. The usual adult dosage is 2 g daily.
3. This drug must be diluted with 20 mL sterile water for injection.
4. After dilution, this drug may be stored in the refrigerator for 96 hours (4 days).
5. The label does not say whether the vial is single or multiple use, nor whether the total daily dosage should be divided into two or more doses, and whether additional dilution is needed before administering the medication. To answer these questions, further investigation using the package insert or a medication reference book is necessary.

Example 2 Answers

1. The vial contains 1 g of ampicillin.
2. The drug may be administered via IM and IV routes.
3. The usual dosage is 250 to 500 mg every 6 hours for patients who weigh more than 40 kg.
4. The diluent is sterile water for injection.
5. The amount of diluent to add is 3.5 mL for an IM injection.
6. The final concentration is 250 mg/mL.
7. The dosage is 2 mL:

$$\text{mL} = \frac{1 \text{ mL}}{250 \text{ mg}} \times 500 \text{ mg} = \frac{1 \text{ mL} \times 500}{250} = 2 \text{ mL}$$

Example 3 Answers

1. The vial contains 250 mg of ceftriaxone.
2. The diluent is sterile water for injection or 0.9 percent sodium chloride solution.
3. 2.4 mL
4. 100 mg/mL
5. 50 to 100 mL
6. Refrigerate after mixing.

Example 4 Answers

1. 20 mL diluent.
2. 4 mL diluent.
3. $\text{mL} = \dfrac{1 \text{ mL}}{100,000 \text{ units}} \times 500,000 \text{ units} = \dfrac{1 \text{ mL} \times 500,000}{100,000} = 5 \text{ mL}$

Example 5 Answers

1. 4.8 mL diluent
2. 3.6 mL diluent
3. 2.3 mL diluent
4. $\text{mL} = \dfrac{1 \text{ mL}}{250 \text{ mg}} \times 500 \text{ mg} = \dfrac{1 \text{ mL} \times 500}{250} = 2 \text{ mL}$

Chapter Post-Test

(answers in Unit 4)

Calculations

Calculate the volume (in mL's) that the nurse should draw into the syringe. Round the final answer to the nearest tenth mL.

1. A provider orders acetazolimide <u>500 mg</u>, IV, every 12 hours. The pharmacy provides acetazolimide in vials containing 500 mg. The vial label states that the contents should be reconstituted with 5 mL sterile water for injection for a final concentration of 100 mg/mL.

2. A provider orders azithromycin 250 mg, IV, daily. Azithromycin comes in vials containing 500 mg. It must be reconstituted with 4.8 mL of sterile water for injection for a final concentration of 100 mg/mL.

3. A provider orders cefoxitin 500 mg IV every 8 hours. Cefoxitin comes in vials containing 2 g and must be reconstituted with 10 mL bacteriostatic water for injection for a final concentration of 200 mg/mL.

4. A provider orders vancomycin <u>500 mg</u>, IV, daily. The medication is mixed as directed on the label for a concentration of 0.05 g/mL. (See Fig. 10-3.)

5. A provider orders penicillin G <u>750,000</u> units, IM, every 6 hours. The vial of ~~5 million~~ units will be reconstituted with <u>8.2 mL</u> of diluent to yield <u>500,000</u> units/mL.

Reading Label

Refer to the label for oxacillin in Figure 10-8.

6. What is the total amount of oxacillin in the vial?
   _____

7. What is the usual dosage of oxacillin?
   _____

8. How much diluent is added for IM injections?
   _____

9. How much diluent is added for IV use?
   _____

10. What is the concentration of the solution after reconstitution for the IM dose?
    _____

11. What is the concentration of the solution after reconstitution for the IV dose?
    _____

12. How long should the vial be shaken after reconstitution? _____

13. If it is refrigerated, how long is the reconstituted solution stable? _____
    _____

14. A provider orders oxacillin 300 mg, IM, every 6 hours. How many mL of oxacillin will the nurse draw up in the syringe? _____
    _____

15. A provider orders oxacillin 500 mg, IV, every 4 hours. How many mL of oxacillin will the nurse draw up in the syringe? _____
    _____

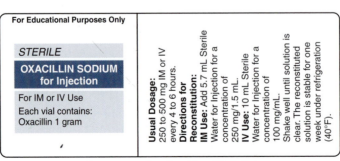

Figure 10-8 Simulated Oxacillin Label

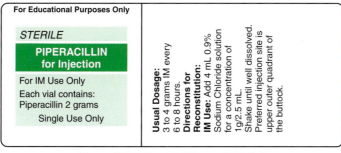

Figure 10-9 Simulated Piperacillin Label

Refer to the label for piperacillin in Figure 10-9.

16. What is the total amount of piperacillin in the vial?

_____

17. What is the usual dosage of piperacillin?

_____

18. How much diluent is added for IM injections?

_____

19. Can this piperacillin formulation be used for IV?

_____

_____

20. What is the concentration of the solution after reconstitution? _____

_____

21. How long should the vial be shaken after reconstitution? _____

_____

22. A provider orders piperacillin 1 g, IM, every 6 hours. How many mL of piperacillin will the nurse draw up in the syringe? Round the final answer to the nearest tenth mL.

_____

23. A provider orders piperacillin 500 mg, IM, every 4 hours. How many mL of piperacillin will the nurse draw up in the syringe? Round the final answer to the nearest tenth mL.

_____

Multiple Choice

Select all correct answers.

24. Care must be taken in mixing reconstituted drugs because
   a. vigorous shaking may deactivate certain proteins in the drug.
   b. overmixing the medication may alter the pH of the drug.
   c. a few particles of powder should remain in the vial for evidence that the drug was mixed correctly.
   d. foam in the vial can delay administration of the drug.

25. A nurse is preparing to reconstitute a multiple-strength medication. Which of the following will influence the nurse's selection of diluent volume?
   a. the patient's current fluid status
   b. the patient's medical history
   c. the patient's allergies
   d. the patient's other medications

Answers to Practice Questions

Reconstituting Medications

1. d

2. a and b

3. a, b, and c

4. b

5. Accidental needlestick, contamination of medication or diluent during preparation, selecting the wrong diluent, administering the wrong dose due to errors during preparation.

Reconstituting Single- and Multiple-Dose Medications

1. 2 g

2. 1 g every 8 to 12 hours

3. sterile water for injection

4. 10 mL

5. 200 mg/mL

6. $mL = \dfrac{1\ mL}{200\ \cancel{mg}} \times \dfrac{1000\ \cancel{mg}}{1\ g} \times 1\ g$

   $= \dfrac{1\ mL \times 1000}{200} = 5\ mL$

7. 10 mL

8. 1.8 mL

9. $mL = \dfrac{1\ mL}{500,000\ \cancel{units}} \times 1,000,000\ \cancel{units}$

   $= \dfrac{1\ mL \times 1,000,000}{500,000} = 2\ mL$

10. 600 mg

11. 300 mg every 6 to 8 hours

12. sterile water for injection

13. 5.8 mL

14. 100 mg/mL

15. $mL = \dfrac{1\ mL}{100\ \cancel{mg}} \times 400\ \cancel{mg}$

    $= \dfrac{1\ mL \times 400}{100} = 4\ mL$

Chapter 11
Calculations Using Weight and Body Surface Area

Glossary

Body Surface Area (BSA): The calculated total surface area of a human body.

Objectives

After completing this chapter, the learner will be able to—
1. Calculate drug dosages based on body weight.
2. Calculate body surface area using pounds and inches.
3. Calculate body surface area using kilograms and centimeters.
4. Calculate drug dosages based on body surface area.

Calculating Dosages Based on Body Weight

Medications may be prescribed based on an individual's body weight. Before calculating a dosage based on weight make sure to weigh the patient using a dependable scale. Do not rely on the weight that the patient states—home scales may not be accurate and patients may under- or overestimate their actual weight.

Ask a pharmacist or another nurse to verify your calculations prior to administering medications based on body weight. If your calculations do not match those written in the provider's order, obtain clarification from the prescribing provider.

Example 1: A provider orders bivalirudin (Angiomax) 0.75 mg/kg, IV, one dose today. The patient weighs 74.6 kg. Calculate the dosage (mg) of bivalirudin (Angiomax) that the nurse should administer. Round the answer to the nearest whole mg.

1. Set up the equation using dimensional analysis and inserting the given quantities for the dosage (0.75 mg/kg).

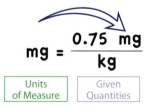

$$mg = \frac{0.75 \text{ mg}}{kg}$$

| Units of Measure | Given Quantities |

2. Enter the given quantity for the patient's weight.

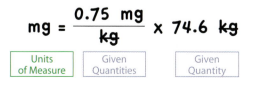

$$mg = \frac{0.75 \text{ mg}}{kg} \times 74.6 \text{ kg}$$

| Units of Measure | Given Quantities | Given Quantity |

3. Solve the equation.

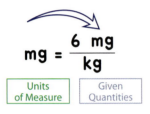

$$mg = \frac{0.75 \ mg}{kg} \times 74.6 \ kg = 55.9 \ mg = 56 \ mg$$

| Units of Measure | Given Quantities | Given Quantity |

The nurse should administer 56 mg of bivalirudin (Angiomax).

Example 2: A provider orders aminophylline 6 mg/kg IV, every 8 hours. The patient weighs 65 kg. Calculate the dosage (in mg) of aminophylline the nurse should administer. Round the answer to the nearest whole mg.

1. Set up the equation using dimensional analysis and inserting the given quantities for the dosage (6 mg/kg).

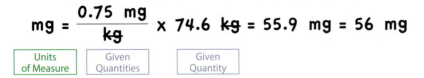

$$mg = \frac{6 \ mg}{kg}$$

| Units of Measure | Given Quantities |

2. Enter the given quantity for the patient's weight.

$$mg = \frac{6 \ mg}{kg} \times 65 \ kg$$

| Units of Measure | Given Quantities | Given Quantity |

3. Solve the equation.

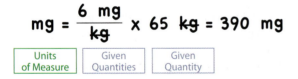

$$mg = \frac{6 \ mg}{kg} \times 65 \ kg = 390 \ mg$$

| Units of Measure | Given Quantities | Given Quantity |

The nurse should administer 390 mg aminophylline. The nurse may also need to calculate the volume of medication to withdraw from the vial (see Example 3).

For Example 3, refer to the directions in Examples 1 and 2.

Example 3: A provider orders rifampin (Rifadin) 5 mg/kg, IV, every 12 hours for 4 days. The patient weighs 84.1 kg.

Calculate the dosage (in mg) of rifampin (Rifadin) that the nurse should administer. Round to the nearest whole mg.

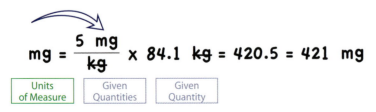

$$mg = \frac{5 \ mg}{kg} \times 84.1 \ kg = 420.5 = 421 \ mg$$

| Units of Measure | Given Quantities | Given Quantity |

The nurse should administer 421 mg of rifampin (Rifadin).

Example 4: Using the dosage of rifampin (Rifadin) calculated in Example 3, calculate the volume (mL) of rifampin (Rifadin) that the nurse should administer, given that the pharmacy supplies rifampin (Rifadin) in a 40-mL vial that contains 25 mg/mL. Round to the nearest tenth mL.

1. Set up the dimensional analysis equation to solve for mL, and insert the first set of given quantities—the concentration of the rifampin (25 mg/mL).

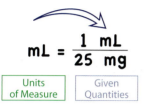

$$mL = \frac{1\ mL}{25\ mg}$$

Units of Measure	Given Quantities

2. Insert the next given quantity—the dosage to be administered (calculated in the first step).

$$mL = \frac{1\ mL}{25\ \cancel{mg}} \times 421\ \cancel{mg}$$

Units of Measure	Given Quantities	Given Quantity

3. Solve the equation.

$$mL = \frac{1\ mL}{25\ \cancel{mg}} \times 421\ \cancel{mg} = 16.84 = 16.8\ mL$$

Units of Measure	Given Quantities	Given Quantity

The nurse should administer 16.8 mL of rifampin (Rifadin).

Note: A common mistake in dosage calculations is assuming that all information offered in a question must be included in the calculation. For instance, in Example 3—

1. The question asks about the number of mL to be removed from the vial for *each administered dose*. Therefore, the frequency of dosing (every 12 hours or twice daily) is irrelevant in this case. The question does not ask how many mg or mL of medication the patient is getting *each day*, but *each dose*.
2. The total volume of the vial (40 mL) is also immaterial information. It is useful only for determining if one vial will provide enough medication for the prescribed dose.
3. The number of days that the medication is to be given (4 days) is also of no importance since we are calculating mg and mL needed per dose, not over the entire course of the prescription.

When calculating dosages, it is vital to know what information is relevant, and what information can be disregarded. Read the question carefully, and use analysis to set up the equation properly to help reduce errors.

Example 5: A provider orders amikacin (Amikin) 7.5 mg/kg, IV, every 12 hr. The pharmacy supplies amikacin (Amikin) in a vial that contains 50 mg/mL. The patient weighs 76 kg. How many mL of amikacin (Amikin) should the nurse withdraw from the vial? Round the answer to the nearest tenth mL.

1. Set up the equation using dimensional analysis and inserting the first set of given quantities—the concentration of amikacin (50 mg/mL).

Note: The actual dosage (in mg) is not specifically calculated in this equation, but it is incorporated into the equation.

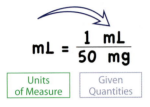

2. Insert the next set of given quantities—the prescribed dosage (7.5 mg/kg):

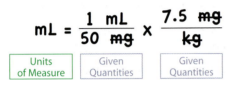

3. Insert the last given quantity—the patient's weight (76 kg).

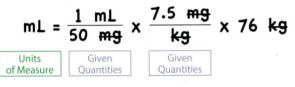

4. Solve the equation.

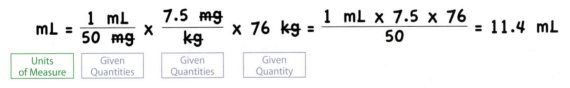

The nurse should administer 11.4 mL of amikacin (Amikin).

For Example 6, refer to the directions in Example 5.

Example 6: A provider orders argatroban 350 mcg/kg, IV, one dose today. The pharmacy supplies argatroban in a premixed bag that contains 1 mg/mL. The patient weighs 68 kg. How many mL of argatroban should the nurse administer? Round the answer to the nearest tenth mL.

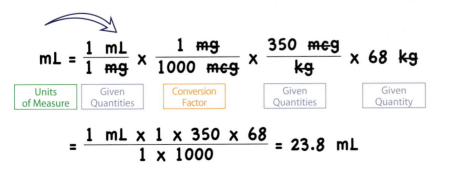

> **Note:** The nurse will have to use two vials of argatroban, since the calculated dosage of 23.8 mL is greater than the amount of drug in one vial (20 mL).

Practice Calculating Dosages Based on Body Weight

(answers on page 195)

Calculate these dosages (mg, mcg, or IU) based on body weight. Round to the nearest whole mg, mcg, or IU.

1. A provider orders lepirudin (Refludan) 0.4 mg/kg, IV, one dose only. The patient weighs 91.6 kg.

2. A provider orders asparaginase (Elspar) 1000 IU/kg, IV, once daily for 10 days. The patient weighs 54 kg.

3. A provider orders bevacizumab (Avastin) 15 mg/kg, IV, one dose, every three weeks. The patient weighs 80 kg.

4. A provider orders oprelvekin (Neumega) 50 mcg/kg, subcut, daily. The patient weighs 72.5 kg.

5. A provider orders phosphenytoin 15 mg/kg, IV, once daily. The patient weighs 57 kg.

Calculate the volume (mL) of medication to be administered. Round the answer to the nearest tenth mL.

6. A provider orders epoetin (Procrit) 100 units/kg, subcut, three times per week on Monday, Wednesday, and Saturday. The pharmacy supplies epoetin in a vial that contains 10,000 units/mL. The patient weighs 48 kg.

7. A provider orders fluorouracil (Adrucil) 12 mg/kg, IV, daily for 4 days. The pharmacy supplies fluorouracil in a vial that contains 50 mg/mL. The patient weighs 87 kg.

8. A provider orders rifampin (Rifadin) 10 mg/kg, IV, once daily. The pharmacy supplies rifampin in a vial that contains 60 mg/mL after reconstitution. The patient weighs 51 kg.

9. A provider orders infliximab (Remicade) 3 mg/kg, IV, one dose today. The pharmacy supplies infliximab in a vial that contains 100 mg/mL. The patient weighs 56 kg.

10. A provider orders palifermin (Kepivance) 60 mcg/kg, IV, once daily for 3 days. The pharmacy supplies palifermin in a vial that contains 5 mg/mL. The patient weighs 64.3 kg.

Calculating Body Surface Area

Most chemotherapy agents are prescribed using body surface area (BSA). An individual's BSA provides for more accurate dosing when compared to using only the patient's weight because BSA considers the individual's height as well as weight.

Several different formulas can be used to calculate body surface area. One of the most common is the Mosteller formula (Mosteller, 1987). The advantage to using the Mosteller formula is that it is easy to compute. All that is needed is a calculator with a square-root function.

BSA is measured as meters squared, or m^2. Although the units of the answer are metric, BSA can be calculated using weight and height in kilograms and centimeters, as well as pounds and inches. Ensure that an accurate height and weight have been obtained prior to calculating the patient's BSA.

> **Alert!** Notify the provider if your calculations do not match those on the provider's order.

> **Note:** Dimensional analysis cannot be used to calculate body surface area.

Calculating BSA (m^2) Using Kilograms and Centimeters

The formula for BSA using **kilograms (kg) and centimeters (cm)** is

$$m^2 = \sqrt{\frac{\text{weight (kg)} \times \text{height (cm)}}{3600}}$$

Example 1: Calculate the BSA (m²) for an individual with a weight of 85 kg and height of 180 cm.

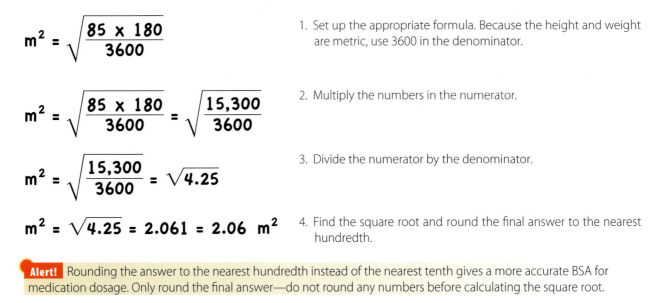

1. Set up the appropriate formula. Because the height and weight are metric, use 3600 in the denominator.

$$m^2 = \sqrt{\dfrac{85 \times 180}{3600}}$$

2. Multiply the numbers in the numerator.

$$m^2 = \sqrt{\dfrac{85 \times 180}{3600}} = \sqrt{\dfrac{15{,}300}{3600}}$$

3. Divide the numerator by the denominator.

$$m^2 = \sqrt{\dfrac{15{,}300}{3600}} = \sqrt{4.25}$$

4. Find the square root and round the final answer to the nearest hundredth.

$$m^2 = \sqrt{4.25} = 2.061 = 2.06 \ m^2$$

Alert! Rounding the answer to the nearest hundredth instead of the nearest tenth gives a more accurate BSA for medication dosage. Only round the final answer—do not round any numbers before calculating the square root.

To compute this BSA using a calculator, follow the sequence in Figure 11-1.

Figure 11-1 BSA Sequence on the Calculator Example 1

Alert! Take extreme care when using a calculator. It is very easy to forget the last step of pressing the square root function button!

For Examples 2 and 3, refer to the directions in Example 1.

Example 2: Calculate the BSA (m²) for an individual with a weight of 56.8 kg and a height of 163 cm. Round the final answer to the nearest hundredth m².

$$m^2 = \sqrt{\dfrac{56.8 \times 163}{3600}} = \sqrt{\dfrac{9258.4}{3600}} = \sqrt{2.571} = 1.603 = 1.60 \ m^2$$

To compute this BSA using a calculator, follow the sequence in Figure 11-2.

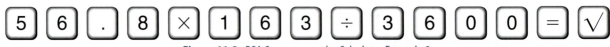

Figure 11-2 BSA Sequence on the Calculator Example 2

Example 3: Calculate the BSA (m²) for an individual with a weight of 100 kg and a height of 187 cm. Round the final answer to the nearest hundredth m².

$$m^2 = \sqrt{\dfrac{100 \times 187}{3600}} = \sqrt{\dfrac{18{,}700}{3600}} = \sqrt{5.194} = 2.279 = 2.28 \ m^2$$

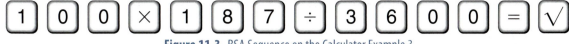

Figure 11-3 BSA Sequence on the Calculator Example 3

To compute this BSA using a calculator, follow the sequence in Figure 11-3.

Practice Calculating BSA (m²) Using Kilograms and Centimeters

(answers on page 196)

*Calculate the BSA in m² for these weight and height combinations. Round the final answer to the nearest **hundredth m²**.*

1. Weight 51 kg; height 150 cm.

2. Weight 71 kg; height 158 cm.

3. Weight 74 kg; height 172 cm.

4. Weight 64 kg; height 167 cm.

5. Weight 60 kg; height 163 cm.

6. Weight 59.4 kg; height 171 cm.

7. Weight 67 kg; height 170 cm.

8. Weight 75 kg; height 175 cm.

9. Weight 80.2 kg; height 184 cm.

10. Weight 54 kg; height 155 cm.

Calculating BSA (m²) Using Pounds and Inches

The formula for BSA using **pounds (lb)** and **inches (in)** is

$$m^2 = \sqrt{\frac{weight\ (lb) \times height\ (in)}{3131}}$$

Note: The only difference between calculating BSA using pounds and inches and using kilograms and centimeters is in the denominator. Notice that in the BSA equation for pounds and inches the denominator is 3131, not 3600.

Example 1:   Calculate the BSA (m²) for an individual with a weight of 167 lb and a height of 69 in.

$$m^2 = \sqrt{\frac{167 \times 69}{3131}}$$

1. Set up the formula.

$$m^2 = \sqrt{\frac{167 \times 69}{3131}} = \sqrt{\frac{11{,}523}{3131}}$$

2. Multiply the numbers in the numerator:

$$m^2 = \sqrt{\frac{11{,}523}{3131}} = \sqrt{3.680}$$

3. Divide the numerator by the denominator:

$$m^2 = \sqrt{3.680} = 1.918 = 1.92\ m^2$$

4. Find the square root and round your answer to the nearest hundredth.

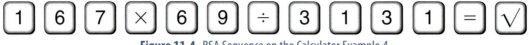

Figure 11-4 BSA Sequence on the Calculator Example 4

To compute this BSA quickly using a calculator, follow the sequence in Figure 11-4.

For Examples 2 and 3, refer to the directions in Example 1.

Example 2: Calculate the BSA (m²) for an individual with a weight of 152 lb and a height of 66 in.

$$m^2 = \sqrt{\frac{152 \times 66}{3131}} = \sqrt{\frac{10{,}032}{3131}} = \sqrt{3.204} = 1.789 = 1.79 \ m^2$$

To compute this BSA using a calculator, follow the sequence in Figure 11-5.

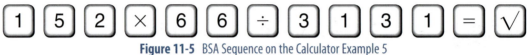

Figure 11-5 BSA Sequence on the Calculator Example 5

Example 3: Calculate the BSA (m²) for an individual with a weight of 161 lb and a height of 64 in.

$$m^2 = \sqrt{\frac{161 \times 64}{3131}} = \sqrt{\frac{10{,}304}{3131}} = \sqrt{3.290} = 1.814 = 1.81 \ m^2$$

To compute this BSA using a calculator, follow the sequence in Figure 11-6.

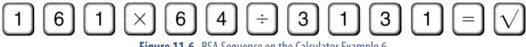

Figure 11-6 BSA Sequence on the Calculator Example 6

Practice Calculating BSA (m²) Using Pounds and Inches

(answers on page 197)

Calculate the BSA in m² for these weight and height combinations. Round the final answer to the nearest hundredth m².

1. Weight 125 lb; height 62 in.

2. Weight 134 lb; height 63 in.

3. Weight 153 lb; height 65 in.

4. Weight 118 lb; height 60 in.

5. Weight 181 lb; height 71 in.

6. Weight 146 lb; height 69 in.

7. Weight 169 lb; height 61 in.

8. Weight 203 lb; height 72 in.

9. Weight 197 lb; height 67 in.

10. Weight 136 lb; height 63 in.

Calculating Medication Dosages Based on Body Surface Area

To calculate dosages based on BSA, multiply the patient's BSA by the prescribed dose. Remember to—

- obtain an accurate, current patient weight.
- have another nurse or pharmacist double-check your calculations.
- communicate with the prescribing provider if your calculations are different from those written in the provider's order.

Example 1:   A provider orders acyclovir (Zovirax) 750 mg/m^2 , IV, three times daily. The patient weighs 75 kg and is 162 cm tall. The pharmacy supplies acyclovir (Zovirax) in a 20-mL vial containing 50 mg/mL.

a. Calculate the dosage (mg) that the nurse should administer. Round to the nearest tenth mg.

   1. Calculate the BSA in m^2.

$$m^2 = \sqrt{\frac{75 \times 162}{3600}} = \sqrt{\frac{12{,}150}{3600}} = \sqrt{3.375} = 1.84 \ m^2$$

   2. Using dimensional analysis principles, calculate the dosage of acyclovir (Zovirax) to be administered. Enter the first set of given quantities (the prescribed dosage of 750 mg/m^2).

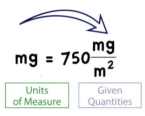

$$mg = 750\frac{mg}{m^2}$$

| Units of Measure | Given Quantities |

   3. Insert the next given quantity—the patient's BSA as calculated in step 1 (1.84 m^2), and solve the equation:

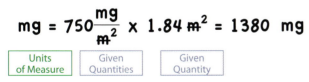

$$mg = 750\frac{mg}{\cancel{m}^2} \times 1.84 \ \cancel{m}^2 = 1380 \ mg$$

| Units of Measure | Given Quantities | Given Quantity |

The nurse will administer 1380 mg of acyclovir (Zovirax) to the patient.

b. Calculate the volume (mL) that the nurse should administer. Round to the nearest tenth mL.

   1. Set up the equation using dimensional analysis. The first set of given quantities will be the concentration of acyclovir (Zovirax).

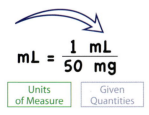

$$mL = \frac{1 \ mL}{50 \ mg}$$

| Units of Measure | Given Quantities |

2. Insert the next given quantity—the dosage of acyclovir (Zovirax) previously calculated (1380 mg).

$$\text{mL} = \frac{1\ \text{mL}}{50\ \cancel{\text{mg}}} \times 1380\ \cancel{\text{mg}}$$

| Units of Measure | Given Quantities | Given Quantity |

3. Solve the equation.

$$\text{mL} = \frac{1\ \text{mL}}{50\ \cancel{\text{mg}}} \times 1380\ \cancel{\text{mg}} = \frac{1\ \text{mL} \times 1380}{50} = 27.6\ \text{mL}$$

| Units of Measure | Given Quantities | Given Quantity |

The nurse should administer 27.6 mL of acyclovir (Zovirax) to the patient. The nurse will need two vials of acyclovir (Zovirax) to draw up the prescribed dose since one vial contains only 20 mL of the medication.

Note: The volume of acyclovir (Zovirax) to administer may be calculated in one equation by inserting the prescribed dosage and patient's BSA. The only drawback to this shortcut is that the actual dosage administered is not evident.

$$\text{mL} = \frac{1\ \text{mL}}{50\ \cancel{\text{mg}}} \times \frac{750\ \cancel{\text{mg}}}{\cancel{\text{m}^2}} \times 1.84\ \cancel{\text{m}^2} = \frac{1\ \text{mL} \times 1380}{50} = 27.6\ \text{mL}$$

| Units of Measure | Given Quantities | Given Quantities | Given Quantity |

For Examples 2–4, refer to the directions in Example 1.

Example 2: A provider orders rituximab (Rituxan) 375 mg/m², IV, once weekly for 4 doses. The patient weighs 82 kg and is 178 cm tall. The pharmacy supplies rituximab in a 500-mg vial with a concentration of 100 mg/mL.

a. Calculate the dosage (mg) that should be administered. Round to the nearest tenth mg.

1: Calculate the BSA in m². The weight and height are given in kilograms and centimeters, so use the denominator *3600*:

$$\text{m}^2 = \sqrt{\frac{82 \times 178}{3600}} = \sqrt{\frac{14{,}596}{3600}} = \sqrt{4.054} = 2.01\ \text{m}^2$$

2. Using dimensional analysis principles, calculate the dosage (mg) of rituximab to be administered.

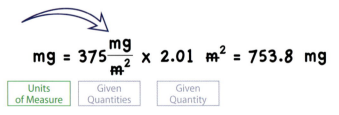

$$\text{mg} = 375\frac{\text{mg}}{\cancel{\text{m}^2}} \times 2.01\ \cancel{\text{m}^2} = 753.8\ \text{mg}$$

| Units of Measure | Given Quantities | Given Quantity |

The nurse should administer 753.8 mg of rituximab (Rituxan).

b. Calculate the volume (mL) to be administered by the nurse. Round to the nearest tenth mL.

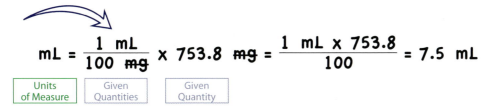

$$mL = \frac{1\ mL}{100\ mg} \times 753.8\ mg = \frac{1\ mL \times 753.8}{100} = 7.5\ mL$$

| Units of Measure | Given Quantities | Given Quantity |

The nurse should administer 7.5 mL of rituximab (Rituxan).

Example 3:   A provider orders docetaxel (Taxotere) 70 mg/m², IV, × 1 dose. The patient weighs 132 lb and is 5 ft 6 in tall. Docetaxel (Taxotere) is supplied in vials containing 80 mg/2 mL.

a. Calculate the dosage (mg) that should be administered. Round to the nearest tenth mg.

1. Calculate the patient's BSA using the denominator 3131 in the equation because weight and height are supplied in pounds and inches. Also change the patient's height to inches before setting up the BSA equation (patient's height = 5 ft × 12 in/ft = 60 in + 6 in = 66 inches).

$$m^2 = \sqrt{\frac{132 \times 66}{3131}} = \sqrt{\frac{8712}{3131}} = \sqrt{2.782} = 1.668 = 1.67\ m^2$$

2. Calculate the dosage (mg) of docetaxel (Taxotere) to be administered.

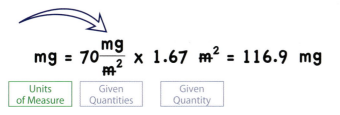

$$mg = 70\frac{mg}{m^2} \times 1.67\ m^2 = 116.9\ mg$$

| Units of Measure | Given Quantities | Given Quantity |

The nurse should administer 116.9 mg of docetaxel (Taxotere).

b. Calculate the volume (mL) to be administered by the nurse. Round to the nearest tenth.

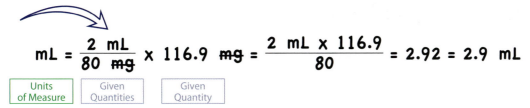

$$mL = \frac{2\ mL}{80\ mg} \times 116.9\ mg = \frac{2\ mL \times 116.9}{80} = 2.92 = 2.9\ mL$$

| Units of Measure | Given Quantities | Given Quantity |

The nurse should administer 2.9 mL of docetaxel (Taxotere).

Example 4:   A provider orders epirubicin (Ellence) 100 mg/m², IV, × 1 dose. The patient weighs 176 lb and is 69 in tall. Epirubicin is supplied in vials containing 200 mg/1 mL.

a. Calculate the dosage (mg) that should be administered. Round to the nearest tenth mg.

1. Calculate the patient's BSA using the denominator 3131 in the equation because weight and height are supplied in pounds and inches.

$$m^2 = \sqrt{\frac{176 \times 69}{3131}} = \sqrt{\frac{12{,}144}{3131}} = \sqrt{3.878} = 1.969 = 1.97 \ m^2$$

2. Calculate the dosage (mg) of epirubicin (Ellence) to be administered. Multiply the patient's BSA by the prescribed dosage.

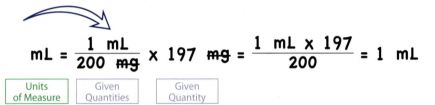

$$mg = 100\frac{mg}{m^2} \times 1.97 \ m^2 = 197 \ mg$$

Units of Measure	Given Quantities	Given Quantity

b. Calculate the volume (mL) to be administered by the nurse. Round to the nearest tenth.

$$mL = \frac{1 \ mL}{200 \ mg} \times 197 \ mg = \frac{1 \ mL \times 197}{200} = 1 \ mL$$

Units of Measure	Given Quantities	Given Quantity

The nurse should administer 1 mL of epirubicin (Ellence).

Practice Calculating Medication Dosages Based on Body Surface Area

(answers on page 198)

Calculate the dosage (mg, mcg, or units) and volume (mL) to be administered for each of these medications. Round m² to nearest hundredth and dosages to the nearest whole mg, mcg, or unit. Round volume to the nearest tenth mL.

1. A provider orders allopurinol 200 mg/m², IV, once daily. The patient weighs 75 kg and is 158 cm in height. Allopurinol is supplied in vials containing 20 mg/mL after reconstitution.

    mg: _____

    mL: _____

2. A provider orders sargramostim (Leukine) 250 mcg/m², IV, once daily for 21 days. The patient weighs 81 kg and is 163 cm in height. Sargramostim (Leukine) is supplied in vials containing 25 mcg/mL after reconstitution.

    mcg: _____

    mL: _____

3. A provider orders bleomycin (Blenoxane) 15 units/m², IV, once daily. The patient weighs 152 lb and is 61 in tall. Bleomycin (Blenoxane) is supplied in vials containing 30 units/5 mL after dilution.

    units: _____

    mL: _____

4. A provider orders pemetrexed (Alimta) 500 mg/m², IV, one dose only today. The patient weighs 195 lb and is 70 in tall. Pemetrexed (Alimta) is supplied in vials containing 100 mg/mL after reconstitution.

   mg: _____

   mL: _____

5. A provider orders cisplatin (Platinol) 20 mg/m², IV, once daily for 5 days. The patient weighs 76 kg and is 179 cm in height. Cisplatin (Platinol) is supplied in vials containing 10 mg/mL.

   mg: _____

   mL: _____

6. A provider orders mitoxantrone (Novantrone) 12 mg/m², IV, once daily for a total of two doses. The patient weighs 55.5 kg and is 155 cm in height. Mitoxantrone (Novantrone) is supplied in vials containing 2 mg/mL.

   mg: _____

   mL: _____

7. A provider orders doxorubicin (Adriamycin PFS) 75 mg/m², IV, one dose only today. The patient weighs 105 lb and is 60 in tall. Doxorubicin (Adriamycin PFS) is supplied in vials containing 20 mg/mL.

   mg: _____

   mL: _____

8. A provider orders fluorouracil (Adrucil) 370 mg/m², IV, one dose only today. The patient weighs 154 lb and is 67 in tall. Fluorouracil (Adrucil) is supplied in vials containing 100 mg/mL.

   mg: _____

   mL: _____

9. A provider orders etoposide (Etopophos) 50 mg/m², IV, once daily for 5 days. The patient weighs 68.3 kg and is 172 cm tall. Etoposide (Etopophos) is supplied in vials containing 20 mg/mL after reconstitution.

   mg: _____

   mL: _____

10. A provider orders mitomycin (Mutamycin) 20 mg/m², IV, once weekly for 6 weeks. The patient weighs 95 kg and is 170 cm in height. Mitomycin (Mutamycin) is supplied in vials containing 10 mg/mL.

    mg: _____

    mL: _____

Read the case study and answer the questions.

Case Study 11–1

Karen Bell is a 64-year-old female with ovarian cancer. She is beginning her chemotherapy. Her provider writes the orders in Figure 11-7.

   1. *Double check the provider's math for the prescribed dosages of Taxol (paclitaxel) and Paraplatin (carboplatin). Are the dosages correct?*
   2. *If the dosages are not correct, what action would you take before administering the chemotherapy agents to the patient?*
   3. *Taxol (paclitaxel) is supplied in vials containing 30 mg/mL. How many mL should the nurse administer with each dose? Round to the nearest tenth mL.*
   4. *Paraplatin (carboplatin) is supplied in vials containing 100 mg/mL. How many mL should the nurse administer with each dose? Round to the nearest tenth mL.*

Date	Physicians' Orders
10/01/18	Regimen Instructions: Taxol (paclitaxel) and Paraplatin
1000	(carboplatin) to be infused every 21 days for 2 cycles following
	completion of radiation therapy:
	1. Taxol (paclitaxel) 320 mg (175 mg/m^2) intravenously,
	over 3 hours.
	2. Paraplatin (carboplatin) 659 mg (360 mg/m^2)
	intravenously, over 30 minutes following paclitaxel.
	Patient weight: 159 lb Height: 66 in
	Premedications:
	1. Dexamethasone 20 mg intravenously, administered at
	12 hours and 6 hours prior to chemotherapy.
	2. Diphenhydramine (Benadryl) 25 mg intravenously prior
	to chemotherapy.
	3. Granisetron (Kytril) 1 mg intravenously prior to
	chemotherapy.
	Post-chemotherapy:
	1. Pegfilgrastim (Neulasta) 5 mg, subcut, 24 hours after
	chemotherapy.
	——————————— *Mary Jones, MD*

Patient label: Karen S. Bell / MR 0826593 / Account 91427895 / Dr. Mary Jones, MD / DOB: 04/16/1945

Figure 11-7 Provider's Order

Key Points

1. The patient's weight and height should be obtained before calculating a drug dosage based on body weight or BSA.
2. Body surface area (BSA) is measured in m^2.
3. BSA can be calculated using either kilograms and centimeters, or pounds and inches.
4. The Mosteller formula for BSA using kilograms and centimeters is

$$m^2 = \sqrt{\frac{\text{weight (kg)} \times \text{height (cm)}}{3600}}$$

5. The Mosteller formula for BSA using pounds and inches is

$$m^2 = \sqrt{\frac{\text{weight (lb)} \times \text{height (in)}}{3131}}$$

6. Calculated dosages should be verified with another licensed nurse or pharmacist before administering the medication.
7. If calculations do not match those in the provider's written order, the discrepancy should be discussed with the prescribing provider.

Reference

1. Mosteller, R.D. (1987). Simplified calculation of body surface area. *The New England Journal of Medicine, 317*(17), 1098 (letter).

Chapter Post-Test

(answers in Unit 4)

Calculations

Calculate these weight-based dosages. Round answers to the nearest whole number.

1. A provider orders lidocaine (Xylocaine) 0.5 mg/kg, IV, STAT. The patient weighs 70.5 kg.

2. A provider orders pancuronium (Pavulon) 0.15 mg/kg, IV, every 20 to 60 minutes as needed to maintain paralysis. The patient weighs 87.2 kg.

3. A provider orders epoetin (Epogen) 50 units/kg, subcut, three times per week. The patient weighs 42 kg.

4. A provider orders eptifibatide (Integrilin) 180 mcg/kg, IV, one dose now. The patient weighs 62.5 kg.

Calculate the volume (mL) of medication to be administered. Round to the nearest tenth mL.

5. A provider orders ondansetron (Zofran) 0.15 mg/kg, IV, 30 minutes before chemotherapy. The pharmacy supplies ondansetron (Zofran) in a vial that contains 2 mg/mL. The patient weighs 63 kg.

6. A provider orders lepirudin (Refludan) 0.4 mg/kg, IV, one dose today only. The pharmacy supplies lepirudin (Refludan) in a vial that contains 50 mg/mL after reconstitution. The patient weighs 91.6 kg.

7. A provider orders pentamidine (Pentam 300) 4 mg/kg, IV, once daily. The pharmacy supplies pentamidine (Pentam) in a vial that contains 100 mg/mL after dilution. The patient weighs 59.8 kg.

8. A provider orders glycopyrrolate (Robinul) 4.4 mcg/kg, IV, one dose pre-operatively. The pharmacy supplies glycopyrrolate (Robinul) in a vial that contains 0.2 mg/mL. The patient weighs 65 kg.

9. A provider orders midazolam (Versed) 0.08 mg/kg, IV, one dose pre-operatively. The pharmacy supplies midazolam (Versed) in a vial that contains 1 mg/mL. The patient weighs 65 kg.

10. A provider orders oprelvekin (Neumega) 50 mcg/kg, subcut once daily. The pharmacy supplies oprelvekin (Neumega) in a vial that contains 5 mg/mL. The patient weighs 60.6 kg.

Calculate the BSA in m^2 for these weight and height combinations. Round the final answer to the nearest hundredth m^2.

11. Weight 128 lb; height 69 in.

12. Weight 144 lb; height 63 in.

13. Weight 196 lb; height 71 in.

14. Weight 130 lb; height 61 in.

15. Weight 205 lb; height 73 in.

16. Weight 67.2 kg; height 158 cm.

17. Weight 88 kg; height 166 cm.

18. Weight 105 kg; height 174 cm.

19. Weight 72.7 kg; height 163 cm.

20. Weight 53 kg; height 152 cm.

Calculate the dosage (mg or units) and volume (mL) to be administered for each of these medications. Round dosages to the nearest whole mg or unit. Round volumes to the nearest tenth mL.

21. A provider orders azacitidine (Vidaza) 75 mg/m², subcut, daily for 7 days. The patient weighs 68 kg and patient's height is 169 cm. Azacitidine (Vidaza) is supplied in vials containing 25 mg/mL after reconstitution.
   a. mg: _____
   b. mL: _____

22. A provider orders docetaxel (Taxotere) 80 mg/m², IV, one dose today. The patient weighs 107 lb and patient's height is 63 in. Docetaxel (Taxotere) is supplied in vials containing 10 mg/mL.
   a. mg: _____
   b. mL: _____

23. A provider orders oxaliplatin (Eloxatin) 85 mg/m², IV, one dose today. The patient weighs 197 lb and patient's height is 71 in. Oxaliplatin (Eloxatin) is supplied in vials containing 50 mg/mL after reconstitution.
   a. mg: _____
   b. mL: _____

24. A provider orders fluorouracil (Adrucil) 300 mg/m², IV, one dose today. The patient weighs 148 lb and patient's height is 65 in. Fluorouracil (Adrucil) is supplied in vials containing 50 mg/mL.
   a. mg: _____
   b. mL: _____

25. A provider orders mitoxantrone (Novantrone) 12 mg/m², IV, once daily for 2 days. The patient weighs 61.4 kg and patient's height is 160 cm. Mitoxantrone (Novantrone) is supplied in vials containing 2 mg/mL.
   a. mg: _____
   b. mL: _____

26. A provider orders rituximab (Rituxan) 375 mg/m², IV, once weekly for 4 weeks. The patient weighs 75.9 kg and patient's height is 159 cm. Rituximab (Rituxan) is supplied in vials containing 100 mg/mL after reconstitution.
   a. mg: _____
   b. mL: _____

27. A provider orders daunorubicin (DaunoXome) 40 mg/m², IV, every 2 weeks. The patient weighs 80 kg and patient's height is 167 cm. Daunorubicin (DaunoXome) is supplied in vials containing 50 mg/mL.
   a. mg: _____
   b. mL: _____

28. A provider orders bleomycin (Blenoxane) 15 units/m², IV, once daily. The patient weighs 123 lb and patient's height is 64 in. Bleomycin (Blenoxane) is supplied in vials containing 30 units/5 mL after dilution.
   a. mg: _____
   b. mL: _____

29. A provider orders irinotecan (Camptosar) 125 mg/m², IV, weekly for 4 weeks. The patient weighs 94.7 kg and patient's height is 188 cm. Irinotecan (Camptosar) is supplied in vials containing 20 mg/mL.
   a. mg: _____
   b. mL: _____

30. A provider orders leucovorin (Wellcovorin) 10 mg/m², IV, every 6 hours. The patient weighs 66 kg and patient's height is 157 cm. Leucovorin (Wellcovorin) is supplied in vials containing 10 mg/mL.
   a. mg: _____
   b. mL: _____

Answers to Practice Questions

Calculating Dosages Based on Body Weight

1. $\text{mg} = \dfrac{0.4 \text{ mg}}{\text{kg}} \times 91.6 \text{ kg} = 36.6 = $ 37 mg

2. $\text{IU} = \dfrac{1000 \text{ IU}}{\text{kg}} \times 54 \text{ kg} = $ 54,000 IU

3. $\text{mg} = \dfrac{15 \text{ mg}}{\text{kg}} \times 80 \text{ kg} = $ 1200 mg

4. $\text{mcg} = \dfrac{50 \text{ mcg}}{\text{kg}} \times 72.5 \text{ kg} = $ 3625 mcg

5. $\text{mg} = \dfrac{15 \text{ mg}}{\text{kg}} \times 57 \text{ kg} = $ 855 mg

6. $\text{mL} = \dfrac{1 \text{ mL}}{10,000 \text{ units}} \times \dfrac{100 \text{ units}}{\text{kg}} \times 48 \text{ kg} = \dfrac{1 \text{ mL} \times 100 \times 48}{10,000} = 0.48 = $ 0.5 mL

7. $\text{mL} = \dfrac{1 \text{ mL}}{50 \text{ mg}} \times \dfrac{12 \text{ mg}}{\text{kg}} \times 87 \text{ kg} = \dfrac{1 \text{ mL} \times 12 \times 87}{50} = 20.88 = $ 20.9 mL

8. $\text{mL} = \dfrac{1 \text{ mL}}{60 \text{ mg}} \times \dfrac{10 \text{ mg}}{\text{kg}} \times 51 \text{ kg} = \dfrac{1 \text{ mL} \times 10 \times 51}{60} = $ 8.5 mL

9. $\text{mL} = \dfrac{1 \text{ mL}}{100 \text{ mg}} \times \dfrac{3 \text{ mg}}{\text{kg}} \times 56 \text{ kg} = \dfrac{1 \text{ mL} \times 3 \times 56}{100} = 1.68 = $ 1.7 mL

10. $\text{mL} = \dfrac{1 \text{ mL}}{5 \text{ mg}} \times \dfrac{1 \text{ mg}}{1000 \text{ mcg}} \times \dfrac{60 \text{ mcg}}{\text{kg}} \times 64.3 \text{ kg}$

$\qquad = \dfrac{1 \text{ mL} \times 1 \times 60 \times 64.3}{5 \times 1000} = 0.77 = $ 0.8 mL

Calculating BSA (m²) Using Kilograms and Centimeters

1. $m^2 = \sqrt{\dfrac{51 \times 150}{3600}} = \sqrt{\dfrac{7650}{3600}} = \sqrt{2.125} = 1.457 = 1.46 \ m^2$

2. $m^2 = \sqrt{\dfrac{71 \times 158}{3600}} = \sqrt{\dfrac{11{,}218}{3600}} = \sqrt{3.116} = 1.765 = 1.77 \ m^2$

3. $m^2 = \sqrt{\dfrac{74 \times 172}{3600}} = \sqrt{\dfrac{12{,}728}{3600}} = \sqrt{3.536} = 1.880 = 1.88 \ m^2$

4. $m^2 = \sqrt{\dfrac{64 \times 167}{3600}} = \sqrt{\dfrac{10{,}688}{3600}} = \sqrt{2.968} = 1.723 = 1.72 \ m^2$

5. $m^2 = \sqrt{\dfrac{60 \times 163}{3600}} = \sqrt{\dfrac{9780}{3600}} = \sqrt{2.716} = 1.648 = 1.65 \ m^2$

6. $m^2 = \sqrt{\dfrac{59.4 \times 171}{3600}} = \sqrt{\dfrac{10{,}157.4}{3600}} = \sqrt{2.821} = 1.679 = 1.68 \ m^2$

7. $m^2 = \sqrt{\dfrac{67 \times 170}{3600}} = \sqrt{\dfrac{11{,}390}{3600}} = \sqrt{3.163} = 1.778 = 1.78 \ m^2$

8. $m^2 = \sqrt{\dfrac{75 \times 175}{3600}} = \sqrt{\dfrac{13{,}125}{3600}} = \sqrt{3.645} = 1.909 = 1.91 \ m^2$

9. $m^2 = \sqrt{\dfrac{80.2 \times 184}{3600}} = \sqrt{\dfrac{14{,}756.8}{3600}} = \sqrt{4.099} = 2.024 = 2.02 \ m^2$

10. $m^2 = \sqrt{\dfrac{54 \times 155}{3600}} = \sqrt{\dfrac{8370}{3600}} = \sqrt{2.325} = 1.524 = 1.52 \ m^2$

Calculating BSA (m²) Using Pounds and Inches

1. $m^2 = \sqrt{\dfrac{125 \times 62}{3131}} = \sqrt{\dfrac{7750}{3131}} = \sqrt{2.475} = 1.573 = 1.57\ m^2$

2. $m^2 = \sqrt{\dfrac{134 \times 63}{3131}} = \sqrt{\dfrac{8442}{3131}} = \sqrt{2.696} = 1.642 = 1.64\ m^2$

3. $m^2 = \sqrt{\dfrac{153 \times 65}{3131}} = \sqrt{\dfrac{9945}{3131}} = \sqrt{3.176} = 1.782 = 1.78\ m^2$

4. $m^2 = \sqrt{\dfrac{118 \times 60}{3131}} = \sqrt{\dfrac{7080}{3131}} = \sqrt{2.261} = 1.503 = 1.5\ m^2$

5. $m^2 = \sqrt{\dfrac{181 \times 71}{3131}} = \sqrt{\dfrac{12,851}{3131}} = \sqrt{4.104} = 2.026 = 2.03\ m^2$

6. $m^2 = \sqrt{\dfrac{146 \times 69}{3131}} = \sqrt{\dfrac{10,074}{3131}} = \sqrt{3.217} = 1.793 = 1.79\ m^2$

7. $m^2 = \sqrt{\dfrac{169 \times 61}{3131}} = \sqrt{\dfrac{10,309}{3131}} = \sqrt{3.292} = 1.814 = 1.81\ m^2$

8. $m^2 = \sqrt{\dfrac{203 \times 72}{3131}} = \sqrt{\dfrac{14,616}{3131}} = \sqrt{4.668} = 2.160 = 2.16\ m^2$

9. $m^2 = \sqrt{\dfrac{197 \times 67}{3131}} = \sqrt{\dfrac{13,199}{3131}} = \sqrt{4.215} = 2.053 = 2.05\ m^2$

10. $m^2 = \sqrt{\dfrac{136 \times 63}{3131}} = \sqrt{\dfrac{8568}{3131}} = \sqrt{2.736} = 1.654 = 1.65\ m^2$

Calculating Medication Dosages Based on Body Surface Area

1. $m^2 = \sqrt{\dfrac{75 \times 158}{3600}} = \sqrt{3.291} = 1.81\ m^2$

   a. $mg = 200\dfrac{mg}{m^2} \times 1.81\ m^2 = 362\ mg$

   b. $mL = \dfrac{1\ mL}{20\ mg} \times 362\ mg = 18.1\ mL$

2. $m^2 = \sqrt{\dfrac{81 \times 163}{3600}} = \sqrt{3.667} = 1.91\ m^2$

   a. $mcg = 250\dfrac{mcg}{m^2} \times 1.91\ m^2 = 478\ mcg$

   b. $mL = \dfrac{1\ mL}{25\ mcg} \times 478\ mcg = 19.1\ mL$

3. $m^2 = \sqrt{\dfrac{152 \times 61}{3131}} = \sqrt{2.961} = 1.72\ m^2$

   a. $units = 15\dfrac{units}{m^2} \times 1.72\ m^2 = 26\ units$

   b. $mL = \dfrac{5\ mL}{30\ units} \times 26\ units = 4.3\ mL$

4. $m^2 = \sqrt{\dfrac{195 \times 70}{3131}} = \sqrt{4.359} = 2.09\ m^2$

   a. $mg = 500\dfrac{mg}{m^2} \times 2.09\ m^2 = 1045\ mg$

   b. $mL = \dfrac{1\ mL}{100\ mg} \times 1045\ mg = 10.5\ mL$

5. $m^2 = \sqrt{\dfrac{76 \times 179}{3600}} = \sqrt{3.778} = 1.94\ m^2$

   a. $mg = 20\dfrac{mg}{m^2} \times 1.94\ m^2 = 39\ mg$

   b. $mL = \dfrac{1\ mL}{10\ mg} \times 39\ mg = 3.9\ mL$

6. $m^2 = \sqrt{\dfrac{55.5 \times 155}{3600}} = \sqrt{2.389} = 1.55 \ m^2$

   a. $mg = 12\dfrac{mg}{m^2} \times 1.55 \ m^2 = 19 \ mg$

   b. $mL = \dfrac{1 \ mL}{2 \ mg} \times 19 \ mg = 9.5 \ mL$

7. $m^2 = \sqrt{\dfrac{105 \times 60}{3131}} = \sqrt{2.012} = 1.42 \ m^2$

   a. $mg = 75\dfrac{mg}{m^2} \times 1.42 \ m^2 = 107 \ mg$

   b. $mL = \dfrac{1 \ mL}{20 \ mg} \times 107 \ mg = 5.4 \ mL$

8. $m^2 = \sqrt{\dfrac{154 \times 67}{3131}} = \sqrt{3.295} = 1.82 \ m^2$

   a. $mg = 370\dfrac{mg}{m^2} \times 1.82 \ m^2 = 673 \ mg$

   b. $mL = \dfrac{1 \ mL}{100 \ mg} \times 673 \ mg = 6.7 \ mL$

9. $m^2 = \sqrt{\dfrac{68.3 \times 172}{3600}} = \sqrt{3.263} = 1.81 \ m^2$

   a. $mg = 50\dfrac{mg}{m^2} \times 1.81 \ m^2 = 91 \ mg$

   b. $mL = \dfrac{1 \ mL}{20 \ mg} \times 91 \ mg = 4.6 \ mL$

10. $m^2 = \sqrt{\dfrac{95 \times 170}{3600}} = \sqrt{4.486} = 2.12 \ m^2$

   a. $mg = 20\dfrac{mg}{m^2} \times 2.12 \ m^2 = 42 \ mg$

   b. $mL = \dfrac{1 \ mL}{10 \ mg} \times 42 \ mg = 4.2 \ mL$

■ *Answers to Case Study 11–1*

1. *Ms. Bell's BSA is 1.83 m².*

$$m^2 = \sqrt{\frac{159 \times 66}{3131}} = \sqrt{3.351} = 1.83 \ m^2$$

Based on a BSA of 1.83 m², the prescribed dose of Taxol (paclitaxel) (320 mg) is correct.

$$mg = 1.83 \ \cancel{m^2} \times 175\frac{mg}{\cancel{m^2}} = 320 \ mg$$

The prescribed dose of Paraplatin (carboplatin) (659 mg) is correct:

$$mg = 1.83 \ \cancel{m^2} \times 360\frac{mg}{\cancel{m^2}} = 659 \ mg$$

2. *If the prescribed dosages are different from the calculated dosages, the nurse should call the physician to resolve the discrepancies in the order.*

3. *The nurse should administer 53.3 mL of Taxol (paclitaxel):*

$$mL = \frac{1 \ mL}{30 \ \cancel{mg}} \times 320 \ \cancel{mg} = 10.7 \ mL$$

4. *The nurse should administer 65.9 mL of Paraplatin (carboplatin):*

$$mL = \frac{1 \ mL}{100 \ \cancel{mg}} \times 659 \ \cancel{mg} = 6.6 \ mL$$

Answers to Practice Questions

Chapter 12

Intravenous Delivery Systems and Equipment

Glossary

Central venous catheter: An intravenous catheter that is placed in a large blood vessel, such as the subclavian vein in the chest.

Drop factor: The calibrated number of drops per mL for intravenous tubing.

Electrolytes: Ions (for example, sodium, potassium, and chloride) that are necessary for normal cell function.

Epidural space: In the spine, the space between the dura mater and the vertebrae.

Flow rate: The amount of fluid infused into a vein over a specified period of time.

Infiltration: The permeation of fluid out of a vein into the surrounding tissues.

Infusion: The introduction of fluids into the body through a vein for therapeutic purposes.

Intrathecal space: The fluid-filled space surrounding the spinal cord.

Maintenance fluids: Intravenous fluids prescribed to maintain normal fluid balance in the body.

Macrodrip tubing: Intravenous tubing with a drop factor of 10, 15, or 20 drops per mL.

Microdrip tubing: Intravenous tubing with a drop factor of 60 drops per mL.

Oncotic pressure: The pressure exerted by plasma proteins that tend to pull water from intracellular and interstitial spaces into the circulatory system.

Peripheral intravenous catheter: An intravenous catheter placed in an extremity such as an arm or a leg.

Replacement fluids: Intravenous fluids prescribed to replace fluids lost through injury or illness.

Vesicant: A substance that damages tissues.

Viscosity: The degree to which a fluid is thick and sticky. Fluids that are viscous have a high resistance to flow.

Objectives

After completing this chapter, the learner will be able to—

1. Explain the purposes of IV therapy.
2. Differentiate between peripherally placed and centrally placed IV catheters.
3. Compare and contrast crystalloid and colloid IV fluids.
4. Explain the necessary checks and safety precautions that must be taken before infusing IV fluids.
5. Discuss the purposes of primary and secondary IV administration sets.
6. Describe the differences between manual gravity flow infusions and infusions using electronic drip controllers, infusion pumps, and syringe pumps.
7. Identify the necessary components of an IV label.
8. Explain the function and safety features of a patient-controlled analgesia pump.

Introduction to IV Therapy

Intravenous (IV) therapy is the infusion of fluids into the vein for the purpose of providing blood or blood products, water, medications, and nutrients (vitamins, minerals, electrolytes, carbohydrates, proteins, and fatty acids). IV infusions are used to correct dehydration, to improve electrolyte balance, to provide nourishment for individuals who cannot eat, or to give medications. Maintenance fluids are prescribed to maintain the body's basal metabolic needs (that is, to replenish fluid loss due to metabolism and water loss through normal body functions). They are ordered for patients who are unable to drink an adequate amount of fluids. Replacement fluids are given to replace fluid lost through bleeding, burns, diarrhea, or vomiting.

IV fluids and medications are administered into the vein through an IV catheter. A catheter that is placed into a vein on a limb is called a *peripheral intravenous catheter* (Fig. 12-1). Peripheral IV catheters may be placed by nurses. Access devices that are placed into a large blood vessel, such as the jugular vein in the neck, or the subclavian vein in the chest, is called a *central venous catheter* (Fig. 12-2). Central venous catheters are usually placed by surgeons. Specialized central lines called peripherally inserted central catheters (PICC lines) may be placed by specially trained RNs (Fig. 12-3).

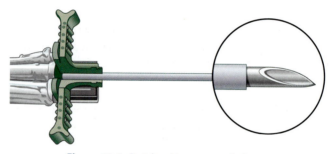

Figure 12-1 Peripheral Intravenous Catheter

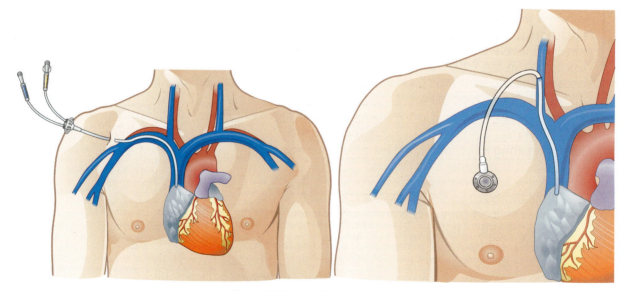

Figure 12-2 Central Venous Catheters

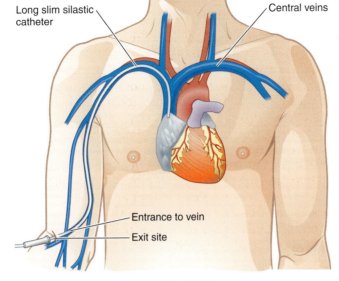

Long slim silastic
catheter

Central veins

Entrance to vein

Exit site

Figure 12-3 PICC Line

IV fluids may be infused continuously or intermittently. A continuous IV is prescribed for patients who need fluid, electrolyte, or nutrient supplementation over a relatively long period of time (days to weeks). The fluid is infused at a prescribed flow rate (Fig. 12-4).

Date	Physicians' Orders	
08/15/18	IV Fluids: D$_5$W/0.45% normal saline to infuse at 125 mL/hr.	Thelma Johnson / MR 00382991 / Account A9184028 / Dr. Martin Haddad, MD / DOB: 10/3/1936
1750	——————— M. Haddad, MD	

In this order, the provider has written the flow rate in mL/hr.

Date	Physicians' Orders	
08/15/18	IV Fluids: Infuse 1 L normal saline over 8 hours continuously.	Thelma Johnson / MR 00382991 / Account A9184028 / Dr. Martin Haddad, MD / DOB: 10/3/1936
1750	——————— M. Haddad, MD	

In this order, the provider has supplied the volume and time of infusion.
The nurse must calculate the mL/hr flow rate.

Figure 12-4 Sample Provider Order for a Continuous IV

Intermittent infusions are used when patients do not need additional fluid or nutrients but require IV medications to be administered periodically (Fig. 12-5). After the medication has been administered, the IV catheter is immediately flushed with saline or heparin to maintain its patency until the next time the medication is due.

Date	Physicians' Orders
08/15/18	Ceftriaxone 1 g IV every 12 hours.
1750	—————————— M. Haddad, MD

Thelma Johnson
MR 00382991
Account A9184028
Dr. Martin Haddad, MD
DOB: 10/3/1936

In this order, the medication ceftriaxone will be administered every 12 hours, and the nurse is responsible for calculating the rate of administration. The flow rate depends on the amount of fluid the medication is mixed with and how long the medication should take to infuse.

Figure 12-5 Sample Provider Order for an Intermittent IV

Types of IV Fluids

IV fluids can be divided into two main groups: crystalloids and colloids.

Crystalloids

Crystalloids are liquids containing dissolved substances, such as sodium or chloride. Some crystalloid solutions also contain dextrose, which provides the body with carbohydrates. Crystalloids are prescribed to treat dehydration and to correct certain electrolyte imbalances. Examples of crystalloid solutions include the following:

- 0.9% sodium chloride solution, (normal saline)
- 0.45% sodium chloride solution
- 5% dextrose solution (D_5W)
- 5% dextrose in 0.45% sodium chloride solution
- 10% dextrose solution ($D_{10}W$)
- Ringer's lactate (also called RL, lactated Ringer's, or LR)
- Plasma-Lyte R

Colloids

Colloids are fluids that contain large, undissolved particles, such as proteins, carbohydrates, fats, or animal collagen (gelatin). These particles increase the oncotic pressure within the blood vessels, which pulls excess fluid from cells and surrounding tissues into the bloodstream (Fig. 12-6). Colloids work by expanding plasma volume and are prescribed for patients who are bleeding when blood products are not immediately available. Albumin may also be prescribed for patients who have protein deficiencies that cause severe swelling. Commonly prescribed colloids include the following:

- 5% Albumin
- 25% Albumin
- Dextran 70
- Dextran 40
- Hetastarch

Safety Precautions

Follow these precautions before infusing any IV solution:

1. Check the provider's order to ensure that the correct type of fluid has been selected. Because IV fluids are considered to be medications, follow the six rights and three checks before beginning an infusion.

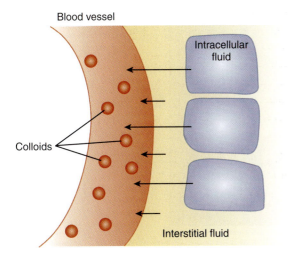

Blood vessel

Intracellular fluid

Colloids

Interstitial fluid

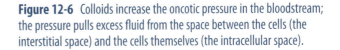

Figure 12-6 Colloids increase the oncotic pressure in the bloodstream; the pressure pulls excess fluid from the space between the cells (the interstitial space) and the cells themselves (the intracellular space).

2. Inspect the outer wrapping for tears or puncture marks. If the wrapping has been compromised, follow the facility's policy for disposing of the bag.
3. Check the manufacturer's expiration date on the bag. Do not use an expired bag of solution. Remove it from the storage container and send it to the pharmacy for disposal.
4. Remove the bag from the outer wrapper. Check the bag for puncture marks or leaks. The bag may feel slightly damp from condensation collected during the sterilization process, but should not be leaking fluid.
5. Inspect the solution to see if it is discolored or contains any solid matter.
6. Apply the appropriate labels to the bag as required by the facility's policy.

Most IV fluids come in sterile plastic infusion bags; however, some IV fluids, such as 5% or 25% albumin, are packaged in glass bottles. Some fluids may require special tubing or filters. Others may require special handling during use. Read any accompanying directions in the package insert before beginning the infusion if the fluid or equipment is unfamiliar.

Essential Equipment for IV Therapy

Equipment needed to start an IV infusion (after the catheter has been placed and the IV solution selected) includes the IV administration set (tubing); a controller, infusion pump, or syringe pump; and all necessary labels. If a controller or IV pump is not available, IV fluids may be gravity controlled; however, this practice is used only in certain circumstances.

IV Administration Sets

An IV administration set is the tubing through which IV fluid is infused. Administration sets are referred to as primary or secondary depending upon the purpose of the IV infusion.

Primary IV Administration Sets

A primary IV administration set is the tubing used to infuse the main IV solution. (Fig. 12-7). Primary tubing is fairly long—anywhere from 39 inches to 100 inches—which allows the patient to move freely. The appearance of primary IV tubing varies from manufacturer to manufacturer, but all IV tubing have common features:

- At one end of the tubing is the insertion spike, a sharp, pointed piece of rigid plastic designed to puncture the plastic membrane over the entry port of the IV bag.
- Below the spike is the drip chamber, and inside it is a small metal or plastic tube that allows fluid from the infusion bag to enter the drip chamber freely. This tube, which varies

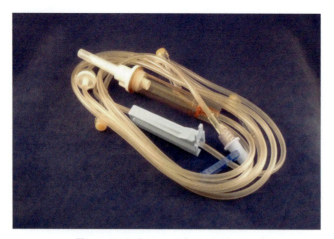

Figure 12-7 Primary Administration Set

in size depending on the manufacturer, determines the "drop factor" of the tubing. Each milliliter of fluid that collects in the drip chamber contains a known quantity of drops. Common tubing drop factors are 10 drops per mL (gtt/mL), 15 gtt/mL, 20 gtt/mL, and 60 gtt/mL. Tubing with drop factors of 10, 15, and 20 gtt/mL are known as macrodrip tubing. Tubing with a drop factor of 60 gtt/mL is known as microdrip tubing, which is most commonly used in the critical care or pediatric setting when very small or precise amounts of fluids or medications are administered.

• The remainder of the tubing, from the drip chamber to the far end (the hub) that attaches to the patient's IV catheter, usually features at least one roller clamp or slide clamp, and one or two injection ports. Injection ports allow secondary administration sets to be attached to the primary administration set, and provide access to the IV site for giving medications. Tubing designed for insertion into infusion pumps will have some type of chamber or specialized section that allows the pump to propel fluid through the tubing toward the patient.

Alert! Purge any air from the IV tubing before connecting it to the hub of the patient's IV catheter. Follow the directions on the tubing wrapper and the facility's policy for priming IV tubing.

Secondary IV Administration Sets

Secondary IV administration sets are shorter than primary administration sets and are used to infuse medications that are needed intermittently (such as antibiotics) or continuously (such as insulin) but at a very slow infusion rate (Fig. 12-8). Secondary infusion sets also have a spiked end and a roller clamp, but may not have extra infusion ports. Secondary IV sets may also be called piggyback sets because they piggyback onto primary IV tubing.

IV Infusion Devices

IV fluids may be administered via drip controller, infusion pump, or syringe pump. Fluids may also be administered manually (that is, without a pump). The manual method is covered in the section "Infusing IV Fluids Using Manual Gravity Flow."

Drip Controllers

Drip controllers operate by gravity flow. A sensor counts the number of drops that are falling in the drip chamber. Drip controllers have fallen out of favor because of the widespread use of the safer and more accurate infusion pump, which is the preferred method of infusing fluids in most facilities.

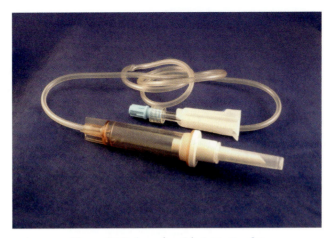

Figure 12-8 Secondary Administration Set

Infusion Pumps

IV infusion pumps use pressure instead of gravity to instill fluids into veins (Fig. 12-9). Infusion pumps work by compressing a section of the IV tubing or a specialized pumping chamber to propel fluid forward through the tubing. Most pumps offer multiple safety features, such as pressure alarms and air detection sensors. Pumps are able to regulate flow rate better than drip controllers—an important feature when the IV fluid is thick and viscous or the IV catheter is extremely small. Unlike controllers, IV pumps can overcome mild resistance to flow by slightly increasing pressure. "Smart" pumps are programmable IV pumps that contain dosage calculation software, which helps reduce the risk of medication errors.

Infusion pumps are not without dangers. Pumps will continue to infuse fluids into the patient's extremity as long as the pressure of the surrounding tissue does not exceed the pressure of the pump. Infiltration can cause damage if caustic medications (called vesicants) leak into surrounding tissues. A patient's IV site should be monitored regularly to ensure that the site is not red, swollen, or leaking fluid. Follow the rights of medication administration to ensure the right medication is infusing at the right rate to the right patient. Double-check the dosage of any potentially harmful medications with another nurse or pharmacist.

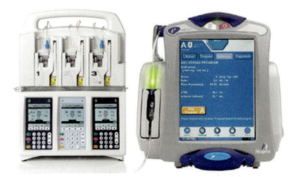

Figure 12-9 Infusion Pumps. Symbiq Infusion System (Hospira) and Plum A+ 3 Infusion System (Hospira)

Syringe Pumps

Syringe pumps are electronic or battery-operated devices designed to infuse small volumes of medications contained in a syringe instead of an IV bag. Some syringe pumps are separate devices that work independently of the IV pump that is infusing the primary fluid. Other syringe pumps are integrated into the main IV pump or come as an attachment to the main IV pump.

Practice IV Therapy, Fluids, and Infusion Devices

(answers on page 217)

Select the best answer.

1. The primary purpose for infusing replacement fluids is to:
   a. provide medications.
   b. replace fluids and electrolytes lost through burns, vomiting, or diarrhea.
   c. maintain fluids and electrolytes lost through normal metabolism.
   d. replace electrolytes only.

2. An IV catheter that is placed in a vein on the hand is called a:
   a. central venous catheter.
   b. Foley catheter
   c. peripheral venous catheter.
   d. peripherally inserted central catheter.

3. A provider writes this order: "Infuse 0.9% sodium chloride solution intravenously at 150 mL/hr." What type of IV infusion is this?
   a. an intermittent IV infusion
   b. a continuous IV infusion

4. A provider writes this order: "Infuse 5% dextrose solution, IV, at 125 mL/hr." Dextrose is an example of which type of fluid?
   a. crystalloid
   b. blood product
   c. electrolyte solution
   d. colloid

5. The nurse retrieves an infusion bag of Ringer's lactate from storage. The bag of solution expired two days ago. What is the appropriate action by the nurse?
   a. Remove the bag from storage and return it to the pharmacy.
   b. Move the bag to the back of the storage bin so no one else will use it.
   c. Infuse the IV solution—IV fluid may still be used up to one week beyond the expiration date.
   d. Infuse the IV solution, but monitor the patient closely for adverse effects.

6. IV tubing with a drop factor of 10 gtt/mL is an example of:
   a. microdrip tubing.
   b. macrodrip tubing.

7. Which of the following electronic infusion devices infuses fluid by gravity flow?
   a. infusion pump
   b. syringe pump
   c. drip controller

Labeling IV Fluids and Tubing

IV bags and tubing should be labeled clearly and according to facility policy. Proper labeling of IV fluids reduces the risk of administering the fluid to the wrong patient. Tubing is labeled as a reminder to nurses to change the tubing and reduce the likelihood of bacterial colonization.

Labeling IV Fluids

IV infusion bags containing medication that was added after manufacturing should be labeled with the following information (Fig. 12-10):

- patient identification information
- the name of the fluid (Example: 0.9% sodium chloride, 5% dextrose/0.45% sodium chloride)
- the name and dosage of additives or medications (Example: ampicillin 500 mg, 20 mEq potassium chloride)
- the flow rate of the infusion (Example: gtt/min or mL/hr)
- the date and time the IV bag was opened (Most IV fluids expire within 24 to 96 hours of the bag's being spiked.)
- the initials of the nurse who prepared the IV fluid

Note: Some medications become unstable after mixing with IV fluids, so the IV mixture may expire in a few hours instead of a few days. Be certain to hang the correct bag at the correct time.

INTRAVENOUS SOLUTION ADDITIVES

PATIENT: _____ ROOM NUMBER: _____
DATE: _____ TIME: _____ BY: _____

SOLUTION:

ADDITIVES:

FLOW RATE: _____ ML/HR
EXPIRATION DATE: _____ TIME: _____

This label must be affixed to all infusion fluids containing additional information.

Figure 12-10 Sample IV Fluid Label

Labeling IV Tubing

IV tubing expires within 24 to 96 hours after removal from its sterile packaging, depending on the fluid being infused. For example, tubing that has infused fat emulsions (lipids) must be changed every 24 hours, whereas IV tubing used to infuse 0.9% normal saline solution may be changed every 96 hours. Refer to your facility's policies for changing tubing.

IV tubing should be labeled with the following information:

- date and time tubing was opened
- expiration date and time
- initials of the nurse

IV tubing does not need to have patient identification on it since it is not specific to the patient (Fig. 12-11).

IV TUBING CHANGE

START DATE:_____ HR: _____
DISCARD DATE:_____ HR: _____
RN INITIALS:_____

Figure 12-11 Sample IV Tubing Label

Infusing IV Fluids Using Manual Gravity Flow

Fluids that are administered manually (that is, without the use of an electronic infusion device) utilize only gravity to instill solutions. The rate at which fluid flows through the IV line depends on numerous factors:

- the height of the IV bag in relation to the IV site on the patient (the higher the bag, the faster the flow rate)
- the size of the IV tubing (the smaller the tubing, the slower the flow rate)
- increased resistance to flow caused by—
  - the roller clamp being in a closed position
  - kinks in the IV tubing
  - increased viscosity of the IV fluid
  - a small IV catheter
  - a small vein
  - the presence of clots in the IV catheter

Gravity flow infusions are measured in drops per minute (gtt/min). To initiate an IV infusion using gravity flow, the roller clamp is opened in small increments every 15 to 30 seconds. The nurse counts the number of drops falling inside the drip chamber until the desired flow rate is achieved. Some IV tubing has a specialized dial or device that helps to regulate the drip rate rather than relying strictly on the roller clamp position.

The flow rate should be monitored frequently, because something as simple as a change in the position of the patient's arm or hand can change an IV flow rate if the IV is infusing manually. A time tape (see Fig. 12-12) can be applied to the IV bag to assist the nurse in recognizing whether the infusion is running too fast or too slow. When the infusion is started, the nurse writes the time on the time tape. For every hour that passes by, the fluid level in the bag should decrease by a predictable amount. The nurse compares the amount of fluid that should have infused with the amount of fluid that has actually infused and adjusts the drip rate up or down (Fig. 12-13). See Table 12-1 for tips on troubleshooting a gravity flow IV.

The advantage of manual gravity flow infusions is that no specialized equipment is needed. However, gravity flow infusions are time intensive for the nurse and carry a high risk of overloading the patient with fluids if the flow rate increases, or failure to hydrate the patient adequately if the flow rate decreases.

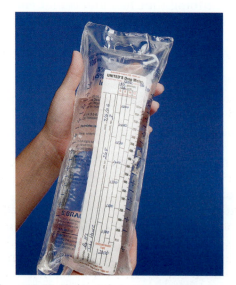

Figure 12-12 Marking Infusion Times on a Time Tape

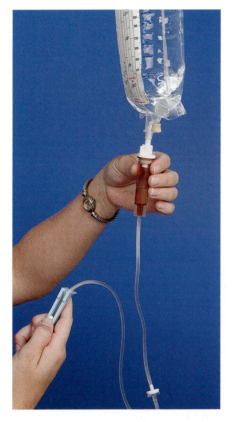

Figure 12-13 Nurse Adjusting the Flow Rate of a Gravity Flow IV

Table 12-1	Troubleshooting a Gravity Flow IV	
To Increase the Flow Rate:		**To Decrease the Flow Rate:**
Raise the height of the infusion bag.		Lower the height of the infusion bag (must be above patient to infuse, however).
Open the roller clamp.		
Reposition the patient's extremity in extended position to reduce resistance to flow.		Close the roller clamp.
Assess the patient's IV site and catheter for patency.		

Other Types of Infusion Devices

Several other types of specialized infusion pumps are used in healthcare facilities, including patient-controlled analgesia pumps and pain pumps.

Patient-Controlled Analgesia Pumps

Patient-controlled analgesia (PCA) refers to a pain control system regulated by the patient, allowing the patient to receive medication when desired. Patients who have had surgery or are in moderate to severe pain from a medical condition may be prescribed PCAs.

PCAs are infusion pumps that deliver a small amount of pain medication, such as morphine sulfate (Astramorph), fentanyl (Sublimaze), or hydromorphone (Dilaudid), to the patient on demand—that is, when the patient pushes a button. An advantage of the PCA is that small frequent doses of pain medication provide a more steady blood level of medication than large, intermittent doses. Large doses tend to peak early and wear off before the next scheduled dose, leaving the patient in pain. Figures 12-14 and 12-15 provide examples of a PCA provider standing order and nursing flow sheet.

Patient Controlled Analgesia Orders

Date: Time:

1. PCA Orders:

• Select the medication from the table below:

Parameters	☐ Hydromorphone		☐ Morphine		☐ Fentanyl		☐ Other	
	Concentration: 0.2 mg/mL		Concentration: 1 mg/mL		Concentration: 10 mcg/mL		Concentration:	
	Reference	Order	Reference	Order	Reference	Order	Reference	Order
Initial Loading Dose (Bolus)	0.2–0.8 mg		0.1–10 mg		20–40 mcg			
PCA Dose	0.1–0.3 mg		0.5–2 mg		5–20 mcg			
Lockout Interval	5–10 min		5–10 min		4–8 min			
One-Hour Limit	0.5–3 mg		5–15 mg		50–150 mcg			
Continuous/Basal Rate	0.1–1 mg/hr		0.1–5 mg/hr		10–50 mcg/hr			
For Breakthrough Pain	1–2 mg intravenously every 2 hr as needed		2–5 mg intravenously every 2 hr as needed		10–25 mcg intravenously every 2 hr as needed			

• No other analgesics or sedatives unless ordered by the PCA prescriber (see #3 below).

2. Patient Monitoring:

• Vital signs (temp, pulse, BP, respiratory rate, and oxygen saturation):

  • Every 2 hours after PCA initiation for the first 4 hours, then every 4 hours.

  • Oxygen saturation continuously for patients receiving a continuous/basal rate.

• Pain level:

  • Every 2 hours after PCA initiation for the first 4 hours, then every 4 hours.

• Sedation level:

  • Every 2 hours after PCA initiation for the first 4 hours, then every 4 hours.

3. Additional Medications:

• For respiratory rate less than 8:

  • Naloxone (Narcan) 0.4 mg intravenously for respiratory rate less than 8.

  • **STOP PCA.**

  • Notify provider.

• For nausea/vomiting:

  • Phenergan 6.25 to 12.5 mg intravenously every 6 hr as needed.

• For itching:

  • Diphenhydramine 25 mg by mouth or intravenously every 6 hr as needed.

• Supplemental Analgesia:

  • Ketorolac (Toradol) 15 mg intramuscularly or intravenously every 6 hr as needed for breakthrough pain.

Provider's Signature: Noted by (Nurse's Signature):

Date: Time: Date: Time:

Patient Identification Sticker

Patient Controlled Analgesia Standing Orders

White: Medical Record   Pink: Pharmacy   Yellow: Nursing

Figure 12-14 Sample PCA Provider Standing Order

Medications can be infused with a PCA into a peripheral vein or through a thin catheter placed in the epidural space in the spine. A peripheral PCA is attached to the patient's primary IV line through an infusion port on the tubing closest to the patient. RNs have the authority to set up and monitor peripheral PCAs in most facilities. The epidural PCA is inserted by a nurse anesthetist or anesthesiologist. Although the catheter is inserted by the anesthetist, the RN is responsible for monitoring the patient while receiving epidural pain medications.

Date: _____

Medication: _____ Concentration: _____

Patient Status									
Time:									
Vital Signs:	T HR RR P SaO₂	T HR RR P SaO₂	T HR RR P SaO₂	T HR RR P SaO₂	T HR RR P SaO₂	T HR RR P SaO₂	T HR RR P SaO₂	T HR RR P SaO₂	T HR RR P SaO₂
Pain Score (1–10 scale):									
Location:									
Quality:									
LOC:									
PCA Use									
PCA Dose:									
Lockout Interval:									
Basal Rate:									
Injection Attempts:									
# Received:									
# Partials:									
1 Hour Dose Limit:									
Nurse's Initials:									

Total amt (mg) left in syringe at end of shift: _____ mg

Nurse's signature:_____ Witness: _____ **RN**

Programming

Programming*: _____ RN /_____ RN   Time: _____

*Two RNs must validate initial PCA programming and any subsequent changes in programming including verification of medication and concentration, PCA dose, basal rate (if applicable), lockout interval, and one-hour dose limit.

Syringe Changes		
Time: _____ Medication: _____ Concentration: _____ Nurse's signature: _____ RN Verified by:_____ RN	Time: _____ Medication: _____ Concentration: _____ Nurse's signature: _____ RN Verified by:_____ RN	Time: _____ Medication: _____ Concentration: _____ Nurse's signature: _____ RN Verified by:_____ RN

Wastage	
Amount wasted: _____ Nurse's signature: _____ RN Witness: _____ RN	Amount wasted: _____ Nurse's signature: _____ RN Witness: _____ RN

Key: LOC
0 = Unarousable; 1 = Arouses to deep pain; 2 = Arouses with difficulty; 3 = Easily aroused; 4 = Awake and alert

Patient Identification Sticker	
	PCA Nursing Flowsheet

Figure 12-15 Sample PCA Nursing Flow Sheet

Safety features of the PCA pump include a programmed lockout interval during which the patient will not receive a dose of medication no matter how many times the button is pushed. The machines can also be programmed to limit the quantity of narcotics that the patient receives during a designated period to reduce the risk of overdose. PCA machines are locked to prevent access to the syringe of medication and to prevent changes to the program by unauthorized individuals.

The most important safeguard against improper use of the PCA is the nurse. Nurses must understand which patients are appropriate candidates for a PCA. Patients who are unable to understand how a PCA works or are incapable of pushing a button because of physical limitations are not good candidates for a PCA. Nurses need to monitor patients using a PCA frequently to ensure that their pain is controlled, yet they are not showing signs of respiratory depression or overdose. Most important, nurses need to provide adequate patient and family teaching about the PCA. Patients should be shown how to activate the PCA button, when to push the button, and how to notify the nurse if their pain is not well controlled. Family members should be instructed never to push the PCA button on behalf of the patient. When individuals other than the patient push the PCA button, the risk of an overdose is greatly increased because other individuals may not recognize the early signs of an impending overdose.

Pain Pumps

Providers may order other types of pain pumps for patients who have undergone surgery or who suffer from chronic pain syndromes. Specialized infusion pumps can deliver medications such as narcotics into subcutaneous or intramuscular tissue. Some pumps infuse narcotics, local anesthetics, or a combination of both into surgical sites, joints (knees, hips, or shoulders), or epidural or intrathecal spaces. Pumps may be surgically implanted into the body or may be clipped to a belt or trouser waistband.

Key Points

1. IV fluids are prescribed to provide fluids, electrolytes, nutrients, blood products, or medications.

2. Necessary equipment and supplies for IV therapy include an IV access device (IV catheter), IV fluid or medication, tubing, and an infusion device (if available).

3. IV fluids may be infused intermittently or continuously, depending upon the medical needs of the patient.

4. IV fluids can be divided into two categories: crystalloids and colloids. Crystalloids provide water, electrolytes, and/or glucose. Colloids provide large particles in solution that act to increase the oncotic pressure within the vessels in order to pull excess fluid from the tissues.

5. Before any solution is infused, the nurse needs to check the manufacturer's expiration date, inspect the outer wrapper and the bag for leaks or tears, examine the solution for discoloration or the presence of particles, and label the bag appropriately.

6. The primary IV administration set is used to infuse the main IV solution.

7. The secondary IV administration set is used to infuse additional IV solutions that are needed intermittently, or are infusing at a very slow rate.

8. IVs may be administered using an electronic infusion device (drip controller, infusion pump, or syringe pump) or by gravity flow with manual adjustment of rate.

9. IV bags and IV tubing should be labeled according to facility policy.

10. Patient-controlled analgesia (PCA) pumps are devices that infuse narcotics and/or local anesthetics into veins or around the spine to control pain. Nursing responsibilities include being familiar with the features of the pump, instructing the patient and family about the pump and how it works, and monitoring the patient's medical status while the patient is using the pump.

Chapter Post-Test

(answers in Unit 4)

Multiple Choice

Select the best answer.

1. The purpose of IV therapy is to:
   a. provide blood.
   b. treat diseases.
   c. correct electrolyte imbalances.
   d. all of the above.

2. A nurse is changing a patient's expired IV tubing. Which of the following information does not need to be written on the tubing label?
   a. the date the tubing was changed
   b. the new expiration date
   c. patient identification information
   d. the initials of the nurse

3. The nurse is going to use a macrodrip administration set. Which of the following drop factors is considered to be macrodrip set?
   a. 10 gtt/mL
   b. 15 gtt/mL
   c. 60 gtt/mL
   d. both a and b

4. Which of the following factors can slow the rate at which fluids are infusing into the patient when using manual gravity flow?
   a. a kink in the IV tubing
   b. hanging the IV bag high above the patient
   c. opening the roller clamp
   d. using a large IV catheter

5. Which of the following statements is not true regarding the nurse's responsibilities when monitoring a patient with a PCA?
   a. The nurse needs to teach the patient about the PCA and how it works.
   b. The nurse must understand how the PCA functions.
   c. The nurse needs to show the patient's family how to push the button of the PCA when the patient is sleeping.
   d. The nurse must know which patients are good candidates for a PCA.

6. Which of the following statements is an advantage of a manual gravity flow IV?
   a. It is time intensive for the nurse.
   b. It does not require any equipment or electricity.
   c. It reduces the risk of accidental overhydration.
   d. The flow rate is not affected by resistance to flow.

7. Which of the following items should be written on the label of an IV bag containing medication?
   a. patient identification information
   b. name of the fluid infusing
   c. name and dosage of the medication added to the bag
   d. all of the above.

8. The purpose of a PCA is to allow the:
   a. nurse to control the amount of pain medication the patient receives.
   b. patient to regulate the timing of pain medication received.
   c. patient's family to control the timing of pain medication received.
   d. patient to receive as much pain medication as he or she wants.

9. The lockout interval on a PCA is designed to:
   a. prevent the patient from receiving too much medication in too short a period.
   b. limit the quantity of medication a patient receives.
   c. prevent the patient from pushing the PCA button.
   d. prevent the nurse from programming the PCA.

10. Maintenance fluids are prescribed to:
    a. replace fluid and electrolytes lost with excessive vomiting.
    b. replace blood lost through bleeding.
    c. replenish fluids lost through normal metabolism and bodily functions.
    d. replenish blood protein levels.

11. Microdrip tubing has a drop factor of:
    a. 10 gtt/mL.
    b. 15 gtt/mL.
    c. 20 gtt/mL.
    d. 60 gtt/mL.

12. The nurse is inspecting an IV bag. Which of the following findings would alert the nurse to discard the bag?
    a. The IV bag is slightly damp when the outer wrapper is removed.
    b. The IV solution in the bag is clear.
    c. The IV solution has small flecks of matter floating in it.
    d. The IV solution expires six months from now.

13. A provider writes the following order: Infuse D_5W at 125 mL/hr. The provider wants the IV to run:
    a. continuously.
    b. intermittently.

14. A provider writes the following order: Moxifloxacin 400 mg, IV, once daily. The provider wants the IV to run:
    a. continuously.
    b. intermittently.

15. Ringer's lactate is an example of what type of fluid?
    a. colloid
    b. crystalloid

16. 5% Albumin is an example of what type of fluid?
    a. colloid
    b. crystalloid

17. The nurse is preparing to infuse an intermittent IV medication. The patient has an IV of 0.9% normal saline solution infusing at 125 mL/hr. Which of the following administration sets should the nurse select to administer the medication?
    a. primary administration set
    b. secondary administration set

True or False

Choose the best answer.

18. Colloid fluids contain dissolved ions, such as sodium or chloride.   True   False

19. Crystalloid solutions are commonly known as plasma volume expanders.   True   False

20. The nurse must follow the six rights and three checks when preparing to infuse IV fluids.   True   False

21. An RN may place all types of central venous catheters.   True   False

22. Infusion pumps can overcome a slight resistance to flow, unlike drip controllers.   True   False

23. A danger of the infusion pump is that it can infuse fluids into the tissue surrounding the vessel, causing tissue damage.   True   False

24. The patient's IV site should be inspected intermittently for redness, swelling, or leaking.   True   False

25. An RN may insert a peripheral IV catheter.   True   False

Answers to Practice Questions

IV Therapy, Fluids, and Infusion Devices

1. b

2. c

3. b

4. a

5. a

6. b

7. c

Chapter 13
Intravenous Calculations

✂ Glossary

Drop Factor: The calibration of IV tubing described as the number of drops contained in 1 mL of fluid; abbreviated as gtt/mL.

Objectives

After completing this chapter, the learner will be able to—
1. Calculate mL/hr flow rates for continuous IV fluids infused using an electronic device.
2. Calculate mL/hr flow rates for intermittent IV fluids infused using an electronic device.
3. Calculate infusion and completion times for IV fluids infused using an electronic device.
4. Calculate gtt/min flow rates for IV fluids infused under manual control.
5. Calculate infusion and completion times for IV fluids infused under manual control using a time tape.

Calculating Flow Rates for IV Infusions

Most IV fluids are infused using a mL/hr flow rate that is programmed into a pump or controller. Smart infusion pumps can be programmed to infuse IV medications with flow rates based on prescribed dosages, such as mg/min or mcg/min. Per-minute flow rates are used to infuse cardiac drugs and medications that must be titrated in small increments. The process of calculating dosage-based flow rates is covered in Chapter 17, "Critical Care Dosage Calculations."

Calculating mL/hr Flow Rates for Continuous IV Fluids

Both IV pumps and controllers use mL/hr flow rates. Providers may order maintenance or replacement fluids directly (for example, "Infuse 0.9% sodium chloride solution at 125 mL/hr") or indirectly (for example, "Infuse 1 L 0.9% sodium chloride over 8 hours"). The indirect order requires that the nurse calculate the mL/hr flow rate. Pumps and controllers used for adults are usually set to deliver whole mL/hr (for example, 100 mL/hr or 150 mL/hr). Some medications and pumps used for children can be programmed to deliver partial mL/hr flow rates (for example, 24.3 mL/hr or 55.6 mL/hr).

Example 1: The provider order reads: "Infuse D$_5$W, 1 L over 10 hours." The nurse should set the pump or controller to what mL/hr flow rate? Round the flow rate to the nearest whole number.

1. Set up the equation using dimensional analysis principles. Notice that the units contained in the answer must be mL/hr, but mL is not in the information offered in the question. The missing information should be a clue that a conversion factor is needed.

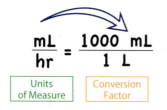

$$\frac{mL}{hr} = \frac{1000 \ mL}{1 \ L}$$

Units of Measure   Conversion Factor

2. Insert the given quantities. In this example, it is the amount of fluid (1 L) and the time over which the fluid is to be infused.

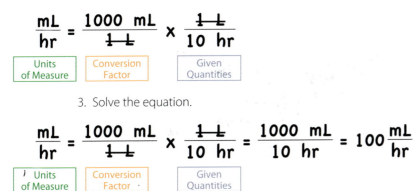

3. Solve the equation.

$$\frac{mL}{hr} = \frac{1000 \; mL}{1 \; L} \times \frac{1 \; L}{10 \; hr} = \frac{1000 \; mL}{10 \; hr} = 100 \frac{mL}{hr}$$

Units of Measure Conversion Factor Given Quantities

Shortcut: Convert the volume in L to mL first, before dividing by the infusion time. This will eliminate the need for a conversion factor in the equation.

$$\frac{mL}{hr} = \frac{1000 \; mL}{10 \; hr} = 100 \frac{mL}{hr}$$

Units of Measure Given Quantities

Note: The only information that is needed to calculate a mL/hr flow rate is the volume of liquid to be infused (mL) and the time of the infusion (hr).

For Examples 2–5, refer to the directions in Example 1.

Example 2: The provider order reads: "Infuse LR, 500 mL over 2 hours." The nurse should set the pump or controller to what mL/hr flow rate? Round the flow rate to the nearest whole number.

$$\frac{mL}{hr} = \frac{500 \; mL}{2 \; hr} = 250 \frac{mL}{hr}$$

Note: In this example, the volume to be infused is given as mL, so no conversion factor is necessary in the equation.

Example 3: The provider order reads: "Infuse 0.9% sodium chloride solution, 2 L over 24 hours." The nurse should set the pump or controller to what mL/hr flow rate? Round the flow rate to the nearest whole number.

$$\frac{mL}{hr} = \frac{1000 \; mL}{1 \; L} \times \frac{2 \; L}{24 \; hr} = \frac{1000 \; mL \times 2}{1 \times 24 \; hr} = \frac{2000 \; mL}{24 \; hr} = 83.3 \frac{mL}{hr} = 83 \frac{mL}{hr}$$

Example 4: The provider order reads: "Infuse D$_5$W, 1.5 L over 8 hours." The nurse should set the pump or controller to what mL/hr flow rate? Round the flow rate to the nearest whole number.

$$\frac{mL}{hr} = \frac{1000 \; mL}{1 \; L} \times \frac{1.5 \; L}{8 \; hr} = \frac{1000 \; mL \times 1.5}{1 \times 8 \; hr} = \frac{1500 \; mL}{8 \; hr} = 187.5 = 188 \frac{mL}{hr}$$

Example 5: The provider order reads: "Infuse 0.45% sodium chloride solution, 750 mL over 6 hours." The nurse should set the pump or controller to what mL/hr flow rate? Round the flow rate to the nearest whole number.

$$\frac{mL}{hr} = \frac{750\ mL}{6\ hr} = 125\ \frac{mL}{hr}$$

Practice Calculating mL/hr Flow Rates for Continuous IV Fluids

(answers on page 245)

Calculate the mL/hr flow rate for these continuous infusions. Round the answers to the nearest whole number.

1. Infuse LR, 1250 mL over 8 hours.

2. Infuse 0.9% sodium chloride solution, 250 mL over 2 hours.

3. Infuse D_5W, 1000 mL over 12 hours.

4. Infuse $D_{10}W$, 500 mL over 4 hours.

5. Infuse D_5W/0.9% sodium chloride solution, 750 mL over 5 hours.

6. Infuse 0.45% sodium chloride solution, 1 L over 4 hours.

7. Infuse D_5W/0.45% sodium chloride solution, 800 mL over 12 hours.

8. Infuse 0.9% sodium chloride solution, 2.5 L over 15 hours.

9. Infuse D_5W/LR, 2 L over 18 hours.

10. Infuse LR, 300 mL over 1.5 hours.

Calculating mL/hr Flow Rates for Intermittent IV Fluids

Calculating the mL/hr flow rate for intermittent IV fluids (also called IV *piggybacks*, or *IVPB* for short) follows the same procedure as calculating larger volume IVs. The only difference is that intermittent IVs usually contain medications and are infused over short periods of time.

Example 1: The provider order reads: "Infuse 350 mg ganciclovir (Cytovene IV) diluted in 100 mL NS over 60 minutes." The nurse should set the pump at what mL/hr flow rate? Round the flow rate to the nearest whole number.

1. Set up the equation using dimensional analysis. Insert the given quantities relating to the volume of fluid and time of infusion.

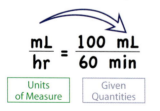

$$\frac{mL}{hr} = \frac{100\ mL}{60\ min}$$

| Units of Measure | Given Quantities |

2. Insert the conversion factor needed to convert minutes into hours, and solve the equation.

$$\frac{mL}{hr} = \frac{100\ mL}{60\ min} \times \frac{60\ min}{1\ hr} = 100\ \frac{mL}{hr}$$

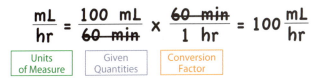

Units of Measure   Given Quantities   Conversion Factor

Note: In this example, the question seems to have three relevant pieces of information: the dosage of ganciclovir, the volume of the IV bag, and the time of infusion. However, the dosage of ganciclovir is not needed to calculate the flow rate. Although the dosage should be checked for accuracy, it is not relevant to calculating how fast the fluid should be infused. The only information needed is the volume of fluid and the infusion time.

For Examples 2–5, refer to the directions in Example 1.

Example 2: The provider order reads: "Infuse 500 mg azithromycin (Zithromax) diluted in 250 mL NS over 3 hours." The nurse should set the pump at what mL/hr flow rate? Round the flow rate to the nearest whole number.

$$\frac{mL}{hr} = \frac{250\ mL}{3\ hr} = 83.3 = 83\ \frac{mL}{hr}$$

Note: No conversion factor is needed in this example since the time given is already in hours.

Example 3: The provider order reads: "Infuse 250 mg ampicillin diluted in 50 mL NS over 20 minutes." The nurse should set the pump at what mL/hr flow rate? Round to the nearest whole number.

$$\frac{mL}{hr} = \frac{50\ mL}{20\ min} = \frac{60\ min}{1\ hr} = \frac{50\ mL \times 60}{20\ hr} = \frac{3000\ mL}{20\ hr} = 150\ \frac{mL}{hr}$$

Example 4: The provider order reads: "Infuse moxifloxacin (Avelox) 400 mg diluted in 250 mL 0.8% sodium chloride solution over 60 minutes." The nurse should set the pump at what mL/hr flow rate? Round the flow rate to the nearest whole number.

$$\frac{mL}{hr} = \frac{250\ mL}{60\ min} \times \frac{60\ min}{1\ hr} = 250\ \frac{mL}{hr}$$

Example 5: The provider order reads: "Infuse metronidazole (Flagyl RTU IV) 500 mg diluted in 100 mL NS over 60 minutes." The nurse should set the pump at what mL/hr flow rate? Round the flow rate to the nearest whole number.

$$\frac{mL}{hr} = \frac{100\ mL}{60\ min} \times \frac{60\ min}{1\ hr} = 100\ \frac{mL}{hr}$$

Note: See also Box 13-1.

■ Box 13-1 IVPB Hints

1. The mL/hr flow rate for an IVPB that is to be infused over 60 minutes is the same as the volume of the bag.
   Example: *Infuse 100 mL over 60 minutes.*

$$\frac{mL}{hr} = \frac{100\ mL}{1\ hr} = 100\ \frac{mL}{hr}$$

2. The mL/hr flow rate for an IVPB to be infused over 30 minutes is double the volume of the IV bag.
   Example: *Infuse 100 mL over 30 minutes.*

$$\frac{mL}{hr} = \frac{100\ mL}{30\ \cancel{min}} \times \frac{60\ \cancel{min}}{1\ hr} = 200\ \frac{mL}{hr}$$

3. The mL/hr flow rate for an IVPB to run over 15 minutes is four times the volume of the IV bag.
   Example: *Infuse 100 mL over 15 minutes.*

$$\frac{mL}{hr} = \frac{100\ mL}{15\ \cancel{min}} \times \frac{60\ \cancel{min}}{1\ hr} = 400\ \frac{mL}{hr}$$

Practice Calculating mL/hr Flow Rates for Intermittent IV Fluids

(answers on page 246)

Calculate the mL/hr flow rate for these intermittent infusions. Round the answer to the nearest whole number.

1. Infuse cefipime (Maxipime) 1 g diluted in 50 mL 0.9% sodium chloride solution over 30 minutes.

2. Infuse ifosfamide (Ifex) 1.7 g diluted in 100 mL lactated Ringer's solution over 45 minutes.

3. Infuse leucovorin calcium (Wellcovorin) 225 mg diluted in 500 mL D_5W solution over 2 hours.

4. Infuse mycophenolate mofetil (CellCept) 1 g diluted in 140 mL D_5W solution over 2 hours.

5. Infuse penicillin G (Pfizerpen) 5 million units diluted in 100 mL 0.9% sodium chloride solution over 30 minutes.

6. Infuse ondansetron (Zofran) 32 mg diluted in 50 mL 0.9% sodium chloride solution over 15 minutes.

7. Infuse nafcillin 1 g diluted in 100 mL 0.9% sodium chloride solution over 45 minutes.

8. Infuse acetazolamide (Diamox) 250 mg diluted in 250 mL 0.45% sodium chloride solution over 4 hours.

9. Infuse cefazolin (Ancef) 1 g diluted in 100 mL 0.9% sodium chloride solution over 30 minutes.

10. Infuse bivalirudin (Angiomax) 150 mg diluted in 50 mL D_5W solution over 4 hours.

Calculating mL/hr Flow Rates for Syringe Pumps

Calculating the flow rate for medications infused via a syringe pump requires the same process as calculating flow rates for IV bag pumps and controllers, except that the fluid is inside a syringe, not an IV bag. Medications administered to children or medications that require very small volumes of diluents may be infused using a syringe pump.

Note: Many syringe pumps may be programmed to deliver medications in flow rates other than mL/hr, such as units/min or mcg/min.

Example 1:   The provider order reads: "Infuse ampicillin 100 mg diluted in 5 mL sterile water over 15 minutes using a syringe pump." The nurse should set the pump at what mL/hr flow rate? Round the flow rate to the nearest tenth.

Set up the equation as shown in "Calculating mL/hr Flow Rates for Intermittent IV Fluids." Since syringe pumps are used to deliver medications in less than 1 hour, a conversion factor for minutes to hours is needed, unless the pump can be programmed to deliver mL/min.

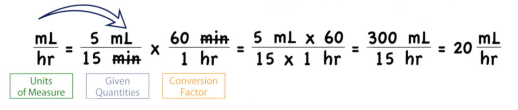

$$\frac{mL}{hr} = \frac{5\ mL}{15\ min} \times \frac{60\ min}{1\ hr} = \frac{5\ mL \times 60}{15 \times 1\ hr} = \frac{300\ mL}{15\ hr} = 20\frac{mL}{hr}$$

Units of Measure	Given Quantities	Conversion Factor

Note: Remember that the dosage of medication in the liquid is not a relevant part of the flow rate equation.

For Examples 2–5, refer to the directions in Example 1.

Example 2:   The provider order reads: "Infuse vancomycin (Vancocin) 45 mg diluted in 5 mL NS over 60 minutes using a syringe pump." The nurse should set the pump at what mL/hr flow rate? Round the flow rate to the nearest tenth.

$$\frac{mL}{hr} = \frac{5\ mL}{60\ min} \times \frac{60\ min}{1\ hr} = \frac{5\ mL}{1\ hr} = 5\frac{mL}{hr}$$

Example 3:   The provider order reads: "Infuse gentamicin 28 mg diluted in 10 mL D_5W over 45 minutes using a syringe pump." The nurse should set the pump at what mL/hr flow rate? Round the flow rate to the nearest tenth.

$$\frac{mL}{hr} = \frac{10\ mL}{45\ min} \times \frac{60\ min}{1\ hr} = \frac{10\ mL \times 60}{45 \times 1\ hr} = \frac{600\ mL}{45\ hr} = 13.33 = 13.3\frac{mL}{hr}$$

Example 4:   The provider order reads: "Infuse digoxin (Lanoxin) 0.5 mg diluted in 4 mL sterile water over 5 minutes using a syringe pump." The nurse should set the pump at what mL/hr flow rate? Round the flow rate to the nearest tenth.

$$\frac{mL}{hr} = \frac{4\ mL}{5\ min} \times \frac{60\ min}{1\ hr} = \frac{4\ mL \times 60}{5 \times 1\ hr} = \frac{240\ mL}{5\ hr} = 48\frac{mL}{hr}$$

Example 5:   The provider order reads: "Infuse morphine sulfate 2 mg diluted in 5 mL NS over 3 minutes using a syringe pump." The nurse should set the pump at what mL/hr flow rate? Round the flow rate to the nearest tenth.

$$\frac{mL}{hr} = \frac{5\ mL}{3\ min} \times \frac{60\ min}{1\ hr} = \frac{5\ mL \times 60}{3 \times 1\ hr} = \frac{300\ mL}{3\ hr} = 100\frac{mL}{hr}$$

Practice Calculating mL/hr Flow Rates for Syringe Pumps

(answers on page 247)

Calculate the mL/hr flow rate for these infusions. Round the answer to the nearest whole number.

1. Infuse folic acid 1 mg diluted in 10 mL 0.9% sodium chloride solution over 5 minutes using a syringe pump.

2. Infuse pantoprazole (Protonix) 40 mg diluted in 10 mL 0.9% sodium chloride solution over 2 minutes using a syringe pump.

3. Infuse aminophylline 300 mg diluted in 12 mL 0.9% sodium chloride solution over 20 minutes using a syringe pump.

4. Infuse methylprednisolone (Solu-Medrol) 250 mg diluted in 20 mL bacteriostatic water over 15 minutes using a syringe pump.

5. Infuse ondansetron (Zofran) 4 mg diluted in 5 mL 0.9% sodium chloride solution over 5 minutes using a syringe pump.

6. Infuse hydromorphone 1.5 mg diluted in 10 mL 0.9% sodium chloride solution over 10 minutes using a syringe pump.

7. Infuse oxacillin 250 mg diluted in 5 mL 0.9% sodium chloride solution over 10 minutes using a syringe pump.

8. Infuse butorphanol (Stadol) 1 mg diluted in 4 mL 0.9% sodium chloride solution over 5 minutes using a syringe pump.

9. Infuse gemcitabine (Gemzar) 1250 mg diluted in 25 mL 0.9% sodium chloride solution over 30 minutes using a syringe pump.

10. Infuse meperidine (Demerol) 75 mg diluted in 10 mL 0.9% sodium chloride solution over 7 minutes using a syringe pump.

Calculating Infusion and Completion Times for mL/hr Flow Rates

At times, the nurse may need to know the time when the current infusion will be complete. For example, if a nurse is infusing 340 mL of red blood cells to a patient at 125 mL/hr, how long will the transfusion take? Because red blood cells must be infused in less than 4 hours, the nurse must be sure that the current flow rate is fast enough to infuse the cells in the allotted time. To calculate the infusion time of an IV, the nurse needs to know the present flow rate and the volume of fluid to be infused. The infusion time may be expressed in hours or minutes, or a combination of both, depending on the prescribed flow rate and total volume of fluid. For maintenance fluids (those infusing longer than 1 hour), use hours as the unit of measure. For IV fluids infusing for a short time (less than one hour), use minutes as the unit of measure.

The completion time is determined by adding the infusion time to the current time. Most healthcare facilities utilize military time (the 24-hour clock) to document time. See Appendix C for instructions on adding military time.

Example 1: Calculate the infusion time for an IV that is infusing at 100 mL/hr with 300 mL of fluid left in the IV bag. The current time is 1120 (11:20 a.m.). When will this IV be completed?

To calculate the infusion time, follow these steps:

1. Set up the equation using dimensional analysis principles. Insert the first set of given quantities. In this example, it is the flow rate of the infusion.

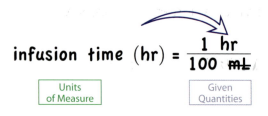

$$\text{infusion time (hr)} = \frac{1 \text{ hr}}{100 \text{ mL}}$$

Units of Measure   Given Quantities

2. Multiply the first set of given quantities by the second given quantity (the volume of remaining fluid to be infused). Solve the equation.

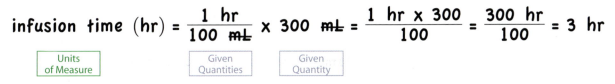

$$\text{infusion time (hr)} = \frac{1 \text{ hr}}{100 \text{ mL}} \times 300 \text{ mL} = \frac{1 \text{ hr} \times 300}{100} = \frac{300 \text{ hr}}{100} = 3 \text{ hr}$$

Units of Measure   Given Quantities   Given Quantity

A volume of 300 mL running at 100 mL/hr will take 3 hours to infuse.

To calculate the completion time, add the infusion time to the current time.

$$\text{completion time} = 1120 + 3 \text{ hr} = 1420 \ (2{:}20 \text{ p.m.})$$

Current Time   Infusion Time

For Examples 2–5, refer to the directions in Example 1.

Example 2: Calculate the infusion time for an IV that is infusing at 125 mL/hr with 1000 mL of fluid left in the IV bag. The current time is 1745 (5:45 p.m.). When will this IV be completed?

$$\text{infusion time (hr)} = \frac{1 \text{ hr}}{125 \text{ mL}} \times 1000 \text{ mL} = \frac{1 \text{ hr} \times 1000}{125} = \frac{1000 \text{ hr}}{125} = 8 \text{ hr}$$

$$\text{completion time} = 1745 + 8 \text{ hr} = 0145 \ (1{:}45 \text{ a.m.})$$

Note: In the first two examples, the time to infuse the IV is in full hours. If the calculated infusion time ends in a decimal point (that is, a partial hour), calculate the minutes as well (see Examples 3–5). For increased accuracy in calculating minutes, the infusion time has rounded to the nearest hundredth.

Example 3: Calculate the infusion time for an IV that is infusing at 150 mL/hr with 800 mL of fluid left in the IV bag. The current time is 0620 (6:20 a.m.). When will this IV be completed?

$$\text{infusion time (hr)} = \frac{1 \text{ hr}}{150 \text{ mL}} \times 800 \text{ mL} = \frac{1 \text{ hr} \times 800}{150} = \frac{800 \text{ hr}}{150} = 5.33 \text{ hr}$$

In this example, *0.33 hours must be converted into minutes*. To do so, set up the equation using dimensional analysis, solving for *minutes*.

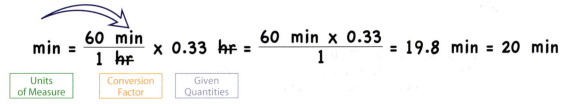

$$\text{min} = \frac{60 \text{ min}}{1 \text{ hr}} \times 0.33 \text{ hr} = \frac{60 \text{ min} \times 0.33}{1} = 19.8 \text{ min} = 20 \text{ min}$$

Units of Measure   Conversion Factor   Given Quantities

The total infusion time for this IV is 5 hours and 20 minutes.

Note: Any decimal point when calculating minutes should be rounded to the nearest whole number, since timing an infusion to the nearest second is not necessary.

$$\text{completion time} = 0620 + 5 \text{ hr, } 20 \text{ min} = 1140 \ (11{:}40 \text{ a.m.})$$

Example 4: Calculate the infusion time for an IV that is infusing at 83 mL/hr with 500 mL of fluid left in the IV bag. The current time is 2105 (9:05 p.m.). When will this IV be completed?

$$\text{infusion time (hr)} = \frac{1 \text{ hr}}{83 \text{ mL}} \times 500 \text{ mL} = \frac{1 \text{ hr} \times 500}{83} = \frac{500 \text{ hr}}{83} = 6.02 \text{ hr}$$

To convert *0.02* hours into minutes:

$$\text{min} = \frac{60 \text{ min}}{1 \text{ hr}} \times 0.02 \text{ hr} = \frac{60 \text{ min} \times 0.02}{1} = 1.2 \text{ min} = 1 \text{ min}$$

The total infusion time for this IV is 6 hours and 1 minute.

$$\text{completion time} = 2105 + 6 \text{ hr, } 1 \text{ min} = 0306 \text{ (3:06 a.m.)}$$

Example 5: Calculate the infusion time for an IV that is infusing at 30 mL/hr with 650 mL of fluid left in the IV bag. The current time is 0035 (12:35 a.m.). When will this IV be completed?

$$\text{infusion time (hr)} = \frac{1 \text{ hr}}{30 \text{ mL}} \times 650 \text{ mL} = \frac{1 \text{ hr} \times 650}{30} = \frac{650 \text{ hr}}{30} = 21.67 \text{ hr}$$

To convert *0.67* hours into minutes:

$$\text{min} = \frac{60 \text{ min}}{1 \text{ hr}} \times 0.67 \text{ hr} = \frac{60 \text{ min} \times 0.67}{1} = 40.2 \text{ min} = 40 \text{ min}$$

The total infusion time for this IV is 21 hours and 40 minutes.

$$\text{completion time} = 0035 + 21 \text{ hr, } 40 \text{ min} = 2215 \text{ (10:15 p.m.)}$$

Practice Calculating Infusion and Completion Times for mL/hr Flow Rates

(answers on page 248)

Calculate the infusion and completion times for these IVs.

1. An IV is infusing at 125 mL/hr with 900 mL of fluid left in the IV bag. The current time is 0855 (8:55 a.m.).

2. An IV is infusing at 67 mL/hr with 275 mL of fluid left in the IV bag. The current time is 1325 (1:25 p.m.).

3. An IV is infusing at 175 mL/hr with 700 mL of fluid left in the IV bag. The current time is 1622 (4:22 p.m.).

4. An IV is infusing at 21 mL/hr with 150 mL of fluid left in the IV bag. The current time is 1930 (7:30 p.m.).

5. An IV is infusing at 150 mL/hr with 500 mL of fluid left in the IV bag. The current time is 2208 (10:08 p.m.).

6. An IV is infusing at 80 mL/hr with 650 mL of fluid left in the IV bag. The current time is 0540 (5:40 a.m.).

7. An IV is infusing at 50 mL/hr with 950 mL of fluid left in the IV bag. The current time is 1200 (12:00 p.m.).

8. An IV is infusing at 25 mL/hr with 250 mL of fluid left in the IV bag. The current time is 1849 (6:49 p.m.).

9. An IV is infusing at 200 mL/hr with 1000 mL of fluid left in the IV bag. The current time is 1427 (2:27 p.m.).

10. An IV is infusing at 73 mL/hr with 425 mL of fluid left in the IV bag. The current time is 2300 (11:00 p.m.).

Calculating gtt/min Flow Rates for IV Fluids Under Manual Control

IV infusions may be controlled manually when an IV pump or controller is not available. The nurse regulates the flow rate by counting the drops of IV fluid falling inside the drip chamber over 1 minute (gtt/min). The flow is adjusted by opening or closing the roller clamp.

IV infusions under manual control need careful monitoring because they have no built-in warning systems alerting the nurse to subtle changes in patient condition. IV catheters placed near elbow or wrist joints may become temporarily occluded when the arm is bent, thereby slowing the flow rate. Conversely, when the arm is straightened, the flow rate may increase. Hanging IV bags high above the patient can also increase the flow rate. Hanging the bag level with the patient can slow or stop the infusion. See Box 13-2.

To calculate the flow rate, the nurse needs the following information:

1. The drop factor of the tubing, which can be found on the tubing package. Standard drop factors for tubing are 10 gtt/mL, 15 gtt/mL, 20 gtt/mL, and 60 gtt/mL.
2. The fluid volume to be infused (as ordered by the provider).
3. The length of time for infusing the fluid (as ordered by the provider).

■ Box 13-2   Adjusting IV Infusions Under Manual Control

An IV fluid that is infusing too fast or too slowly may need to be adjusted to bring the IV back on schedule. However, risks may be involved. Before adjusting the flow rate, the nurse should ask these questions:

1. Will changing the IV flow rate have unintended consequences for this patient? The patient may become overloaded with fluid if he or she receives a large amount in a small period of time. Fluid overloading may affect the patient's blood pressure or breathing.
2. Will changing the IV flow rate mean that the patient will not receive the medication at the intended rate? A medication that infuses too quickly or too slowly may result in adverse drug reactions and may affect the timing of future doses.
3. Will changing the flow rate of a fluid containing a medication be considered a change in the dosage administered to the patient? If the answer is yes, then the provider must be notified, and a new order obtained.

If no consequences to altering the flow rate of the IV fluid are identified, then proceed with these steps:

1. Determine the volume of fluid remaining.
2. Identify the length of time available for the fluid to be infused.
3. Calculate the new gtt/min flow rate.
4. Adjust the flow rate of the infusion using the roller clamp and adjust the height of the infusion bag, if necessary. The IV bag must be higher than the patient's IV site to flow.

Example: *An IV infusion under manual control is behind schedule. The nurse estimates that 300 mL are left in the bag. The fluid must be infused over the next 2 hours. The tubing drop factor is 20 gtt/mL. No risk factors to the patient have been identified.*

1. *Calculate the new flow rate (gtt/min):*

$$\text{gtt/min} = \frac{\text{gtt}}{\text{min}} = \frac{20 \text{ gtt}}{1 \text{ mL}} \times \frac{300 \text{ mL}}{2 \text{ hr}} \times \frac{1 \text{ hr}}{60 \text{ min}} = \frac{20 \text{ gtt} \times 300}{2 \times 60 \text{ min}} = 50 \frac{\text{gtt}}{\text{min}}$$

2. *Open the roller clamp to allow the drops to fall faster into the drip chamber, and check that the infusion bag is placed higher than the patient's IV site.*

Example 1: An IV of 1 L D$_5$W/0.45% sodium chloride solution is to be infused over 8 hours. The IV tubing has a drop factor of 20 gtt/mL. Calculate the gtt/min flow rate.

1. Set up the equation using dimensional analysis. The first given quantity in the equation is the drop factor of the tubing (20 gtt/mL).

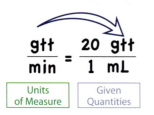

$$\frac{gtt}{min} = \frac{20\ gtt}{1\ mL}$$

| Units of Measure | Given Quantities |

2. Insert the conversion factor for mL/L.

$$\frac{gtt}{min} = \frac{20\ gtt}{1\ mL} \times \frac{1000\ mL}{1\ L}$$

| Units of Measure | Given Quantities | Conversion Factor |

3. Enter the next set of given quantities—the volume of the prescribed IV fluid (1 L) and the time that the fluid is to infuse (8 hr).

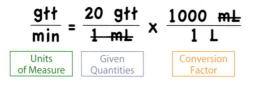

$$\frac{gtt}{min} = \frac{20\ gtt}{1\ mL} \times \frac{1000\ mL}{1\ L} \times \frac{1\ L}{8\ hr}$$

| Units of Measure | Given Quantities | Conversion Factor | Given Quantities |

4. Insert the factor to change hours into minutes.

$$\frac{gtt}{min} = \frac{20\ gtt}{1\ mL} \times \frac{1000\ mL}{1\ L} \times \frac{1\ L}{8\ hr} \times \frac{1\ hr}{60\ min}$$

| Units of Measure | Given Quantities | Conversion Factor | Given Quantities | Conversion Factor |

5. Solve the equation for gtt/min.

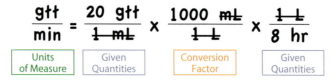

$$\frac{gtt}{min} = \frac{20\ gtt}{1\ mL} \times \frac{1000\ mL}{1\ L} \times \frac{1\ L}{8\ hr} \times \frac{1\ hr}{60\ min} = \frac{20\ gtt \times 1000}{8 \times 60\ min}$$

$$= \frac{20,000\ gtt}{480\ min} = 41.7 = 42\ \frac{gtt}{min}$$

Note: The final answer must be rounded to the nearest whole number since it is impossible to count a partial drop.

For Examples 2–5, refer to the directions in Example 1.

Example 2: An IV of 250 mL lactated Ringer's solution is to be infused over 2 hours. The IV tubing has a drop factor of 15 gtt/mL. Calculate the gtt/min flow rate.

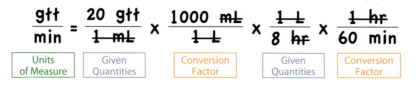

$$\frac{gtt}{min} = \frac{15\ gtt}{1\ mL} \times \frac{250\ mL}{2\ hr} \times \frac{1\ hr}{60\ min} \times \frac{15\ gtt \times 250}{2 \times 60\ min}$$

$$= \frac{3750\ gtt}{120\ min} = 31.3 = 31\ \frac{gtt}{min}$$

Example 3: An IV of 2 L 0.9% sodium chloride solution is to be infused over 24 hours. The IV tubing has a drop factor of 10 gtt/mL. Calculate the gtt/min flow rate.

$$\frac{gtt}{min} = \frac{10\ gtt}{1\ mL} \times \frac{1000\ mL}{1\ L} \times \frac{2\ L}{24\ hr} \times \frac{1\ hr}{60\ min} = \frac{10\ gtt \times 1000 \times 2}{1 \times 24 \times 60\ min}$$

$$= \frac{20{,}000\ gtt}{1440\ min} = 13.9 = 14\ \frac{gtt}{min}$$

Example 4: An IV of 300 mL Normosol-R solution is to be infused over 6 hours. The IV tubing has a drop factor of 60 gtt/mL. Calculate the gtt/min flow rate.

$$\frac{gtt}{min} = \frac{60\ gtt}{1\ mL} \times \frac{300\ mL}{6\ hr} \times \frac{1\ hr}{60\ min} \times \frac{60\ gtt \times 300}{6 \times 60\ min}$$

$$= \frac{18{,}000\ gtt}{360\ min} = 50\ \frac{gtt}{min}$$

Example 5: An IV of 750 mL D_5W/0.9% sodium chloride solution is to be infused over 8 hours. The IV tubing has a drop factor of 10 gtt/mL. Calculate the gtt/min flow rate.

$$\frac{gtt}{min} = \frac{10\ gtt}{1\ mL} \times \frac{750\ mL}{8\ hr} \times \frac{1\ hr}{60\ min} \times \frac{10\ gtt \times 750}{8 \times 60\ min}$$

$$= \frac{7500\ gtt}{480\ min} = 15.6 = 16\ \frac{gtt}{min}$$

Practice Calculating gtt/min Flow Rates for IV Fluids Under Manual Control

(answers on page 250)

Calculate the gtt/min flow rate for these IV fluids under manual control.

1. An IV of 1000 mL 0.9% sodium chloride solution is to be infused over 10 hours. The IV tubing has a drop factor of 15 gtt/mL.

2. An IV of 500 mL D_5W solution is to be infused over 4 hours. The IV tubing has a drop factor of 10 gtt/mL.

3. An IV of 1000 mL lactated Ringer's solution is to be infused over 6 hours. The IV tubing has a drop factor of 20 gtt/mL.

4. An IV of 100 mL 0.45% sodium chloride solution is to be infused over 2 hours. The IV tubing has a drop factor of 60 gtt/mL.

5. An IV of 750 mL D_5W solution is to be infused over 8 hours. The IV tubing has a drop factor of 15 gtt/mL.

6. An IV of 1000 mL 0.9% sodium chloride solution is to be infused over 12 hours. The IV tubing has a drop factor of 20 gtt/mL.

7. An IV of 500 mL D_5W/0.9% sodium chloride solution is to be infused over 3 hours. The IV tubing has a drop factor of 20 gtt/mL.

8. An IV of 300 mL 0.45% sodium chloride solution is to be infused over 90 minutes. The IV tubing has a drop factor of 10 gtt/mL.

9. An IV of 1500 mL Lactated Ringer's solution is to be infused over 15 hours. The IV tubing has a drop factor of 10 gtt/mL.

10. An IV of 50 mL D_5W/0.9% sodium chloride solution is to be infused over 60 minutes. The IV tubing has a drop factor of 60 gtt/mL.

Calculating gtt/min Flow Rates From mL/hr Flow Rates

A gtt/min flow rate can easily be calculated from a mL/hr flow rate. The only additional information needed is the drop factor of the tubing.

Example 1:   Calculate the gtt/min flow rate for a fluid infusing at 100 mL/hr. The drop factor of the tubing is 20 gtt/mL.

1. Set up the equation using dimensional analysis. The first given quantity in the equation is the drop factor of the tubing (20 gtt/mL).

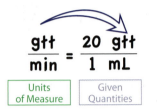

$$\frac{gtt}{min} = \frac{20\ gtt}{1\ mL}$$

| Units of Measure | Given Quantities |

2. Insert the second set of given quantities—the flow rate in mL/hr.

$$\frac{gtt}{min} = \frac{20\ gtt}{1\ mL} \times \frac{100\ mL}{1\ hr}$$

| Units of Measure | Given Quantities | Given Quantities |

3. Insert the factor to convert hours into minutes.

$$\frac{gtt}{min} = \frac{20\ gtt}{1\ mL} \times \frac{100\ mL}{1\ hr} \times \frac{1\ hr}{60\ min}$$

| Units of Measure | Given Quantities | Given Quantities | Conversion Factor |

4. Solve the equation for gtt/min.

$$\frac{gtt}{min} = \frac{20\ gtt}{1\ mL} \times \frac{100\ mL}{1\ hr} \times \frac{1\ hr}{60\ min} = \frac{20\ gtt \times 100}{1 \times 60\ min}$$

$$= \frac{2000\ gtt}{60\ min} = 33.3 = 33\ \frac{gtt}{min}$$

For Examples 2–5, refer to the directions in Example 1.

Example 2:   Calculate the gtt/min flow rate for a fluid infusing at 125 mL/hr. The drop factor of the tubing is 15 gtt/mL.

$$\frac{gtt}{min} = \frac{15\ gtt}{1\ mL} \times \frac{125\ mL}{1\ hr} \times \frac{1\ hr}{60\ min} = \frac{15\ gtt \times 125}{1 \times 60\ min}$$

$$= \frac{1875\ gtt}{60\ min} = 31.3 = 31\ \frac{gtt}{min}$$

Example 3: Calculate the gtt/min flow rate for a fluid infusing at 150 mL/hr. The drop factor of the tubing is 20 gtt/mL.

$$\frac{gtt}{min} = \frac{20\ gtt}{1\ mL} \times \frac{150\ mL}{1\ hr} \times \frac{1\ hr}{60\ min} = \frac{20\ gtt \times 150}{1 \times 60\ min} = \frac{3000\ gtt}{60\ min} = 50\ \frac{gtt}{min}$$

Example 4: Calculate the gtt/min flow rate for a fluid infusing at 50 mL/hr. The drop factor of the tubing is 10 gtt/mL.

$$\frac{gtt}{min} = \frac{10\ gtt}{1\ mL} \times \frac{50\ mL}{1\ hr} \times \frac{1\ hr}{60\ min} = \frac{10\ gtt \times 50}{1 \times 60\ min} = \frac{500\ gtt}{60\ min} = 8.3 = 8\ \frac{gtt}{min}$$

Example 5: Calculate the gtt/min flow rate for a fluid infusing at 200 mL/hr. The drop factor of the tubing is 20 gtt/mL.

$$\frac{gtt}{min} = \frac{20\ gtt}{1\ mL} \times \frac{200\ mL}{1\ hr} \times \frac{1\ hr}{60\ min} = \frac{20\ gtt \times 200}{1 \times 60\ min}$$

$$= \frac{4000\ gtt}{60\ min} = 66.7 = 67\ \frac{gtt}{min}$$

Practice Calculating gtt/min Flow Rates From mL/hr Flow Rates

(answers on page 251)

Calculate the gtt/min flow rate for these IV fluids infusing in mL/hr.

1. An IV fluid is infusing at 125 mL/hr. The drop factor of the tubing is 10 gtt/mL.
2. An IV fluid is infusing at 150 mL/hr. The drop factor of the tubing is 20 gtt/mL.
3. An IV fluid is infusing at 63 mL/hr. The drop factor of the tubing is 15 gtt/mL.
4. An IV fluid is infusing at 15 mL/hr. The drop factor of the tubing is 60 gtt/mL.
5. An IV fluid is infusing at 175 mL/hr. The drop factor of the tubing is 20 gtt/mL.
6. An IV fluid is infusing at 50 mL/hr. The drop factor of the tubing is 10 gtt/mL.
7. An IV fluid is infusing at 160 mL/hr. The drop factor of the tubing is 15 gtt/mL.
8. An IV fluid is infusing at 83 mL/hr. The drop factor of the tubing is 20 gtt/mL.
9. An IV fluid is infusing at 21 mL/hr. The drop factor of the tubing is 60 gtt/mL.
10. An IV fluid is infusing at 250 mL/hr. The drop factor of the tubing is 10 gtt/mL.

Calculating Infusion and Completion Times for gtt/min Flow Rates

To calculate the infusion time for an IV that is being manually controlled, the drip rate, volume of fluid to be infused, and the tubing drop factor must be known. The completion time is computed in the same manner as mL/hr flow rates. See "Calculating Infusion and Completion Times for mL/hr Flow Rates."

Example 1: Calculate the infusion and completion times for an IV that is infusing at 64 gtt/min; 1000 mL of fluid remain in the IV bag. The drop factor of the tubing is 10 gtt/mL. The current time is 0200 (2:00 a.m.).

To calculate the infusion time, follow these steps:

1. Set up the equation using dimensional analysis principles. Insert the first set of quantities. In this example, it is a conversion factor for time.

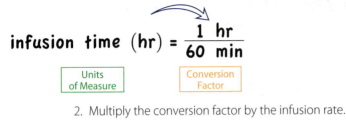

$$\text{infusion time (hr)} = \frac{1 \text{ hr}}{60 \text{ min}}$$

Units of Measure · Conversion Factor

2. Multiply the conversion factor by the infusion rate.

$$\text{infusion time (hr)} = \frac{1 \text{ hr}}{60 \text{ min}} \times \frac{1 \text{ min}}{64 \text{ gtt}}$$

Units of Measure · Conversion Factor · Given Quantities

3. Insert the next set of given quantities—the drop factor of the tubing.

$$\text{infusion time (hr)} = \frac{1 \text{ hr}}{60 \text{ min}} \times \frac{1 \text{ min}}{64 \text{ gtt}} \times \frac{10 \text{ gtt}}{1 \text{ mL}}$$

4. Insert the last given quantity—the amount of fluid to be infused (1000 mL).

$$\text{infusion time (hr)} = \frac{1 \text{ hr}}{60 \text{ min}} \times \frac{1 \text{ min}}{64 \text{ gtt}} \times \frac{10 \text{ gtt}}{1 \text{ mL}} \times 1000 \text{ mL}$$

Units of Measure · Conversion Factor · Given Quantities · Given Quantities · Given Quantity

5. Solve the equation.

$$\text{infusion time (hr)} = \frac{1 \text{ hr}}{60 \text{ min}} \times \frac{1 \text{ min}}{64 \text{ gtt}} \times \frac{10 \text{ gtt}}{1 \text{ mL}} \times 1000 \text{ mL}$$

$$= \frac{1 \text{ hr} \times 10 \times 1000}{60 \times 64} = \frac{10,000 \text{ hr}}{3840} = 2.6 \text{ hr}$$

At a flow rate of 64 gtt/min, it will take 2.6 hours to infuse 1000 mL.

6. Convert *0.6* hours into minutes.

$$\text{min} = \frac{60 \text{ min}}{1 \text{ hr}} \times 0.6 \text{ hr} = \frac{60 \text{ min} \times 0.6}{1} = 36 \text{ min}$$

The total infusion time is 2 hours and 36 minutes.

To calculate the completion time, add the IV infusion time to the current time.

completion time = 0200 + 2 hr, 36 min = 0436 (4:36 a.m.)

Current Time · Infusion Time

For Examples 2–5, refer to the directions in Example 1.

Example 2: Calculate the infusion time for an IV that is infusing at 31 gtt/min; 750 mL of fluid remain in the IV bag. The drop factor of the tubing is 15 gtt/mL. The current time is 0005 (12:05 a.m.).

$$\text{infusion time (hr)} = \frac{1\ hr}{60\ min} \times \frac{1\ min}{31\ gtt} \times \frac{15\ gtt}{1\ mL} \times 750\ mL$$

$$= \frac{1\ hr \times 15 \times 750}{60 \times 31} = \frac{11{,}250\ hr}{1860} = 6.05\ hr$$

Convert *0.5* hours into minutes:

$$min = \frac{60\ min}{1\ hr} \times 0.05\ hr = \frac{60\ min \times 0.05}{1} = 3\ min$$

The total infusion time for this IV is 6 hours and 3 minutes.

$$\text{completion time} = 0005 + 6\ hr,\ 3\ min = 0608\ (6{:}08\ a.m.)$$

Example 3: Calculate the infusion time for an IV that is infusing at 21 gtt/min; 150 mL of fluid remain in the IV bag. The drop factor of the tubing is 60 gtt/mL. The current time is 1945 (7:45 p.m.).

$$\text{infusion time (hr)} = \frac{1\ hr}{60\ min} \times \frac{1\ min}{21\ gtt} \times \frac{60\ gtt}{1\ mL} \times 150\ mL$$

$$= \frac{1\ hr \times 150}{21} = \frac{150\ hr}{21} = 7.14\ hr$$

Convert *0.14* hours into minutes.

$$min = \frac{60\ min}{1\ hr} \times 0.14\ hr = \frac{60\ min \times 0.14}{1} = 8.4 = 8\ min$$

The total infusion time for this IV is 7 hours and 8 minutes.

$$\text{completion time} = 1945 + 7\ hr,\ 8\ min = 0253\ (2{:}53\ a.m.)$$

Example 4: Calculate the infusion time for an IV that is infusing at 48 gtt/min; 500 mL of fluid remain in the IV bag. The drop factor of the tubing is 20 gtt/mL. The current time is 2210 (10:10 p.m.).

$$\text{infusion time (hr)} = \frac{1\ hr}{60\ min} \times \frac{1\ min}{48\ gtt} \times \frac{20\ gtt}{1\ mL} \times 500\ mL$$

$$= \frac{1\ hr \times 20 \times 500}{60 \times 48} = \frac{10{,}000\ hr}{2880} = 3.47\ hr$$

Convert *0.47* hours into minutes:

$$min = \frac{60\ min}{1\ hr} \times 0.47\ hr = \frac{60\ min \times 0.47}{1} = 28.2 = 28\ min$$

The total infusion time for this IV is 3 hours and 28 minutes.

$$\text{completion time} = 2210 + 3\ hr,\ 28\ min = 0138\ (1{:}38\ a.m.)$$

Example 5: Calculate the infusion time for an IV that is infusing at 60 gtt/min; 300 mL of fluid remain in the IV bag. The drop factor of the tubing is 60 gtt/mL. The current time is 0455 (4:55 a.m.).

$$\text{infusion time (hr)} = \frac{1 \text{ hr}}{60 \text{ min}} \times \frac{1 \text{ min}}{60 \text{ gtt}} \times \frac{60 \text{ gtt}}{1 \text{ mL}} \times 300 \text{ mL}$$

$$= \frac{1 \text{ hr} \times 300}{60} = \frac{300 \text{ hr}}{60} = 5 \text{ hr}$$

The total infusion time for this IV is exactly 5 hours.

$$\text{completion time} = 0455 + 5 \text{ hr} = 0955 \text{ (9:55 a.m.)}$$

Practice Calculating Infusion and Completion Times for gtt/min Flow Rates

(answers on page 252)

Calculate the infusion and completion times for these IVs.

1. An IV is infusing at 28 gtt/min; 125 mL of fluid remain in the IV bag. The drop factor of the tubing is 60 gtt/mL. The current time is 1215 (12:15 p.m.).

2. An IV is infusing at 42 gtt/min; 425 mL of fluid remain in the IV bag. The drop factor of the tubing is 15 gtt/mL. The current time is 0300 (3:00 a.m.).

3. An IV is infusing at 54 gtt/min; 150 mL of fluid remain in the IV bag. The drop factor of the tubing is 10 gtt/mL. The current time is 1620 (4:20 p.m.).

4. An IV is infusing at 12 gtt/min; 525 mL of fluid remain in the IV bag. The drop factor of the tubing is 15 gtt/mL. The current time is 2025 (8:25 p.m.).

5. An IV is infusing at 15 gtt/min; 250 mL of fluid remain in the IV bag. The drop factor of the tubing is 60 gtt/mL. The current time is 0545 (5:45 a.m.).

6. An IV is infusing at 26 gtt/min; 225 mL of fluid remain in the IV bag. The drop factor of the tubing is 15 gtt/mL. The current time is 2350 (11:50 p.m.).

7. An IV is infusing at 18 gtt/min; 100 mL of fluid remain in the IV bag. The drop factor of the tubing is 60 gtt/mL. The current time is 01:10 (1:10 a.m.).

8. An IV is infusing at 48 gtt/min; 475 mL of fluid remain in the IV bag. The drop factor of the tubing is 10 gtt/mL. The current time is 1415 (2:15 p.m.).

9. An IV is infusing at 32 gtt/min; 350 mL of fluid remain in the IV bag. The drop factor of the tubing is 20 gtt/mL. The current time is 0700 (7:00 a.m.).

10. An IV is infusing at 36 gtt/min; 950 mL of fluid remain in the IV bag. The drop factor of the tubing is 15 gtt/mL. The current time is 1740 (5:40 p.m.).

Preparing Time Tapes for Manually Controlled Infusions

After the gtt/min flow rate and the infusion time have been calculated, a time tape can be prepared to assist the nurse in monitoring the infusion (see Figure 13-1). Time tapes are available commercially, but one can be made at the bedside. See Box 13-3.

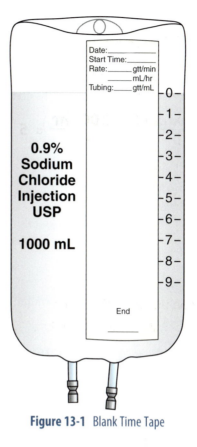

Date:_____
Start Time:_____
Rate:_____ gtt/min
_____ mL/hr
Tubing:_____ gtt/mL

0 –
1 –
2 –
3 –
4 –
5 –
6 –
7 –
8 –
9 –

0.9%
**Sodium
Chloride
Injection
USP**

1000 mL

End

_____

Figure 13-1 Blank Time Tape

■ Box 13-3 *Making a Time Tape*

1. Cut a length of tape (white paper tape works well) that is slightly shorter than the length of the infusion bag.
2. Place the tape on the bag to the left of the volume level markings.
3. Determine the flow rate of the IV in gtt/min and mL/hr. Then write the gtt/min flow rate on the tape so that other nurses can monitor the IV when the primary nurse is out of the patient's room. The mL/hr flow rate is necessary to determine the amount of fluid that will be gone after each hour has elapsed and the time when the IV is to end.
4. Using a marking pen, write the date, start time, flow rate, and tubing drop factor at the top of the tape. Be careful not to write on the IV bag itself as some bags may absorb ink. At the bottom of the tape, write the time that the infusion is expected to be complete; add the date if the infusion continues into the next day.
5. Make hash marks on the tape where the fluid should be for each infusion hour and note that time. Those marks and times allow the nurse to see if the fluid is infusing at the predicted rate.

Note: The hash marks are estimates of the actual fluid remaining in the bag at a given time. It is impossible to be exact.

Example 1:   The nurse starts an infusion of 1000 mL of 0.9% sodium chloride solution at 0330 (3:30 a.m.). The infusion is to run over 8 hours. No electronic infusion device is available, so the fluid will be infused under manual control. The tubing drop factor is 15 gtt/mL.

1. Calculate both the gtt/min and the mL/hr flow rates.
   a. gtt/min flow rate:

$$\frac{gtt}{min} = \frac{15\ gtt}{1\ mL} \times \frac{1000\ mL}{8\ hr} \times \frac{1\ hr}{60\ min} = \frac{15\ gtt \times 1000}{8 \times 60\ min}$$

$$= \frac{15{,}000\ gtt}{480\ min} = 31.25 = 31\ \frac{gtt}{min}$$

b. mL/hr flow rate:

$$\frac{mL}{hr} = \frac{1000\ mL}{8\ hr} = 125\ \frac{mL}{hr}$$

2. Determine the ending time of the infusion by adding the current time to the infusion time.

$$\underset{\text{Current Time}}{0330} + \underset{\text{Infusion Time}}{8\ hr} = 1130\ (11{:}30\ \text{a.m.})$$

If the infusion started at 0330, and there are no delays or difficulties with the flow, the IV infusion should end at 1130 a.m.

3. Calculate the amount of fluid that has been infused and the remaining fluid in the bag for each hour of the infusion.

At 0430:
a. Amount of fluid infused:
The mL infused is equal to the flow rate (mL/hr) multiplied by the number of hours elapsed. Use dimensional analysis to set up the equation:

$$mL\ infused = \underset{\text{Flow Rate}}{\frac{125\ mL}{hr}} \times \underset{\text{Elapsed Time}}{1\ hr} = 125\ mL$$

b. Remaining fluid:
Subtract the mL infused from the original volume of the infusion.

$$mL\ left = \underset{\substack{\text{Original} \\ \text{Volume}}}{1000\ mL} - \underset{\substack{\text{Volume} \\ \text{Infused}}}{125\ mL} = 875\ mL$$

At 0530:
a. Amount of fluid infused:

$$mL\ infused = \frac{125\ mL}{hr} \times 2\ hr = 250\ mL$$

b. Remaining fluid:

$$mL\ left = 1000\ mL - 250\ mL = 750\ mL$$

At 0630:
a. Amount of fluid infused:

$$mL\ infused = \frac{125\ mL}{hr} \times 3\ hr = 375\ mL$$

b. Remaining fluid:

$$mL\ left = 1000\ mL - 375\ mL = 625\ mL$$

At 0730:
a. Amount of fluid infused:

$$\text{mL infused} = \frac{125 \text{ mL}}{\text{hr}} \times 4 \text{ hr} = 500 \text{ mL}$$

b. Remaining fluid:

$$\text{mL left} = 1000 \text{ mL} - 500 \text{ mL} = 500 \text{ mL}$$

At 0830:
a. Amount of fluid infused:

$$\text{mL infused} = \frac{125 \text{ mL}}{\text{hr}} \times 5 \text{ hr} = 625 \text{ mL}$$

b. Remaining fluid:

$$\text{mL left} = 1000 \text{ mL} - 625 \text{ mL} = 375 \text{ mL}$$

At 0930:
a. Amount of fluid infused:

$$\text{mL infused} = \frac{125 \text{ mL}}{\text{hr}} \times 6 \text{ hr} = 750 \text{ mL}$$

b. Remaining fluid:

$$\text{mL left} = 1000 \text{ mL} - 750 \text{ mL} = 250 \text{ mL}$$

At 1030:
a. Amount of fluid infused:

$$\text{mL infused} = \frac{125 \text{ mL}}{\text{hr}} \times 7 \text{ hr} = 875 \text{ mL}$$

b. Remaining fluid:

$$\text{mL left} = 1000 \text{ mL} - 875 \text{ mL} = 125 \text{ mL}$$

At 1130:
a. Amount of fluid infused:

$$\text{mL infused} = \frac{125 \text{ mL}}{\text{hr}} \times 8 \text{ hr} = 1000 \text{ mL}$$

b. Remaining fluid:

$$\text{mL left} = 1000 \text{ mL} - 1000 \text{ mL} = 0 \text{ mL}$$

4. Complete the time tape in Figure 13-2, marking the remaining level of fluid for each hour that has passed.

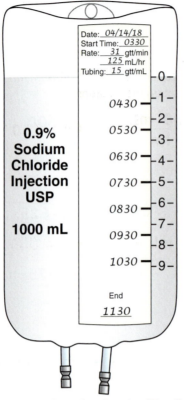

Date: _04/14/18_
Start Time: _0330_
Rate: _31_ gtt/min
_125_ mL/hr
Tubing: _15_ gtt/mL

0

0430 — 1
2
0530 — 3
0630 — 4
0730 — 5
6
0830 — 7
0930 — 8
1030 — 9

End
_1130_

0.9%
Sodium
Chloride
Injection
USP

1000 mL

Figure 13-2 Example 1: Completed Time Tape

Example 2: The nurse starts an infusion of 1000 mL of 0.45% sodium chloride solution at 1545. The infusion is ordered to run at 150 mL/hr. No electronic infusion device is available, so the fluid will be infused under manual control. The tubing drop factor is 20 gtt/mL.

1. Calculate the gtt/min flow rate. See "Calculating the gtt/min Flow Rate From a mL/hr Flow Rate."

$$\frac{gtt}{min} = \frac{20 \ gtt}{1 \ mL} \times \frac{150 \ mL}{1 \ hr} \times \frac{1 \ hr}{60 \ min} = \frac{3000 \ gtt}{60 \ min} = 50 \ \frac{gtt}{min}$$

2. Calculate the total time of the infusion.
   a. Total time of infusion (hr) =

$$\frac{1 \ hr}{150 \ mL} \times 1000 \ mL = \frac{1000 \ hr}{150} = 6.6\overline{6} = 6.67 \ hr$$

   b. Convert *0.67* hours to minutes.

$$min = \frac{60 \ min}{1 \ hr} \times 0.67 \ hr = 40 \ min$$

The total time of infusion is 6 hours and 40 minutes.

3. Determine the ending time of the infusion by adding the total time of infusion to the beginning time of the infusion.

$$1545 + 6 \ hr \ 40 \ min = 2225$$

The infusion should end at 2225 (10:25 p.m.).

4. For each hour of the infusion, calculate the amount of fluid that has been infused and the remaining fluid in the bag.

At 1645:

a. Amount of fluid infused:

The mL infused is equal to the flow rate (mL/hr) multiplied by the number of hours elapsed. Use dimensional analysis to set up the equation.

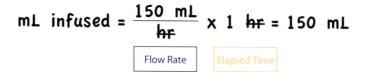

$$\text{mL infused} = \frac{150 \text{ mL}}{\text{hr}} \times 1 \text{ hr} = 150 \text{ mL}$$

Flow Rate   Elapsed Time

b. Remaining fluid:

Subtract the mL infused from the original volume of the infusion.

$$\text{mL left} = 1000 \text{ mL} - 150 \text{ mL} = 850 \text{ mL}$$

Original Volume   Volume Infused

At 1745:

a. Amount of fluid infused:

$$\text{mL infused} = \frac{150 \text{ mL}}{\text{hr}} \times 2 \text{ hr} = 300 \text{ mL}$$

b. Remaining fluid:

$$\text{mL left} = 1000 \text{ mL} - 300 \text{ mL} = 700 \text{ mL}$$

At 1845:

a. Amount of fluid infused:

$$\text{mL infused} = \frac{150 \text{ mL}}{\text{hr}} \times 3 \text{ hr} = 450 \text{ mL}$$

b. Remaining fluid:

$$\text{mL left} = 1000 \text{ mL} - 450 \text{ mL} = 550 \text{ mL}$$

At 1945:

a. Amount of fluid infused:

$$\text{mL infused} = \frac{150 \text{ mL}}{\text{hr}} \times 4 \text{ hr} = 600 \text{ mL}$$

b. Remaining fluid:

$$\text{mL left} = 1000 \text{ mL} - 600 \text{ mL} = 400 \text{ mL}$$

At 2045:

a. Amount of fluid infused:

$$\text{mL infused} = \frac{150 \text{ mL}}{\text{hr}} \times 5 \text{ hr} = 750 \text{ mL}$$

b. Remaining fluid:

$$\text{mL left} = 1000 \text{ mL} - 750 \text{ mL} = 250 \text{ mL}$$

At 2145:

a. Amount of fluid infused:

$$mL\ infused = \frac{150\ mL}{hr} \times 6\ hr = 900\ mL$$

b. Remaining fluid:

$$mL\ left = 1000\ mL - 900\ mL = 100\ mL$$

After 6 hours and 25 minutes (at 2225), the remaining 100 mL of fluid should have infused.

5. Complete the time tape in Figure 13-3, making sure to mark the remaining level of fluid for each hour that has passed.

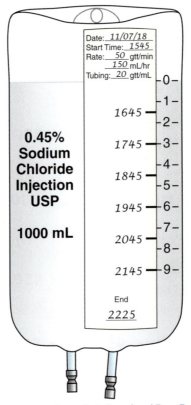

Figure 13-3 Example 2: Completed Time Tape

Practice Preparing Time Tapes for Manually Controlled Infusions

(answers on page 255)

The nurse starts an infusion of 1000 mL of D$_5$W/0.9% sodium chloride solution at 2125. The infusion is to run over 6 hours. No electronic infusion device is available, so the fluid will be infused under manual control. The tubing drop factor is 20 gtt/mL.

1. Calculate the flow rate in mL/hr, rounding to the nearest whole number: _____

2. Calculate the flow rate in gtt/min: _____

3. Determine at what time the infusion will end: _____

For each hour of the infusion, calculate the amount of fluid that has been infused and the remaining fluid in the IV bag.

4. Hour 1: _____

5. Hour 2: _____,

6. Hour 3: _____

7. Hour 4: _____

8. Hour 5: _____

9. Complete the time tape on the bag in Figure 13-4.

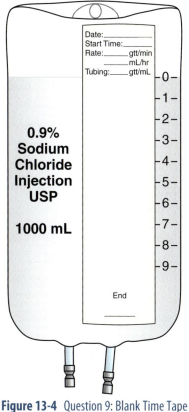

Date:_____
Start Time:_____
Rate:_____ gtt/min
_____ mL/hr
Tubing:_____ gtt/mL

0
1
2
3
4
5
6
7
8
9

0.9% Sodium Chloride Injection USP

1000 mL

End
_____

Figure 13-4 Question 9: Blank Time Tape

Key Points

1. IV fluids administered via electronic pumps, controllers, or syringe pumps are infused using a flow rate of mL/hr.

2. Some pumps can infuse intravenous medications using flow rates based on dosages, such as mg/min, mcg/min, or units/kg/hr.

3. The dosage of the medication in an intermittent IV (also known as an IV piggyback or IVPB) or a syringe, if using a syringe pump, is not used to calculate a mL/hr IV flow rate.

4. If an electronic infusion device is not available, IV fluids may still be infused manually if the drop factor of the IV tubing is known. The most common drop factors are 10 gtt/mL, 15 gtt/mL, 20 gtt/mL, and 60 gtt/mL.

5. IV infusions under manual control require careful monitoring by the nurse. The nurse must periodically count the number of drops of fluid falling into the drip chamber to ensure that the flow rate is correct. A time tape placed on the infusion bag can help the nurse to see if the IV is infusing at the correct time, or if it is significantly ahead or behind schedule.

Chapter Post-Test   *(answers in Unit 4)*

Calculation of Flow Rates in mL/hr

Calculate these flow rates in mL/hr, rounding the flow rate to the nearest whole number.

1. Infuse 450 mL over 7 hours.

2. Infuse 825 mL over 5 hours.

3. Infuse 1000 mL over 3 hours.

4. Infuse 650 mL over 4 hours.

5. Infuse 150 mL over 1 hour.

Calculate the flow rates in mL/hr for these intermittent IV infusions (rounding the flow rate to the nearest whole number).

6. Infuse cefipime (Maxipime) 1.5g diluted in 50 mL 0.9% sodium chloride solution over 45 minutes.

7. Infuse ifosfamide (Ifex) 1 g diluted in 50 mL lactated Ringer's solution over 90 minutes.

8. Infuse leucovorin calcium (Wellcovorin) 200 mg diluted in 250 mL D_5W solution over 2 hours.

9. Infuse mycophenolate mofetil (CellCept) 2 g diluted in 200 mL D_5W solution over 3 hours.

10. Infuse penicillin G (Pfizerpen) 2 million units diluted in 50 mL 0.9% sodium chloride solution over 15 minutes.

Calculate the following flow rates in mL/hr for these syringe pump infusions (rounding the flow rate to the nearest whole number).

11. Infuse ondansetron (Zofran) 4 mg diluted in 10 mL 0.9% sodium chloride solution over 5 minutes.

12. Infuse hydromorphone 1 mg diluted in 5 mL 0.9% sodium chloride solution over 6 minutes.

13. Infuse oxacillin 500 mg diluted in 15 mL 0.9% sodium chloride solution over 10 minutes.

14. Infuse butorphanol (Stadol) 1 mg diluted in 8 mL 0.9% sodium chloride solution over 10 minutes.

15. Infuse gemcitabine (Gemzar) 1 g diluted in 15 mL 0.9% sodium chloride solution over 20 minutes.

Infusion and Completion Times

Calculate the infusion and completion times for these IVs:

16. An IV fluid is infusing at 150 mL/hr; 500 mL of fluid remain in the bag. The current time is 0800.

17. An IV fluid is infusing at 42 mL/hr; 350 mL of fluid remain in the bag. The current time is 1930.

18. An IV fluid is infusing at 130 mL/hr; 475 mL of fluid remain in the bag. The current time is 0100.

19. An IV fluid is infusing at 30 mL/hr; 200 mL of fluid remain in the bag. The current time is 0500.

20. An IV fluid is infusing at 75 mL/hr; 150 mL of fluid remain in the bag. The current time is 1200.

Calculation of Flow Rates in gtt/min

Calculate these flow rates in gtt/min, rounding the flow rate to the nearest whole number.

21. An IV of 1000 mL 0.9% sodium chloride solution is to be infused over 5 hours. The IV tubing has a drop factor of 10 gtt/mL.

22. An IV of 500 mL D_5W solution is to be infused over 3 hours. The IV tubing has a drop factor of 15 gtt/mL.

23. An IV of 750 mL lactated Ringer's solution is to be infused over 7 hours. The IV tubing has a drop factor of 20 gtt/mL.

24. An IV of 250 mL 0.45% sodium chloride solution is to be infused over 12 hours. The IV tubing has a drop factor of 60 gtt/mL.

25. An IV of 1 L D_5W solution is to be infused over 8 hours. The IV tubing has a drop factor of 20 gtt/mL.

Calculate the gtt/min flow rate from these mL/hr flow rates.

26. An IV of D_5W/0.45% sodium chloride solution is infusing at 50 mL/hr. The drop factor of the tubing is 15 gtt/mL.

27. An IV of 0.9% sodium chloride solution is infusing at 160 mL/hr. The drop factor of the tubing is 20 gtt/mL.

28. An IV of $D_{10}W$ solution is infusing at 8 mL/hr. The drop factor of the tubing is 60 gtt/mL.

29. An IV of Plasma-Lyte R solution is infusing at 83 mL/hr. The drop factor of the tubing is 20 gtt/mL.

30. An IV of 0.45% sodium chloride solution is infusing at 90 mL/hr. The drop factor of the tubing is 20 gtt/mL.

Infusion and Completion Times

Calculate infusion and completion times for these IVs.

31. An IV is infusing at 31 gtt/min; 375 mL of fluid remain in the bag. The drop factor of the tubing is 10 gtt/mL. The current time is 1630.

32. An IV is infusing at 45 gtt/min; 250 mL of fluid remain in the bag. The drop factor of the tubing is 15 gtt/mL. The current time is 0500.

33. An IV is infusing at 12 gtt/min; 175 mL of fluid remain in the bag. The drop factor of the tubing is 60 gtt/mL. The current time is 2300.

34. An IV is infusing at 60 gtt/min; 500 mL of fluid remain in the bag. The drop factor of the tubing is 60 gtt/mL. The current time is 0100.

35. An IV is infusing at 38 gtt/min; 950 mL of fluid remain in the bag. The drop factor of the tubing is 10 gtt/mL. The current time is 1430.

Manual Control Flow Rates

The nurse starts an infusion of 1000 mL D_5W/0.9% sodium chloride solution at 2100. The infusion is to run over 8 hours. No electronic pump is available, so the fluid will be infused under manual control. The tubing drop factor is 15 gtt/mL.

36. Calculate the flow rate in mL/hr (rounding to the nearest whole number).

37. Calculate the flow rate in gtt/min.

38. Determine the time the infusion will end.

For each hour of the infusion, calculate the amount of fluid that has been infused and the remaining fluid in the IV bag.

39. Hour 1

40. Hour 2

41. Hour 3

42. Hour 4

43. Hour 5

44. Hour 6

45. Hour 7

46. Hour 8

47. Complete the time tape on the bag in Figure 13-5

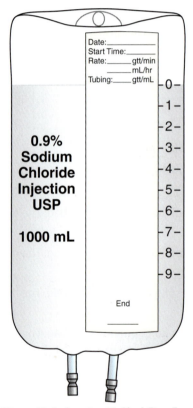

Figure 13-5 Question 47: Blank Time Tape

Answers to Practice Questions

Practice Calculating mL/hr Flow Rates for Continuous IV Fluids

1. $\dfrac{mL}{hr} = \dfrac{1250\ mL}{8\ hr} = 156.25\dfrac{mL}{hr} = 156\ \dfrac{mL}{hr}$

2. $\dfrac{mL}{hr} = \dfrac{250\ mL}{2\ hr} = 125\ \dfrac{mL}{hr}$

3. $\dfrac{mL}{hr} = \dfrac{1000\ mL}{12\ hr} = 83.3 = 83\ \dfrac{mL}{hr}$

4. $\dfrac{mL}{hr} = \dfrac{500\ mL}{4\ hr} = 125\ \dfrac{mL}{hr}$

5. $\dfrac{mL}{hr} = \dfrac{750\ mL}{5\ hr} = 150\ \dfrac{mL}{hr}$

6. $\dfrac{mL}{hr} = \dfrac{1000\ mL}{1\ \cancel{L}} \times \dfrac{1\ \cancel{L}}{4\ hr} = \dfrac{1000\ mL}{4\ hr} = 250\ \dfrac{mL}{hr}$

7. $\dfrac{mL}{hr} = \dfrac{800\ mL}{12\ hr} = 66.7 = 67\ \dfrac{mL}{hr}$

8. $\dfrac{mL}{hr} = \dfrac{1000\ mL}{1\ \cancel{L}} \times \dfrac{2.5\ \cancel{L}}{15\ hr} = \dfrac{1000\ mL \times 2.5}{15\ hr} = 166.7 = 167\ \dfrac{mL}{hr}$

9. $\dfrac{mL}{hr} = \dfrac{1000\ mL}{1\ \cancel{L}} \times \dfrac{2\ \cancel{L}}{18\ hr} = \dfrac{1000\ mL \times 2}{18\ hr} = 111.1 = 111\ \dfrac{mL}{hr}$

10. $\dfrac{mL}{hr} = \dfrac{300\ mL}{1.5\ hr} = 200\ \dfrac{mL}{hr}$

Practice Calculating mL/hr Flow Rates for Intermittent IV Fluids

1. $\dfrac{mL}{hr} = \dfrac{50\ mL}{30\ min} \times \dfrac{60\ min}{1\ hr} = \dfrac{50\ mL \times 60}{30\ hr} = 100\dfrac{mL}{hr}$ or $\dfrac{mL}{hr} = \dfrac{50\ mL}{0.5\ hr} = 100\ \dfrac{mL}{hr}$

2. $\dfrac{mL}{hr} = \dfrac{100\ mL}{45\ min} \times \dfrac{60\ min}{1\ hr} = \dfrac{100\ mL \times 60}{45\ hr} = 133.3 = 133\ \dfrac{mL}{hr}$

3. $\dfrac{mL}{hr} = \dfrac{500\ mL}{2\ hr} = 250\ \dfrac{mL}{hr}$

4. $\dfrac{mL}{hr} = \dfrac{140\ mL}{2\ hr} = 70\ \dfrac{mL}{hr}$

5. $\dfrac{mL}{hr} = \dfrac{100\ mL}{30\ min} \times \dfrac{60\ min}{1\ hr} = \dfrac{100\ mL \times 60}{30\ hr} = 200\ \dfrac{mL}{hr}$

6. $\dfrac{mL}{hr} = \dfrac{50\ mL}{15\ min} \times \dfrac{60\ min}{1\ hr} = \dfrac{50\ mL \times 60}{15\ hr} = 200\ \dfrac{mL}{hr}$

7. $\dfrac{mL}{hr} = \dfrac{100\ mL}{45\ min} \times \dfrac{60\ min}{1\ hr} = \dfrac{100\ mL \times 60}{45\ hr} = 133.3 = 133\ \dfrac{mL}{hr}$

8. $\dfrac{mL}{hr} = \dfrac{250\ mL}{4\ hr} = 62.5 = 63\ \dfrac{mL}{hr}$

9. $\dfrac{mL}{hr} = \dfrac{100\ mL}{30\ min} \times \dfrac{60\ min}{1\ hr} = \dfrac{100\ mL \times 60}{30\ hr} = 200\ \dfrac{mL}{hr}$

10. $\dfrac{mL}{hr} = \dfrac{50\ mL}{4\ hr} = 12.5 = 13\ \dfrac{mL}{hr}$

Practice Calculating mL/hr Flow Rates for Syringe Pumps

1. $\dfrac{mL}{hr} = \dfrac{10\ mL}{5\ \cancel{min}} \times \dfrac{60\ \cancel{min}}{1\ hr} = \dfrac{10\ mL \times 60}{5\ hr} = \dfrac{600\ mL}{5\ hr} = 120\ \dfrac{mL}{hr}$

2. $\dfrac{mL}{hr} = \dfrac{10\ mL}{2\ \cancel{min}} \times \dfrac{60\ \cancel{min}}{1\ hr} = \dfrac{10\ mL \times 60}{2\ hr} = \dfrac{600\ mL}{2\ hr} = 300\ \dfrac{mL}{hr}$

3. $\dfrac{mL}{hr} = \dfrac{12\ mL}{20\ \cancel{min}} \times \dfrac{60\ \cancel{min}}{1\ hr} = \dfrac{12\ mL \times 60}{20\ hr} = \dfrac{720\ mL}{20\ hr} = 36\ \dfrac{mL}{hr}$

4. $\dfrac{mL}{hr} = \dfrac{20\ mL}{15\ \cancel{min}} \times \dfrac{60\ \cancel{min}}{1\ hr} = \dfrac{20\ mL \times 60}{15\ hr} = \dfrac{1200\ mL}{15\ hr} = 80\ \dfrac{mL}{hr}$

5. $\dfrac{mL}{hr} = \dfrac{5\ mL}{5\ \cancel{min}} \times \dfrac{60\ \cancel{min}}{1\ hr} = \dfrac{5\ mL \times 60}{5\ hr} = \dfrac{300\ mL}{5\ hr} = 60\ \dfrac{mL}{hr}$

6. $\dfrac{mL}{hr} = \dfrac{10\ mL}{10\ \cancel{min}} \times \dfrac{60\ \cancel{min}}{1\ hr} = \dfrac{10\ mL \times 60}{10\ hr} = \dfrac{600\ mL}{10\ hr} = 60\ \dfrac{mL}{hr}$

7. $\dfrac{mL}{hr} = \dfrac{5\ mL}{10\ \cancel{min}} \times \dfrac{60\ \cancel{min}}{1\ hr} = \dfrac{5\ mL \times 60}{10\ hr} = \dfrac{300\ mL}{10\ hr} = 30\ \dfrac{mL}{hr}$

8. $\dfrac{mL}{hr} = \dfrac{4\ mL}{5\ \cancel{min}} \times \dfrac{60\ \cancel{min}}{1\ hr} = \dfrac{4\ mL \times 60}{5\ hr} = \dfrac{240\ mL}{5\ hr} = 48\ \dfrac{mL}{hr}$

9. $\dfrac{mL}{hr} = \dfrac{25\ mL}{30\ \cancel{min}} \times \dfrac{60\ \cancel{min}}{1\ hr} = \dfrac{25\ mL \times 60}{30\ hr} = \dfrac{1500\ mL}{30\ hr} = 50\ \dfrac{mL}{hr}$

10. $\dfrac{mL}{hr} = \dfrac{10\ mL}{7\ \cancel{min}} \times \dfrac{60\ \cancel{min}}{1\ hr} = \dfrac{10\ mL \times 60}{7\ hr} = \dfrac{600\ mL}{7\ hr} = 85.7 = 86\ \dfrac{mL}{hr}$

Practice Calculating Infusion and Completion Times for mL/hr Flow Rates

1. infusion time (hr) = $\dfrac{1 \text{ hr}}{125 \text{ mL}}$ x 900 mL = $\dfrac{1 \text{ hr} \times 900}{125}$ = $\dfrac{900 \text{ hr}}{125}$ = **7.2 hr**

   conversion of *.2* hours into minutes:

   min = $\dfrac{60 \text{ min}}{1 \text{ hr}}$ x 0.2 hr = $\dfrac{60 \text{ min} \times 0.2}{1}$ = **12 min**

   completion time = 0855 + 7 hr, 12 min = **1607 (4:07 p.m.)**

2. infusion time (hr) = $\dfrac{1 \text{ hr}}{67 \text{ mL}}$ x 275 mL = $\dfrac{1 \text{ hr} \times 275}{67}$ = $\dfrac{275 \text{ hr}}{67}$ = **4.1 hr**

   conversion of *.1* hours into minutes:

   min = $\dfrac{60 \text{ min}}{1 \text{ hr}}$ x 0.1 hr = $\dfrac{60 \text{ min} \times 0.1}{1}$ = **6 min**

   completion time = 1325 + 4 hr, 6 min = **1731 (5:31 p.m.)**

3. infusion time (hr) = $\dfrac{1 \text{ hr}}{175 \text{ mL}}$ x 700 mL = $\dfrac{1 \text{ hr} \times 700}{175}$ = $\dfrac{700 \text{ hr}}{175}$ = **4 hr**

   completion time = 1622 + 4 hr = **2022 (8:22 p.m.)**

4. infusion time (hr) = $\dfrac{1 \text{ hr}}{21 \text{ mL}}$ x 150 mL = $\dfrac{1 \text{ hr} \times 150}{21}$ = $\dfrac{150 \text{ hr}}{21}$ = **7.14 hr**

   conversion of *.14* hours into minutes:

   min = $\dfrac{60 \text{ min}}{1 \text{ hr}}$ x 0.14 hr = $\dfrac{60 \text{ min} \times 0.14}{1}$ = **8 min**

   completion time = 1930 + 7 hr, 8 min = **0238 (2:38 a.m.)**

5. infusion time (hr) = $\dfrac{1 \text{ hr}}{150 \text{ mL}}$ x 500 mL = $\dfrac{1 \text{ hr} \times 500}{150}$ = $\dfrac{500 \text{ hr}}{150}$ = **3.33 hr**

   conversion of *.33* hours into minutes:

   min = $\dfrac{60 \text{ min}}{1 \text{ hr}}$ x 0.33 hr = $\dfrac{60 \text{ min} \times 0.33}{1}$ = **19.8 = 20 min**

   completion time = 2208 + 3 hr, 20 min = **0128 (1:28 a.m.)**

6. infusion time (hr) = $\frac{1 \text{ hr}}{80 \text{ mL}}$ x 650 mL = $\frac{1 \text{ hr x } 650}{80}$ = $\frac{650 \text{ hr}}{80}$ = 8.13 hr

conversion of .13 hours into minutes:

min = $\frac{60 \text{ min}}{1 \text{ hr}}$ x 0.13 hr = $\frac{60 \text{ min x } 0.13}{1}$ = 7.8 = 8 min

completion time = 0540 + 8 hr, 8 min = 1348 (1:48 p.m.)

7. infusion time (hr) = $\frac{1 \text{ hr}}{50 \text{ mL}}$ x 950 mL = $\frac{1 \text{ hr x } 950}{50}$ = $\frac{950 \text{ hr}}{50}$ = 19 hr

completion time = 1200 + 19 hr = 0700 (7:00 a.m.)

8. infusion time (hr) = $\frac{1 \text{ hr}}{25 \text{ mL}}$ x 250 mL = $\frac{1 \text{ hr x } 250}{25}$ = $\frac{250 \text{ hr}}{25}$ = 10 hr

completion time = 1849 + 10 hr = 0449 (4:49 a.m.)

9. infusion time (hr) = $\frac{1 \text{ hr}}{200 \text{ mL}}$ x 1000 mL = $\frac{1 \text{ hr x } 1000}{200}$ = $\frac{1000 \text{ hr}}{200}$ = 5 hr

completion time = 1427 + 5 hr = 1927 (7:27 p.m.)

10. infusion time (hr) = $\frac{1 \text{ hr}}{73 \text{ mL}}$ x 425 mL = $\frac{1 \text{ hr x } 425}{73}$ = $\frac{425 \text{ hr}}{73}$ = 5.82 hr

conversion of .82 hours into minutes:

min = $\frac{60 \text{ min}}{1 \text{ hr}}$ x 0.82 hr = $\frac{60 \text{ min x } 0.82}{1}$ = 49 min

completion time = 2300 + 5 hr, 49 min = 0449 (4:49 a.m.)

Practice Calculating gtt/min Flow Rates for IV Fluids Under Manual Control

1. $\dfrac{gtt}{min} = \dfrac{15\ gtt}{1\ mL} \times \dfrac{1000\ mL}{10\ hr} \times \dfrac{1\ hr}{60\ min} = \dfrac{15\ gtt \times 1000}{10 \times 60\ min} = \dfrac{15{,}000\ gtt}{600\ min} = 25\ \dfrac{gtt}{min}$

2. $\dfrac{gtt}{min} = \dfrac{10\ gtt}{1\ mL} \times \dfrac{500\ mL}{4\ hr} \times \dfrac{1\ hr}{60\ min} = \dfrac{10\ gtt \times 500}{4 \times 60\ min} = \dfrac{5000\ gtt}{240\ min} = 20.8 = 21\ \dfrac{gtt}{min}$

3. $\dfrac{gtt}{min} = \dfrac{20\ gtt}{1\ mL} \times \dfrac{1000\ mL}{6\ hr} \times \dfrac{1\ hr}{60\ min} = \dfrac{20\ gtt \times 1000}{6 \times 60\ min}$

   $= \dfrac{20{,}000\ gtt}{360\ min} = 55.5 = 56\ \dfrac{gtt}{min}$

4. $\dfrac{gtt}{min} = \dfrac{60\ gtt}{1\ mL} \times \dfrac{100\ mL}{2\ hr} \times \dfrac{1\ hr}{60\ min} = \dfrac{60\ gtt \times 100}{2 \times 60\ min} = \dfrac{6000\ gtt}{120\ min} = 50\ \dfrac{gtt}{min}$

5. $\dfrac{gtt}{min} = \dfrac{15\ gtt}{1\ mL} \times \dfrac{750\ mL}{8\ hr} \times \dfrac{1\ hr}{60\ min} = \dfrac{15\ gtt \times 750}{8 \times 60\ min} = \dfrac{11{,}250\ gtt}{480\ min} = 23.4 = 23\ \dfrac{gtt}{min}$

6. $\dfrac{gtt}{min} = \dfrac{20\ gtt}{1\ mL} \times \dfrac{1000\ mL}{12\ hr} \times \dfrac{1\ hr}{60\ min} = \dfrac{20\ gtt \times 1000}{12 \times 60\ min}$

   $= \dfrac{20{,}000\ gtt}{720\ min} = 27.8 = 28\ \dfrac{gtt}{min}$

7. $\dfrac{gtt}{min} = \dfrac{20\ gtt}{1\ mL} \times \dfrac{500\ mL}{3\ hr} \times \dfrac{1\ hr}{60\ min} = \dfrac{20\ gtt \times 500}{3 \times 60\ min} = \dfrac{10{,}000\ gtt}{180\ min} = 55.6 = 56\ \dfrac{gtt}{min}$

8. $\dfrac{gtt}{min} = \dfrac{10\ gtt}{1\ mL} \times \dfrac{300\ mL}{90\ min} = \dfrac{10\ gtt \times 300}{90\ min} = \dfrac{3000\ gtt}{90\ min} = 33.3 = 33\ \dfrac{gtt}{min}$

9. $\dfrac{gtt}{min} = \dfrac{10\ gtt}{1\ mL} \times \dfrac{1500\ mL}{15\ hr} \times \dfrac{1\ hr}{60\ min} = \dfrac{10\ gtt \times 1500}{15 \times 60\ min}$

   $= \dfrac{15{,}000\ gtt}{900\ min} = 16.7 = 17\ \dfrac{gtt}{min}$

10. $\dfrac{gtt}{min} = \dfrac{60\ gtt}{1\ mL} \times \dfrac{50\ mL}{60\ min} = \dfrac{60\ gtt \times 50}{60\ min} = \dfrac{3000\ gtt}{60\ min} = 50\ \dfrac{gtt}{min}$

Practice Calculating gtt/min Flow Rates From mL/hr Flow Rates

1. $\dfrac{gtt}{min} = \dfrac{10\ gtt}{1\ mL} \times \dfrac{125\ mL}{1\ hr} \times \dfrac{1\ hr}{60\ min} = \dfrac{10\ gtt \times 125}{1 \times 60\ min} = \dfrac{1250\ gtt}{60\ min} = 20.8 = 21\ \dfrac{gtt}{min}$

2. $\dfrac{gtt}{min} = \dfrac{20\ gtt}{1\ mL} \times \dfrac{150\ mL}{1\ hr} \times \dfrac{1\ hr}{60\ min} = \dfrac{20\ gtt \times 150}{1 \times 60\ min} = \dfrac{3000\ gtt}{60\ min} = 50\ \dfrac{gtt}{min}$

3. $\dfrac{gtt}{min} = \dfrac{15\ gtt}{1\ mL} \times \dfrac{63\ mL}{1\ hr} \times \dfrac{1\ hr}{60\ min} = \dfrac{15\ gtt \times 63}{1 \times 60\ min} = \dfrac{945\ gtt}{60\ min} = 15.8 = 16\ \dfrac{gtt}{min}$

4. $\dfrac{gtt}{min} = \dfrac{60\ gtt}{1\ mL} \times \dfrac{15\ mL}{1\ hr} \times \dfrac{1\ hr}{60\ min} = \dfrac{60\ gtt \times 15}{1 \times 60\ min} = \dfrac{900\ gtt}{60\ min} = 15\ \dfrac{gtt}{min}$

5. $\dfrac{gtt}{min} = \dfrac{20\ gtt}{1\ mL} \times \dfrac{175\ mL}{1\ hr} \times \dfrac{1\ hr}{60\ min} = \dfrac{20\ gtt \times 175}{1 \times 60\ min} = \dfrac{3500\ gtt}{60\ min} = 58.3 = 58\ \dfrac{gtt}{min}$

6. $\dfrac{gtt}{min} = \dfrac{10\ gtt}{1\ mL} \times \dfrac{50\ mL}{1\ hr} \times \dfrac{1\ hr}{60\ min} = \dfrac{10\ gtt \times 50}{1 \times 60\ min} = \dfrac{500\ gtt}{60\ min} = 8.3 = 8\ \dfrac{gtt}{min}$

7. $\dfrac{gtt}{min} = \dfrac{15\ gtt}{1\ mL} \times \dfrac{160\ mL}{1\ hr} \times \dfrac{1\ hr}{60\ min} = \dfrac{15\ gtt \times 160}{1 \times 60\ min} = \dfrac{2400\ gtt}{60\ min} = 40\ \dfrac{gtt}{min}$

8. $\dfrac{gtt}{min} = \dfrac{20\ gtt}{1\ mL} \times \dfrac{83\ mL}{1\ hr} \times \dfrac{1\ hr}{60\ min} = \dfrac{20\ gtt \times 83}{1 \times 60\ min} = \dfrac{1660\ gtt}{60\ min} = 27.7 = 28\ \dfrac{gtt}{min}$

9. $\dfrac{gtt}{min} = \dfrac{60\ gtt}{1\ mL} \times \dfrac{21\ mL}{1\ hr} \times \dfrac{1\ hr}{60\ min} = \dfrac{60\ gtt \times 21}{1 \times 60\ min} = \dfrac{1260\ gtt}{60\ min} = 21\ \dfrac{gtt}{min}$

10. $\dfrac{gtt}{min} = \dfrac{10\ gtt}{1\ mL} \times \dfrac{250\ mL}{1\ hr} \times \dfrac{1\ hr}{60\ min} = \dfrac{10\ gtt \times 250}{1 \times 60\ min} = \dfrac{2500\ gtt}{60\ min} = 41.7 = 42\ \dfrac{gtt}{min}$

Practice Calculating Infusion and Completion Times for gtt/min Flow Rates

1. infusion time (hr) = $\dfrac{1 \text{ hr}}{60 \text{ min}} \times \dfrac{1 \text{ min}}{28 \text{ gtt}} \times \dfrac{60 \text{ gtt}}{1 \text{ mL}} \times 125 \text{ mL} = \dfrac{1 \text{ hr} \times 125}{28}$

$= \dfrac{125 \text{ hr}}{28} = 4.46 \text{ hr}$

conversion of .46 hours into minutes:

min = $\dfrac{60 \text{ min}}{1 \text{ hr}} \times 0.46 \text{ hr} = \dfrac{60 \text{ min} \times 0.46}{1} = 28 \text{ min}$

completion time = 1215 + 4 hr, 28 min = 1643 (4:43 p.m.)

2. infusion time (hr) = $\dfrac{1 \text{ hr}}{60 \text{ min}} \times \dfrac{1 \text{ min}}{42 \text{ gtt}} \times \dfrac{15 \text{ gtt}}{1 \text{ mL}} \times 425 \text{ mL} = \dfrac{1 \text{ hr} \times 15 \times 425}{60 \times 42}$

$= \dfrac{6375 \text{ hr}}{2520} = 2.53 \text{ hr}$

conversion of .53 hours into minutes:

min = $\dfrac{60 \text{ min}}{1 \text{ hr}} \times 0.53 \text{ hr} = \dfrac{60 \text{ min} \times 0.53}{1} = 32 \text{ min}$

completion time = 0300 + 2 hr, 32 min = 0532 (5:32 a.m.)

3. infusion time (hr) = $\dfrac{1 \text{ hr}}{60 \text{ min}} \times \dfrac{1 \text{ min}}{54 \text{ gtt}} \times \dfrac{10 \text{ gtt}}{1 \text{ mL}} \times 150 \text{ mL} = \dfrac{1 \text{ hr} \times 10 \times 150}{60 \times 54}$

$= \dfrac{1500 \text{ hr}}{3240} = 0.46 \text{ hr}$

conversion of .46 hours into minutes:

min = $\dfrac{60 \text{ min}}{1 \text{ hr}} \times 0.46 \text{ hr} = \dfrac{60 \text{ min} \times 0.46}{1} = 28 \text{ min}$

completion time = 1620 + 28 min = 1648 (4:48 p.m.)

4. infusion time (hr) = $\dfrac{1 \text{ hr}}{60 \text{ min}} \times \dfrac{1 \text{ min}}{12 \text{ gtt}} \times \dfrac{15 \text{ gtt}}{1 \text{ mL}} \times 525 \text{ mL} = \dfrac{1 \text{ hr} \times 15 \times 525}{60 \times 12}$

$= \dfrac{7875 \text{ hr}}{720} = 10.94 \text{ hr}$

conversion of .94 hours into minutes:

min = $\dfrac{60 \text{ min}}{1 \text{ hr}} \times 0.94 \text{ hr} = \dfrac{60 \text{ min} \times 0.94}{1} = 56 \text{ min}$

completion time = 2025 + 10 hr, 56 min = 0721 (7:21 a.m.)

5. infusion time (hr) = $\dfrac{1 \text{ hr}}{60 \text{ min}}$ x $\dfrac{1 \text{ min}}{15 \text{ gtt}}$ x $\dfrac{60 \text{ gtt}}{1 \text{ mL}}$ x 250 mL = $\dfrac{1 \text{ hr} \times 250}{15}$

$= \dfrac{250 \text{ hr}}{15} = 16.67 \text{ hr}$

conversion of .67 hours into minutes:

min = $\dfrac{60 \text{ min}}{1 \text{ hr}}$ x 0.67 hr = $\dfrac{60 \text{ min} \times 0.67}{1}$ = 40 min

completion time = 0545 + 16 hr, 40 min = 2225 (10:25 p.m.)

6. infusion time (hr) = $\dfrac{1 \text{ hr}}{60 \text{ min}}$ x $\dfrac{1 \text{ min}}{26 \text{ gtt}}$ x $\dfrac{15 \text{ gtt}}{1 \text{ mL}}$ x 225 mL

$= \dfrac{1 \text{ hr} \times 15 \times 225}{60 \times 26} = \dfrac{3375 \text{ hr}}{1560} = 2.16 \text{ hr}$

conversion of .16 hours into minutes:

min = $\dfrac{60 \text{ min}}{1 \text{ hr}}$ x 0.16 hr = $\dfrac{60 \text{ min} \times 0.16}{1}$ = 10 min

completion time = 2350 + 2 hr, 10 min = 0200 (2:00 a.m.)

7. infusion time (hr) = $\dfrac{1 \text{ hr}}{60 \text{ min}}$ x $\dfrac{1 \text{ min}}{18 \text{ gtt}}$ x $\dfrac{60 \text{ gtt}}{1 \text{ mL}}$ x 100 mL

$= \dfrac{1 \text{ hr} \times 100}{18} = \dfrac{100 \text{ hr}}{18} = 5.56 \text{ hr}$

conversion of .56 hours into minutes:

min = $\dfrac{60 \text{ min}}{1 \text{ hr}}$ x 0.56 hr = $\dfrac{60 \text{ min} \times 0.56}{1}$ = 34 min

completion time = 0110 + 5 hr, 34 min = 0644 (6:44 a.m.)

8. infusion time (hr) = $\dfrac{1 \text{ hr}}{60 \text{ min}}$ x $\dfrac{1 \text{ min}}{48 \text{ gtt}}$ x $\dfrac{10 \text{ gtt}}{1 \text{ mL}}$ x 475 mL

$= \dfrac{1 \text{ hr} \times 10 \times 475}{60 \times 48} = \dfrac{4750 \text{ hr}}{2880} = 1.65 \text{ hr}$

conversion of .65 hours into minutes:

min = $\dfrac{60 \text{ min}}{1 \text{ hr}}$ x 0.65 hr = $\dfrac{60 \text{ min} \times 0.65}{1}$ = 39 min

completion time = 1415 + 1 hr, 39 min = 1554 (3:54 p.m.)

9. infusion time (hr) = $\dfrac{1\ hr}{60\ min} \times \dfrac{1\ min}{32\ gtt} \times \dfrac{20\ gtt}{1\ mL} \times 350\ mL$

$= \dfrac{1\ hr \times 20 \times 350}{60 \times 32} = \dfrac{7000\ hr}{1920} = 3.65\ hr$

conversion of .65 hours into minutes:

min = $\dfrac{60\ min}{1\ hr} \times 0.65\ hr = \dfrac{60\ min \times 0.65}{1} = 39\ min$

completion time = 0700 + 3 hr, 39 min = 1039 (10:39 a.m.)

10. infusion time (hr) = $\dfrac{1\ hr}{60\ min} \times \dfrac{1\ min}{36\ gtt} \times \dfrac{15\ gtt}{1\ mL} \times 950\ mL$

$= \dfrac{1\ hr \times 15 \times 950}{60 \times 36} = \dfrac{14,250\ hr}{2160} = 6.6\ hr$

conversion of .6 hours into minutes:

min = $\dfrac{60\ min}{1\ hr} \times 0.6\ hr = \dfrac{60\ min \times 0.6}{1} = 36\ min$

completion time = 1740 + 6 hr, 36 min = 0016 (00:16 a.m.)

Practice Preparing Time Tapes for Manually Controlled Infusions

1. **Flow rate (mL/hr):**

$$\frac{mL}{hr} = \frac{1000 \ mL}{6 \ hr} = 166.7 = 167 \ \frac{mL}{hr}$$

2. **Flow rate (gtt/min):**

$$\frac{gtt}{min} = \frac{20 \ gtt}{1 \ mL} \times \frac{1000 \ mL}{6 \ hr} \times \frac{1 \ hr}{60 \ min} = \frac{20 \ gtt \times 1000}{6 \times 60 \ min} = \frac{20,000 \ gtt}{360 \ min}$$

$$= 55.6 = 56 \ \frac{gtt}{min}$$

3. **Infusion end time:**

2125 + 5 hr 59 min = 0324 (3:24 a.m.)

4. **Hour 1:**

$$mL \ infused = \frac{167 \ mL}{hr} \times 1 \ hr = 167 \ mL$$

mL remaining = 1000 mL − 167 mL = 833 mL

5. **Hour 2:**

$$mL \ infused = \frac{167 \ mL}{hr} \times 2 \ hr = 334 \ mL$$

mL remaining = 1000 mL − 334 mL = 666 mL

6. **Hour 3:**

$$mL \ infused = \frac{167 \ mL}{hr} \times 3 \ hr = 501 \ mL$$

mL remaining = 1000 mL − 501 mL = 499 mL

7. **Hour 4:**

$$mL \ infused = \frac{167 \ mL}{hr} \times 4 \ hr = 668 \ mL$$

mL remaining = 1000 mL − 668 mL = 332 mL

8. **Hour 5:**

mL infused = $\dfrac{167\ mL}{hr}$ x 5 hr = 835 mL

mL remaining = 1000 mL - 835 mL = 165 mL

After 5 hr, 59 min (at 0324) the remaining 165 mL should be infused.

9. **See Figure 13-6.**

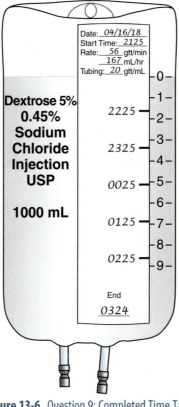

Figure 13-6 Question 9: Completed Time Tape

Unit 2 Post-Test

(answers in Unit 4)

After studying Unit 2, "Medication Administration," answer these questions and solve the problems. In each group, circle the error in notation.

1. 7.0 mg   3.5 g   2.4 cm   8.001 kg

2. 21 kg   26 mcg   1.34 gm   636 mg

3. 5 mg   8.26 Ltr   83 mL   187 mg

Write the correct notation for these quantities.

4. 78 liters _____

5. 440 micrograms _____

6. 80 kilograms _____

7. 19 grams _____

8. 10 fluid ounces _____

Calculate these conversions. Do not round the answers.

9. 82 mcg = _____ mg

10. 2010 mL = _____ L

11. 865 mg = _____ g

12. 0.154 L = _____ mL

13. 0.02 kg = _____ g

14. 4 g = _____ mg

15. 2.102 g = _____ mcg

16. 915 mg = _____ kg

17. 85 mL = _____ L

Calculate these conversions. Round answers to the nearest tenth.

18. 8.2 lb = _____ kg

19. 12 cm = _____ in

20. 2 fl oz = _____ mL

21. 5 tsp = _____ mL

22. 51 kg = _____ lb

23. 18 in = _____ cm

24. 2.6 lb = _____ g

25. 77 mL = _____ fl oz

26. 30 mL = _____ tsp

Choose True or False for each statement.

27. The apothecary system of measure should not be used to prescribe, compound, dispense, or administer medications.   True   False

28. Most medication errors are preventable events.   True   False

29. The abbreviation NPO means "nothing by mouth."   True   False

30. The nurse should document administration of a medication on the Medication Administration Record before it is given.   True   False

31. The nurse should call the provider if a medication order is incomplete or illegible.   True   False

Choose the best answer(s) for each question.

32. What is the purpose of a state's Nurse Practice Act?
    a. to protect the health, safety, and welfare of the public
    b. to protect nurses from legal charges
    c. to protect nurses from violent patients
    d. to punish nurses who make mistakes

33. Which patient identifiers may be used to verify patient identity?
    a. patient's name and bed assignment
    b. patient's name and date of birth
    c. patient's date of birth and room number
    d. patient's name and room number

34. Which dosage is written incorrectly?
    a. 41 mcg
    b. 4.1 mcg
    c. 65.0 mcg
    d. 0.65 mcg

35. Which item is not one of the six rights?
    a. patient
    b. dose
    c. time
    d. physician

36. How often should a drug that is ordered to be administered b.i.d. be given?
    a. once per day
    b. twice per day
    c. three times per day
    d. four times per day

37. Which abbreviation should not be used in charting dosages?
    a. cc
    b. PRN
    c. subcut
    d. mg

38. Which drop factor is considered to be part of a microdrip administration set?
    a. 10 gtt/mL
    b. 15 gtt/mL
    c. 20 gtt/mL
    d. 60 gtt/mL

39. When using manual gravity flow, which factor can increase the rate at which fluids infuse into a patient?
    a. a kink in the IV tubing
    b. hanging the IV bag high above the patient
    c. lowering the IV bag level to the patient's IV site
    d. closing the roller clamp

40. Which item should be written on the label of an IV bag containing medication?
    a. patient identification information
    b. name of the fluid infusing
    c. name and dosage of the medication added to the bag
    d. all of the above

41. Which component is not necessary for a medication order?
    a. the chemical name of the medication
    b. the name of the provider ordering the medication
    c. the name of the patient
    d. the route of administration

42. When receiving a telephone order from a provider, what must the nurse do?
    a. Have another nurse verify the order with the provider.
    b. Read back the order to the provider.
    c. Have the pharmacist co-sign the order.
    d. Ask the provider to come in to write the order—nurses cannot take telephone orders.

Match the abbreviation in Column A with the correct meaning in Column B.

Column A

43. _____ p.c.

44. _____ t.i.d.

45. _____ a.c.

46. _____ PO

47. _____ NKA

48. _____ IM

49. _____ IV

50. _____ q

51. _____ STAT

Column B

a. intravenous

b. no known allergies

c. immediately

d. every

e. after meals

f. orally

g. before meals

h. intramuscular

i. three times per day

Answer the questions for the medication label in each figure.

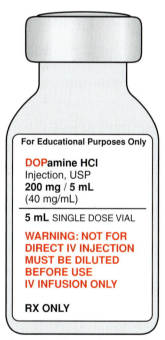

Figure U2PT-1 Medication Label

52. What is the name of the drug in Figure U2PT-1?

53. What is the dosage strength of the drug in Figure U2PT-1?

54. How many mL are in the vial in Figure U2PT-1?

55. Is the vial in Figure U2PT-1 a single- or multiple-dose vial?

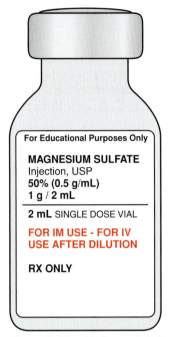

Figure U2PT-2 Medication Label

56. What is the dosage strength of the drug in Figure U2PT-2?

57. Is the vial in Figure U2PT-2 a single- or multiple-dose vial?

58. How many mL are in the vial in Figure U2PT-2?

59. By which two routes may the drug in Figure U2PT-2 be given?

Calculate the volume (mL) of medication that the nurse should administer for these oral medications. Round the answers to the nearest whole mg or mL.

60. The provider orders acetaminophen 320 mg, PO, every 4 hours, PRN fever. The pharmacy provides acetaminophen in a suspension containing 160 mg in 5 mL.

61. The provider orders loperamide 4 mg, PO, after every loose stool. The pharmacy provides loperamide in a liquid containing 4 mg in 5 mL.

62. The provider orders lamivudine 150 mg, PO, every 12 hours. The pharmacy supplies lamivudine in an oral solution containing 10 mg in 1 mL.

Indicate the quantities on the hypodermic syringe in each figure.

63. 0.34 mL (Fig. U2PT-3)

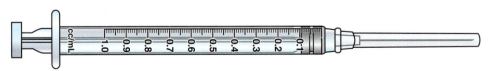

Figure U2PT-3 1-mL Syringe

64. 2.6 mL (Fig. U2PT-4)

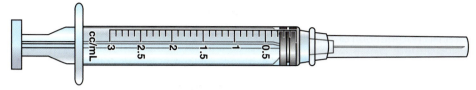

Figure U2PT-4 3-mL Syringe

65. 4.2 mL (Fig. U2PT-5)

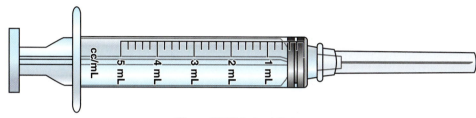

Figure U2PT-5 5-mL Syringe

66. 8.6 mL (Fig. U2PT-6)

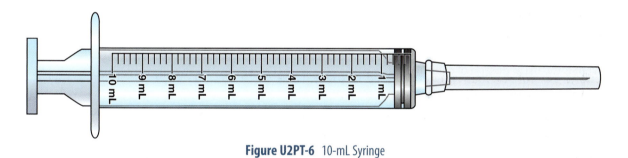

Figure U2PT-6 10-mL Syringe

Calculate the volume (mL) of medication to be administered per dose for these parenteral orders.

67. The provider orders adenosine 1 mg, IV, STAT. The pharmacy provides adenosine in vials containing 3 mg in 1 mL. Round to the nearest hundredth mL.

68. The provider orders procainamide 150 mg, IV, every 5 minutes up to 5 doses. The pharmacy provides procainamide in vials containing 100 mg in 1 mL. Round to the nearest tenth mL.

69. The provider orders labetalol 15 mg, IV, PRN, for systolic blood pressure greater than 160 mm Hg. The pharmacy provides labetalol in vials containing 5 mg in 1 mL. Round to the nearest tenth mL.

Calculate the volume of reconstituted medication (mL) to be administered. Round the answers to the nearest tenth mL.

70. A provider orders acetazolimide 250 mg, IV, every 8 hours. The pharmacy provides acetazolimide in vials containing 500 mg. The vial label states that the contents should be reconstituted with 5 mL sterile water for injection for a final concentration of 100 mg/mL.

71. A provider orders azithromycin 500 mg, IV, daily. Azithromycin comes in vials containing 500 mg. It must be reconstituted with 4.8 mL of sterile water for injection for a final concentration of 100 mg/mL.

72. A provider orders cefoxitin 2 g IV every 12 hours. Cefoxitin comes in vials containing 2 g. It must be reconstituted with 10 mL bacteriostatic water for injection for a final concentration of 200 mg/mL.

Answer these questions for the medication label in Figure U2PT-7.

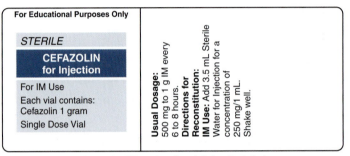

Figure U2PT-7 Simulated Cefazolin Label

73. What is the total amount of cefazolin in the vial?

74. What is the usual dosage of cefazolin?

75. How much diluent is added for IM injections?

76. What is the concentration of the solution after reconstitution for the IM dose?

77. A provider orders cefazolin 750 mg, IM, every 8 hours. How many mL of cefazolin should the nurse draw up in the syringe?

Calculate these weight-based dosages. Round the answers to the nearest whole mg, mcg, or unit.

78. A provider orders pancuronium 0.1 mg/kg, IV, every 20 to 60 minutes as needed to maintain paralysis. The patient weighs 96 kg.

79. A provider orders epoetin (Epogen) 40 units/kg, subcut, 3 times per week. The patient weighs 65 kg.

80. A provider orders oprelvekin (Neumega) 75 mcg/kg, subcut, daily. The patient weighs 60 kg.

Calculate the BSA in m² for these weight and height combinations. Round the final answers to the nearest hundredth m².

81. weight 188 lb, height 72 in

82. weight 125 lb, height 65 in

83. weight 79 kg, height 178 cm

84. weight 64 kg, height 146 cm

Calculate the dosage (mg) and volume of medication (mL) to be administered for these medications. Round the answers to the nearest tenth mg or mL.

85. A provider orders azacitidine 70 mg/m^2, subcut, daily for 7 days. The patient weighs 55 kg and is 151 cm in height. Azacitidine is supplied in vials containing 25 mg/mL after reconstitution.

    a. mg: _____

    b. mL: _____

86. A provider orders docetaxel 30 mg/m^2, IV, daily. The patient weighs 140 lb and is 60 in in height. Docetaxel is supplied in vials containing 10 mg/mL.

    a. mg: _____

    b. mL: _____

Calculate the flow rates (mL/hr) for these IV fluids. Round the answers to the nearest whole number.

87. Infuse 250 mL over 45 minutes.

88. Infuse 800 mL over 6 hours.

89. Infuse 100 mL over 30 minutes.

Calculate the flow rates (mL/hr) for these secondary IV infusions. Round the answers to the nearest whole number.

90. Infuse cefipime 2 g diluted in 100 mL 0.9% sodium chloride solution over 60 minutes.

91. Infuse ifosfamide 500 mg diluted in 50 mL D$_5$W solution over 90 minutes.

92. Infuse ampicillin 500 mg diluted in 50 mL 0.9% sodium chloride solution over 30 minutes.

Calculate the end time for these IVs on an infusion pump.

93. An IV is infusing at 125 mL/hr with 300 mL of fluid left in the IV bag. The current time is 0915.

94. An IV is infusing at 50 mL/hr with 175 mL of fluid left in the IV bag. The current time is 2240.

Calculate these flow rates in gtt/min. Round answers to the nearest whole gtt.

95. A provider orders 1000 mL of 0.9% sodium chloride solution to be infused over 8 hours. The IV tubing drop factor is 15 gtt/mL.

96. A provider orders 500 mL of lactated Ringer's solution to be infused over 4 hours. The IV tubing drop factor is 20 gtt/mL.

97. A provider orders 400 mL of D$_5$W solution to be infused over 90 minutes. The IV tubing drop factor is 10 gtt/mL.

Calculate the end times for these IVs under manual control.

98. An IV is infusing at 25 gtt/min with 350 mL of fluid left in the IV bag. The IV tubing drop factor is 15 gtt/mL. The current time is 1420.

99. An IV is infusing at 38 gtt/min with 250 mL of fluid left in the IV bag. The IV tubing drop factor is 10 gtt/mL. The current time is 0940.

100. An IV is infusing at 42 gtt/min with 800 mL of fluid left in the IV bag. The IV tubing drop factor is 20 gtt/mL. The current time is 2210.

UNIT 3

Special Topics

Chapter 14
Enteral Tube Feedings

Glossary

Aspiration: The accidental drawing of stomach contents into the respiratory tract.
Auscultating: Listening to sounds inside the body, usually with a stethoscope.
Bore: The interior diameter of a tube.
Dumping syndrome: Occurs when the contents of the stomach are rapidly emptied, or dumped, into the small intestine.
Endoscope: A long, thin tube used to visually examine the inside of a hollow organ, such as the stomach, colon, or bladder.
Enteral: By way of the intestine; pertaining to the digestive tract.
Gastric residual volume: The volume of contents (usually an enteral formula) aspirated from the stomach through a patient's feeding tube.
Hang-time: The length of time that a formula is considered safe for administration to the patient.
Isotonic: Describes a solution that contains the same concentration of salt as the cells and blood of the body.
Macronutrient: Nutrients needed in large quantities, such as carbohydrates, proteins, and fats.
Micronutrient: Nutrients needed in small quantities, such as vitamins and minerals.
Nares: The nostrils.

Objectives

After completing this chapter, the learner will be able to—
1. Describe the purpose of enteral nutrition.
2. Differentiate between the various routes of enteral nutrition administration.
3. Describe the different methods of enteral nutrition delivery.
4. Describe the three basic types of formulas.

5. Compare and contrast open and closed systems of enteral nutrition administration.
6. Discuss the nursing care of patients receiving enteral nutrition.
7. Describe the process of administering medications through an enteral tube.
8. Calculate calorie and protein needs for patients.
9. Calculate flow rates for enteral feedings.
10. Calculate dilutions for enteral feedings.

Enteral Nutrition

Enteral nutrition refers to the delivery of nutrients directly into the digestive tract (specifically the stomach, duodenum, or jejunum). Patients who are unable to eat or are eating inadequate amounts, but have a functioning or partially functioning gastrointestinal (GI) tract are candidates for enteral nutrition (see Box 14-1).

Nutrition received enterally is generally preferred over nutrition received intravenously. Nutrients that pass through the intestine stimulate normal gastrointestinal functioning and maintain the intestine's immunity. In addition, nutrients present inside the GI tract stimulate the release of digestive enzymes and hormones that keep it healthy for nutrient absorption. Food inside the gut also helps maintain the intestinal tissue responsible for processing bacteria.

Routes of Administration

Enteral nutrition may be delivered by several routes. Feeding tubes can be placed through the nares into the stomach (called nasogastric tubes) or the duodenum (called nasoenteric tubes), or through the mouth into the stomach (called orogastric tubes). Feeding tubes placed into the GI tract through the nose or mouth are temporary—they stay in for several days to weeks. Enteral tubes can also be placed directly into the stomach or the small intestine through a surgical procedure using an endoscope. These tubes are called *percutaneous endoscopic gastrostomy tubes* or *G-tubes*. The choice of route depends on the reasons why the patient needs a feeding tube and the length of time that the tube is expected to be used (short-term or long-term). See Figure 14-1 for locations and Table 14-1 for the types, sizes, uses, advantages, and disadvantages for each tube type.

Delivery Methods

Enteral feedings may be administered four different ways: bolus, continuous, cyclic, and intermittent. The delivery type depends upon the route of administration (gastric, duodenal, or jejunal), the size of the feeding tube (small bore versus large bore), the availability of equipment, and patient tolerance.

Bolus tube feedings are administered at regular intervals in large quantities over a relatively short period. Bolus feedings are designed to mimic natural mealtimes and are used only for feedings that are instilled into the stomach. A typical bolus feeding consists of administering 200 to 400 mL of

---

■ **Box 14-1 Indications for Enteral Nutrition**

- Risk of aspiration due to a neurological disorder or injury
- Difficulty chewing food or swallowing food or fluids
- Intestinal obstruction
- Coma or altered level of consciousness
- GI tract disorder, injury, or surgery
- Severe burns
- Mechanical ventilation (respirator)
- Malnutrition

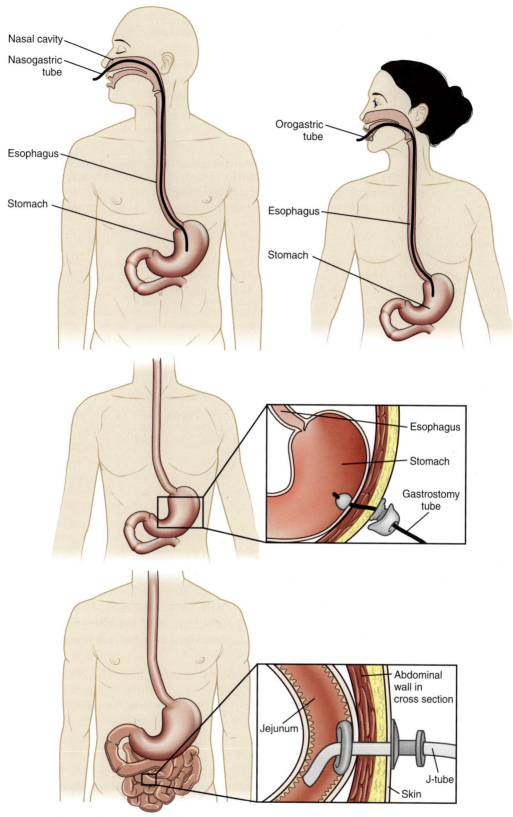

Figure 14-1 Locations of Nasogastric, Orogastric, Gastrostomy, and Jejunostomy Tubes

Table 14-1	Types, Sizes, Uses, Advantages, and Disadvantages of Enteral Tubes			
Type of Tube	**Size**	**Uses**	**Advantages**	**Disadvantages**
Nasogastric (NG) tube	5 to 8 French (The "French" system measures the outside diameter of a tube. 1 French = 0.33 mm.)	Short-term feeding (less than 6 weeks)	• Easily placed by nursing staff. • May be used for bolus, intermittent, and continuous feedings. • Can use more concentrated formula.	• Irritating to the nares and esophagus. • Easily dislodged. • High risk of aspirating feeding into lungs.
Nasoduodenal tube Nasojejunal tube	6 to 10 French	• Short-term feeding • Used when gastric feeding is not possible or is contraindicated	• May provide higher calorie intake. • Associated with lower risk of aspiration.	• Not appropriate for bolus or intermittent feedings because of small volume of intestine. • Formula must be isotonic.
Gastrostomy tube (also known as a percutaneous endoscopic gastronomy [PEG] tube)	12 to 30 French (Selected size will depend upon patient size and surgeon preference.)	Long-term feeding	• More comfortable than NG tube. • Can be hidden under clothing. • May give bolus, intermittent, or continuous feedings. • Reduced risk of aspiration since tube cannot be inserted into trachea. • Can deliver higher volumes of feeding than NG tubes, and are less likely to become clogged. • Can use more concentrated formulas.	• Requires surgical procedure. • Risk of infection at insertion site. • Tube can become dislodged. • Care of stoma required.
Jejunostomy tube (also known as a percutaneous endoscopic jejunostomy [PEJ] tube)	12 to 24 French	Long-term feeding	• More comfortable than NG tube. • Can be hidden under clothing. • Reduced risk of aspiration since tube cannot be inserted into trachea.	• Requires surgical procedure. • Risk of infection at insertion site. • Tube can become dislodged. • Care of stoma required. • Tubes may become clogged easily due to small size.
Gastrojejunostomy tube (also known as percutaneous endoscopic transgastric jejunostomy [PEGJ] tube)	12 to 30 French	Long-term feeding	• Jejunostomy tube is passed through a new or existing gastrostomy opening. • Reduced risk of aspiration.	• Same as jejunostomy tube. • Jejunal portion of tube may migrate back into the stomach.

formula over 15 to 60 minutes 4 to 6 times per day using gravity flow. The disadvantage of bolus feedings is that they tend to cause nausea, vomiting, diarrhea, cramping, and bloating. They also place the patient at higher risk of aspirating stomach contents because of the large amount of fluid present in the stomach.

Continuous feedings deliver a constant amount of formula to the patient using gravity flow or an electronic feeding pump (Fig. 14-2) set at a mL/hour flow rate as prescribed by the provider. Continuous feedings are appropriate for gastric and intestinal (duodenal or jejunal) feedings. Continuous feedings are usually reserved for patients who are very ill. Compared to other types of feedings, continuous feedings cause less GI upset, present a lower risk of aspiration, and may decrease the severity of diarrhea compared to periodic, large-volume feedings. However, continuous feedings result in increased bacterial growth in the stomach due to higher pH levels from the constant presence of formula.

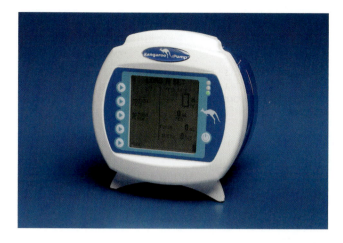

Figure 14-2 Enteral Feeding Pump

Cyclic feedings are similar to continuous feedings except that the formula is infused over a period of 8 to 12 hours, often during the night when the patient is sleeping. The rate of instillation is usually somewhat higher than that of a continuous feeding, since the same amount of formula must be infused in a shorter time. Cyclic feedings may be prescribed for malnourished patients who need supplementation to their oral diet or who are transitioning from continuous feedings to an oral diet.

Intermittent feedings are similar to bolus feedings in that they are administered in equal amounts throughout the day, but use smaller volumes and longer administration times than bolus feedings—usually 250 to 300 mL of formula delivered over one or more hours via gravity flow or electronic feeding pump. Intermittent feedings allow for a 4- to 8-hour period of bowel rest, which allows the stomach pH to return to its acidic state and gives the patient freedom from being attached to tubes.

> **Alert!**
> 1. Enteral formulas can cause death if infused intravenously. Most enteral tubes have bright orange end adapters or connections to differentiate them from intravenous tubing.
> 2. Never use an enteral feeding pump to deliver intravenous fluids or medication, and vice versa.

Types of Formulas

A wide range of enteral formulas are available to meet a variety of patient needs. The choice of formula depends upon the patient's specific nutritional needs, presence of GI tract abnormalities, and specific disease processes, like liver, kidney, or lung disease. Formulas are designed to provide all micro- and macronutrients required by the body, including fiber and additional calories if needed. Formulas are divided into three broad categories by composition: polymeric, monomeric, and disease-specific.

Polymeric formulas contain whole molecules of protein, fats, and carbohydrates and are intended for patients who can tolerate and digest complex molecules properly.

Monomeric formulas are made for patients who cannot digest or absorb whole nutrients. These formulas contain proteins, fats, and carbohydrates that are broken down into easy-to-digest molecules.

Disease-specific formulas are designed for patients with liver, kidney, and pulmonary diseases, and patients with diabetes or impaired immunity. These formulas contain nutrients in amounts or compositions that help compensate for the nutritional imbalances caused by the disease. For example, formulas for individuals with diabetes contain lower amounts of carbohydrates than regular formulas, and formulas made for people with kidney disease contain less protein and less potassium than normal. Some formulas also contain soluble or insoluble fiber to decrease the rate of gastric emptying, add bulk to the stool, and help control diarrhea.

Practice Routes of Administration, Delivery Methods, and Types of Formulas

(answers on page 289)

Match the type of tube with the correct location for its use.

1. Nasoduodenal tube _____

2. Percutaneous transgastric jejunostomy tube _____

3. Nasogastric tube _____

4. Percutaneous gastrostomy tube _____

5. Orogastric tube _____

A. Stomach

B. Duodenum

C. Jejunum

Choose True or False for each statement.

6. Bolus feedings deliver large amounts of formula over 2 to 3 hours.   True   False

7. Continuous feedings are delivered at a constant rate over a long period of time.   True   False

8. Intermittent feedings are administered regularly throughout the day over one or more hours.   True   False

9. Enteral pumps can be used to deliver both enteral and intravenous fluids.   True   False

10. Monomeric formulas contain molecules of fat, carbohydrates, and proteins in a form that is easier to digest.   True   False

Open and Closed Feeding Systems

Most tube-feeding formulas used in hospitals come in ready-to-use 8-ounce cans, 32-ounce cans, and 1- to 1.5-liter ready-to-hang (RTH) bottles. The systems are either open or closed.

Open feeding systems are used for cans of formula. In an open system, formula is administered in one of two ways: (1) enteral feeding syringe (Fig. 14-3) or (2) enteral nutrition bag (Fig. 14-4). Bolus feedings may be given using a 50- or 60-mL enteral feeding syringe. The syringe, with the plunger removed, is attached to the feeding tube, and formula is poured into the syringe. The feeding is regulated by gravity—the higher the syringe is held, the faster the formula flows. The lower the syringe, the more slowly the formula flows. The syringe should be thoroughly rinsed and allowed to air-dry between feedings or according to the facility's policy. The syringe and all associated pieces should be replaced at least every 24 hours. The new syringe kit should be labeled with the date, time, and nurse's initials.

An enteral nutrition bag holds up to 1000 mL of formula, and is typically used for continuous, cyclic, or intermittent feedings, but may be used for large bolus feedings as well. Sterile formulas that have been emptied into a nutrition bag can hang for a maximum of 4 to 8 hours, depending on the facility's policy. The bag itself must be changed every 24 hours and should be thoroughly rinsed with water between intermittent or bolus feedings.

Closed feeding systems refer to enteral feedings administered through RTH bottles. They are considered closed because the bottles containing the formula are sterile. Enteral feed tubing must be used with RTH bottles of formula. This tubing is sterile and should be handled aseptically. Do not use IV tubing in place of enteral feed tubing.

Patients receiving continuous feedings or large quantities of formula are good candidates for RTH bottles (Fig. 14-5). A new bottle with new feeding tubing may hang for up to 48 hours.

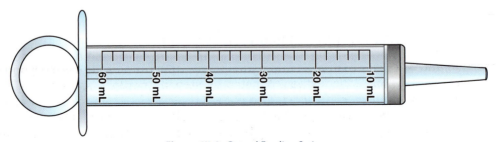

Figure 14-3 Enteral Feeding Syringe

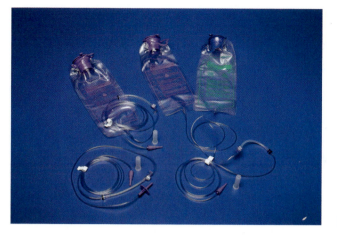

Figure 14-4 Enteral Nutrition Bags

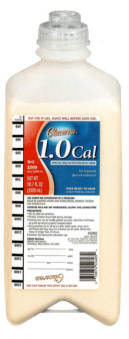

Figure 14-5 Ready-to-Hang Enteral Nutrition Bottle

Powdered Formulas

Powdered formulas are used most commonly for pediatric patients. When preparing a feeding from a powder, follow the manufacturer's directions closely to ensure that the child receives the appropriate quantity of nutrients and water. Before administering a reconstituted formula, agitate the container to mix the solution thoroughly. Reconstituted formulas must be used within 24 hours of mixing. Unused formula should be refrigerated, and formula left at room temperature must be discarded after 4 hours.

Nursing Care for a Patient on Enteral Nutrition

NG-tube insertion and NG-, gastrostomy-, and jejunostomy-tube nursing care are beyond the scope of this book. Refer to a nursing skills textbook for step-by-step instructions on these skills. However, general principles to remember while caring for a patient on tube feeding include the following:

1. Verify the provider's order for the type of formula, route of administration (NG tube, gastrostomy tube, or jejunostomy tube), delivery method (bolus, intermittent, cyclic, or continuous), rate of administration (if a continuous feeding), and frequency (Fig. 14-6).

FORMULA

Pt DOB: _____   Weight: _____

☐ Standard _____ cal/mL   ☐ Reduced carbohydrate _____ cal/mL

☐ High protein   ☐ With fiber

☐ Other: _____

ROUTE AND ACCESS

Route: Access:

☐ Gastric   ☐ Orogastric   ☐ Nasogastric   ☐ Gastrostomy (PEG)

☐ Duodenum   ☐ Nasoduodenal

☐ Jejunum   ☐ Nasojejunal   ☐ Gastrojejunostomy (PEGJ)   ☐ Jejunostomy (PEJ)

METHOD OF ADMINISTRATION

Method: Rate:

☐ Enteral pump   ☐ Initial rate: _____ mL/hr

                    ☐ Advance by _____ mL/hr every _____ hr to a goal of _____ mL/hr.

☐ Gravity-assisted ☐ Initial rate: _____ mL over _____ min _____ times per day.

 (infuse over 30–60 min) ☐ Advance by _____ mL over _____ min each day to a goal of
                    _____ mL feeding over _____ min _____ times daily.

☐ Bolus (syringe)   ☐ Initial _____ mL bolus over _____ min _____ times daily.

                    ☐ Advance by _____ mL each day to a goal of _____ mL feeding
                    over _____ min _____ times daily.

GASTRIC RESIDUAL AND FLUSHING

☐ Check residual every _____ hr.

     ☐ If residual greater than _____ mL, hold feeding for _____ hours and recheck.

     ☐ If residual greater than 500 mL, hold feeding and notify provider.

☐ Flush tube with _____ mL sterile water or NS every _____ hours.

OTHER

☐ Observe for abdominal distension, firmness, or discomfort every _____ hours.

☐ Weigh patient daily.

☐ Strict I&O every 8 hours.

☐ Keep HOB elevated 30 to 45 degrees.

☐ _____

☐ _____

Physician's Signature _____   Date: _____   Time:_____

Noted by:_____ RN   Date: _____   Time:_____

Patient Identification Sticker

**ADULT ENTERAL NUTRITION ORDER FORM
GENERAL HOSPITAL**

Figure 14-6 Sample Enteral Nutrition Order

ENTERAL USE ONLY
General Hospital

Patient: _____ Room Number:_____
Med Record Number: _____

Formula: _____
Additives:_____
Prepared by:_____ Date: _____ Time:_____

Delivery Site

Route: _____

Administration

Method: Bolus   Continuous   Intermittent
                   Rate:_____ mL/hr
Formula Hung by: _____ Date:_____ Time:_____
Expiration Date:_____ Time: _____

Figure 14-7 Sample Enteral Nutrition Label

2. Label the formula administration equipment (bags, bottles, or syringes) with the following information (Fig. 14-7):
   a. patient identifiers (per facility protocol)
   b. type of formula
   c. enteral access site (NG, gastrostomy, or jejunostomy tube)
   d. administration method (bolus, continuous, intermittent, cyclic)
   e. initials of person preparing the feeding
   f. date and time the formula was prepared and hung
3. Maintain aseptic technique while preparing formula and equipment:
   a. Wash hands before handling formula and equipment.
   b. Wipe formula can tops and the screw caps of bottles with alcohol and allow them to dry before opening.
   c. Wear disposable gloves during the preparation and administration of the formula.
   d. Swab the hub of the patient's feeding tube with alcohol swabs prior to accessing.
   e. Wash hands and change gloves between checking gastric residual volume and instilling the feeding.
   f. Follow facility policy regarding the hang-time of enteral feedings.
   g. Discard equipment (syringes, irrigation trays, and enteral bags) as outlined by facility policy.
4. Verify placement of an NG tube prior to administering a feeding. Methods of verification include:
   a. Radiography: The gold standard for verifying placement of a feeding tube is by x-ray. However, this cannot be done prior to every feeding because of the obvious cost and the dangers of repeated exposure to radiation.
   b. Bedside: A combination of the following techniques should be used. Do not rely on just one method.
      i. Aspirating of stomach contents, which are normally greenish-brown in color
      ii. Testing the pH of stomach contents, which are normally acidic (approximately 4.0 pH)
      iii. Injecting a small amount of air (5 to 30 mL) via a feeding syringe while auscultating for whooshing sounds over the stomach
      iv. Testing the tube for the presence of carbon dioxide, which may indicate that the tube is in the trachea instead of the esophagus

5. Elevate the head of the bed 30 to 45 degrees while administering the feeding and for one hour after the feeding to reduce the risk of aspiration.
6. Aspirate for gastric residual volume before every feeding:
   a. Measure the amount of gastric aspirate obtained. Observe the color and consistency of the aspirate for documentation in the patient's record. Return the aspirate to the stomach.

> **Note:** Failing to return gastric aspirate can impair the natural acid-base and electrolyte balance inside the stomach.

   b. Hold the next feeding if the residual volume is more than half the previous feeding volume.
   c. For patients on continuous feedings, monitor for residual volume every 4 hours for critically ill patients, and every 6 to 8 hours for non–critically ill patients (Bankhead et al., 2009). Place the feeding on hold if the residual volume is equal to or greater than the hourly rate.
   d. Document the residual volume aspirated and its disposition (discarded or reinstilled), the administration of any medications, the amount of water used for flushing the tube, the patient's tolerance to the procedure, and any problems that may have occurred (Fig. 14-8).
7. Be prepared to manage complications (Table 14-2).

> **Alert!** Tap water and distilled water may contain contaminants that can harm a very ill or immunocompromised patient. Use sterile water for irrigation or sterile normal saline (0.9% sodium chloride solution) for dissolving medications or irrigating feeding tubes, especially jejunostomy tubes.

| 7-10-2018 1220 | 250 mL Isocal HN bolus administered by gravity into PEG tube via enteral syringe over 20 minutes, after verifying tube placement via x-ray. Pt. tolerated procedure without complaints of nausea or bloating. Denies having diarrhea after feedings. Aspirated 78 mL white, slightly curdled fluid prior to administration of formula. Aspirate returned to stomach. Instilled 100 mL sterile water after feeding. Enteral syringe rinsed with sterile water and air-dried. _____ S. Reed, RN |

Figure 14-8 Sample Documentation

Table 14-2 Enteral Tube Complications and Nursing Interventions

Complication	Intervention
Infection	Use aseptic technique when handling enteral feeding equipment and supplies. Discard formula, administration sets, and supplies per manufacturer's specifications and facility policy. Monitor tube insertion site for signs and symptoms of infection. Monitor patient's vital signs as directed.
Nausea or vomiting	Reduce the flow rate. Check the gastric residual volume. Notify the provider. Anticipate orders for reduced volume of feedings, increased frequency of feedings, or change to continuous feeding. Administer medications such as metoclopramide as ordered to increase GI motility. Administer antiemetics as ordered for nausea. Anticipate change to a less-concentrated formula.
Aspiration of stomach contents into the lungs	Immediately discontinue tube feeding. Suction oral cavity to clear contents. Notify physician for possible chest x-ray and prophylactic antibiotics. Check placement of tube.
Clogged tube	Flush tube with 20 to 30 mL water before and after every feeding or every 4 hours during a continuous feed. Flush tube before, after, and between medications.

Giving Medications Through a Feeding Tube

Patients unable to swallow medications may need to receive them through a feeding tube. However, administering medications through a feeding tube can be risky. NG tubes and jejunostomy tubes clog easily because of their small diameter. In addition, certain medications may form a solid mass when in contact with formula inside the tube, causing the tube to become obstructed. Some medications that are intended to be absorbed in the stomach may be rendered inactive if given through a jejunostomy tube.

General guidelines for administering medication through a feeding tube include these points:

1. Assess the medication for its ability to be instilled into a feeding tube:
   a. Does the medication come in liquid form? Liquids are best for administering through a feeding tube.
   b. If the medication is in a tablet form, ensure that it can be crushed. Some solid medications, like extended- or sustained-release tablets, or those with specialized coatings, should not be crushed. Check with a medication reference book or a pharmacist before crushing tablets.
   c. Before opening a capsule, check with a pharmacist to be sure its contents can be administered through a feeding tube.
   d. Dissolve crushed medications or capsule contents in a plastic medication cup using a small amount of warm sterile water or normal saline. Be sure that all contents of the cup have been emptied. Some medications that do not dissolve well may stick to the sides of the medication cup.
   e. If more than one medication is needed, each medication should be crushed and dissolved in a separate container.
2. Elevate the head of the bed 30 to 45 degrees to reduce the risk of aspiration.
3. Verify placement of the feeding tube in the stomach per the facility's protocol.
4. Check residual volume of stomach contents. Some providers may want the medication held if there is evidence that a large volume of the feeding is not being digested in a certain amount time.
5. Flush the feeding tube with 15 to 60 mL of water, per facility policy and patient's fluid status.
6. Pour the first medication into the syringe and allow it to flow into the tube using gravity, making sure all the medication from the cup has been instilled.
7. Flush the tube with 15 mL of water between each medication if more than one medication is required.
8. After all medications have been administered, flush the tubing with 15 to 60 mL of water, per facility policy and patient's fluid status.
9. Monitor the patient for the desired effects of the medication.
10. Document the medication given, how it was prepared (*crushed* for tablets, *contents emptied* for capsule), the amount of water used to dissolve the medication, the amount of water used to flush the tubing, and the patient's reaction to the medication (Fig. 14-9).

| 4-14-2018 2200 | Pt. BP 187/102; denies headache or visual changes. Labetalol 25 mg tablet crushed, dissolved in 10 mL sterile water, and administered by gravity via PEG tube. Tube flushed before and after medication with 15 mL sterile water. Pt. tolerated procedure without difficulty. PEG tube site intact, without redness, swelling or drainage. _____ S. Reed, RN |
| 4-14-2018 2300 | Pt. BP 150/87. Denies headache or visual changes. _____ S. Reed, RN |

Figure 14-9 Sample Documentation for Medication Administration

Practice Open and Closed Feeding Systems, Powdered Formulas, Nursing Care for a Patient on Enteral Nutrition, and Giving Medications Through a Feeding Tube

(answers on page 289)

Select the best answer for each question.

1. Enteral feeding labels should contain all of the following information except:
   a. patient identifiers.
   b. administration method.
   c. initials of the prescriber.
   d. date and time the formula was hung.

2. An open system enteral nutrition bag should be changed every:
   a. 24 hours.
   b. 48 hours.
   c. 72 hours.
   d. 96 hours.

3. Sterile, ready-to-hang bottles may hang for no longer than:
   a. 4 hours.
   b. 8 hours.
   c. 24 hours.
   d. 48 hours.

4. The nurse is teaching a patient how to reconstitute a powdered formula for enteral feedings. Which of these statements made by the patient indicates the need for additional teaching?
   a. "I can save money by using more water than indicated in the instructions."
   b. "I can store leftover formula in the refrigerator for up to 24 hours.
   c. "I need to thoroughly mix the reconstituted solution before using."
   d. "Formula left at room temperature must be used within four hours."

5. The gold standard for verifying placement of a feeding tube is:
   a. injecting air into the tube and auscultating for whooshing sounds over the stomach.
   b. checking the pH of gastric aspirate.
   c. testing for the presence of carbon monoxide inside the feeding tube.
   d. using radiography (x-ray).

6. Which of these actions shows that the nurse understands the concepts of caring for a patient with a feeding tube?
   a. The nurse aspirates stomach contents to check gastric residual volume right after completing a bolus feeding.
   b. The nurse elevates the head of the bed to 15 degrees during the feeding.
   c. The nurse wipes the formula lid with an alcohol swab prior to opening.
   d. The nurse obtains 100 mL of normal gastric aspirate and discards it.

7. Which of these statements is true regarding the administration of medications through a feeding tube?
   a. All types of medications may be given through a feeding tube.
   b. Dissolve enteric-coated tablets in a small amount of warm water.
   c. Delivering all medications through the feeding tube at the same time is acceptable.
   d. Flush the feeding tube after each medication with 15 to 60 mL sterile water.

Calculating Calorie and Protein Needs for Patients Receiving Enteral Tube Feedings

Tracking the calorie and protein intake of patients receiving enteral nutrition is a function of the registered dietician on staff at most facilities; however, nurses also need to know the intake to assess the patient's nutritional status and to anticipate problems.

The average individual needs 25 to 30 calories per kg of body weight per day and 0.8 g protein per kg of body weight per day. These amounts vary depending on a patient's medical condition, age, current nutritional status, and the presence of other illnesses or injuries.

Example 1: Calculate the daily calorie and protein needs of a patient who weighs 87.5 kg and has normal calorie (25 cal/kg/day) and protein needs. Round to the nearest whole number.

1. Use dimensional analysis to set up the equation for daily calorie needs. Insert the first set of given quantities—the daily calorie requirements needed per kilogram of body weight.

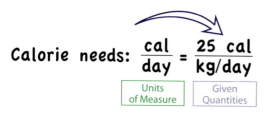

2. Insert the next given quantity—the patient's weight. Solve the equation.

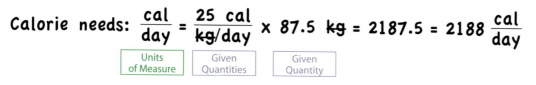

3. Set up the equation for daily protein needs in the same fashion as for calorie needs.

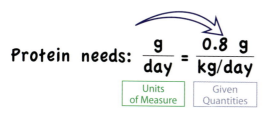

4. Insert the second given quantity (patient weight). Solve the equation.

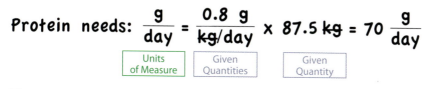

This patient needs 2188 calories and 70 g of protein per day based on current weight.

For Example 2, refer to the directions in Example 1.

Example 2: Calculate the daily calorie and protein needs of a patient who weighs 51 kg and has higher calorie needs (30 cal/kg/day) and normal protein needs. Round to the nearest whole number.

Calorie needs: $\dfrac{cal}{day} = \dfrac{30\ cal}{kg/day} \times 51\ kg = 1530\ \dfrac{cal}{day}$

Protein needs: $\dfrac{g}{day} = \dfrac{0.8\ g}{kg/day} \times 51\ kg = 40.8 = 41\ \dfrac{g}{day}$

This patient requires 1530 calories and 41 g of protein per day.

Example 3: A provider orders an enteral formula for a patient that provides 1500 calories per 1000 mL. The patient weighs 75 kg and has normal calorie needs. How much formula would the patient need per day (mL/day) to meet those caloric needs? Round to the nearest whole number.

1. First, calculate the daily calorie needs for the patient (cal/day).

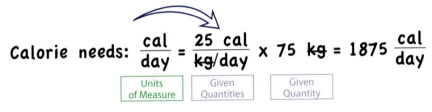

Calorie needs: $\dfrac{cal}{day} = \dfrac{25\ cal}{kg/day} \times 75\ kg = 1875\ \dfrac{cal}{day}$

| Units of Measure | Given Quantities | Given Quantity |

2. Calculate the amount of formula needed per day (mL/day) to meet the patient's requirement for calories. The first set of given quantities is the caloric concentration of the formula.

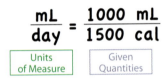

$\dfrac{mL}{day} = \dfrac{1000\ mL}{1500\ cal}$

| Units of Measure | Given Quantities |

3. Insert the next set of given quantities—the daily calorie needs of the patient calculated in step 1.

$\dfrac{mL}{day} = \dfrac{1000\ mL}{1500\ cal} \times \dfrac{1875\ cal}{day} = \dfrac{1,875,000\ mL}{1500\ day} = 1250\ \dfrac{mL}{day}$

| Units of Measure | Given Quantities | Given Quantity |

The patient needs 1250 mL of formula per day to meet his or her caloric needs.

Example 4:   A provider orders an enteral formula for a patient that provides 68 g protein per liter. The patient weighs 84 kg and has normal protein needs. How much formula would the patient need per day (mL/day) to meet those protein needs? Round to the nearest whole number.

1. Calculate the daily protein needs for the patient.

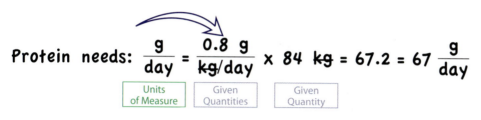

$$\text{Protein needs: } \frac{g}{day} = \frac{0.8\ g}{kg/day} \times 84\ kg = 67.2 = 67\ \frac{g}{day}$$

| Units of Measure | Given Quantities | Given Quantity |

2. Calculate the amount of formula needed per day (mL/day) to meet the patient's requirement for protein.

$$\frac{mL}{day} = \frac{1000\ mL}{68\ g} \times \frac{67\ g}{day} = \frac{67,000\ mL}{68\ day} = 985\ \frac{mL}{day}$$

| Units of Measure | Given Quantities | Given Quantity |

The patient requires 985 mL of formula to provide enough protein for the day.

Practice Calculating Calorie and Protein Needs for Patients Receiving Enteral Feedings

(answers on page 289)

Calculate the daily calorie and protein needs for these patients. Assume that each patient requires normal amounts of calories (25 cal/kg/day) and protein (0.8 g/kg/day). Round the final answer to the nearest whole number.

1. Patient weight: 48.3 kg

2. Patient weight: 97 kg

3. Patient weight: 44.5 kg

4. Patient weight: 62 kg

5. Patient weight: 77 kg

Calculate the daily amount of formula (mL/day) needed for these patients. Assume that each patient requires normal amounts of calories (25 cal/kg/day) and protein (0.8 g/kg/day). Round the final answer to the nearest whole number.

6. Patient weight: 94.6 kg. The formula provides 360 calories per 240 mL.

7. Patient weight: 58.2 kg. The formula provides 16 g protein per 240 mL.

8. Patient weight: 65 kg. The formula provides 3000 calories per 1.5 L.

9. Patient weight 70 kg. The formula provides 50 g protein per 1 L.

10. Patient weight 86.1 kg. The formula provides 1000 calories per 1 L.

Calculating Flow Rates for Enteral Feedings

The nurse is responsible for calculating the flow rate for continuous, cyclic, or intermittent feedings if the provider has not written a specific order for an hourly rate. Nurses should estimate a flow rate even for bolus feedings because if given too quickly, bolus feedings can cause abdominal discomfort such as nausea and bloating.

Example 1:   The nurse is to administer a bolus feeding of 240 mL formula over 15 minutes using a 60-mL enteral syringe. At what mL/min rate should the nurse instill the feeding to ensure that it is administered in the correct amount of time? Round to the nearest whole number.

Set up the equation using dimensional analysis, and fill in the given quantities—the total amount of formula, and the time over which the formula should be administered. Solve the equation.

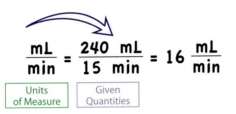

$$\frac{mL}{min} = \frac{240\ mL}{15\ min} = 16\ \frac{mL}{min}$$

Units of Measure   Given Quantities

The nurse should administer the feeding at a rate of 16 mL/min.

Example 2:   The nurse is to administer a bolus feeding of 300 mL over 30 minutes using an enteral nutrition bag and electronic feeding pump. At what mL/hr rate should the nurse set the pump? Round to the nearest whole number.

1. Start by setting up the equation using dimensional analysis and insert the first set of given quantities—the volume of formula and the time of infusion.

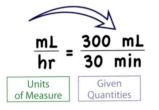

$$\frac{mL}{hr} = \frac{300\ mL}{30\ min}$$

Units of Measure   Given Quantities

2. Since the enteral pump infuses in mL/hr and not mL/min, insert a conversion factor. Solve the equation.

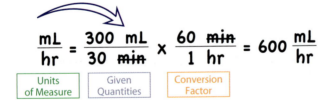

$$\frac{mL}{hr} = \frac{300\ mL}{30\ \cancel{min}} \times \frac{60\ \cancel{min}}{1\ hr} = 600\ \frac{mL}{hr}$$

Units of Measure   Given Quantities   Conversion Factor

Note: This rate may seem high, but remember that this is a feeding, not an intravenous infusion. However, if the patient is not tolerating the feeding, the rate can be slowed.

For Examples 3 and 4, refer to the directions in Examples 1 and 2.

Example 3: The provider orders a feeding of 800 mL of formula to be given over 8 hours via enteral feeding pump while the patient is sleeping. Calculate the mL/hr flow rate. Round to the nearest whole number.

$$\frac{mL}{hr} = \frac{800\ mL}{8\ hr} = 100\ \frac{mL}{hr}$$

Example 4: The provider orders a feeding of 1000 mL of formula to be given over 16 hours via enteral feeding pump. Calculate the mL/hr flow rate. Round to the nearest whole number.

$$\frac{mL}{hr} = \frac{1000\ mL}{16\ hr} = 62.5 = 63\ \frac{mL}{hr}$$

Practice Calculating Flow Rates for Enteral Feedings

(answers on page 290)

Calculate the flow rate for these feedings. Round the final answer to the nearest whole number.

1. The provider orders a feeding of 480 mL of formula to be given over 4 hours via enteral feeding pump. Calculate the mL/hr flow rate.

2. The provider orders a feeding of 240 mL of formula to be given over 30 minutes via enteral feeding pump. Calculate the mL/hr flow rate.

3. The nurse is to administer a bolus feeding of 150 mL to be given over 20 minutes using an enteral feeding syringe. At what mL/min rate should the nurse administer the feeding?

4. The provider orders a feeding of 1.5 L of formula to be given over 24 hours via enteral feeding pump. Calculate the mL/hr flow rate.

5. The provider orders a feeding of 300 mL of formula to be given over 2 hours via enteral feeding pump. Calculate the mL/hr flow rate.

6. The nurse is to administer a bolus feeding of 200 mL to be given over 15 minutes using an enteral feeding syringe. At what mL/hr rate should the nurse administer the feeding?

7. The nurse is to administer a bolus feeding of 240 mL to be given over 20 minutes using an enteral nutrition bag and electronic feeding pump. At what mL/min rate should the nurse set the pump?

8. The provider orders a feeding of 1000 mL of formula to be given over 12 hours via enteral feeding pump. Calculate the mL/hr flow rate.

9. The provider orders a feeding of 720 mL of formula to be given over 8 hours via enteral feeding pump. Calculate the mL/hr flow rate.

10. The provider orders a feeding of 480 mL of formula to be given over 40 minutes via enteral feeding pump. Calculate the mL/hr flow rate.

Diluting Enteral Feedings

In the past, enteral feedings were diluted for patients just starting on feedings to help prevent gastrointestinal discomfort from highly concentrated formulas. At the time, a provider ordered a particular strength formula, such as 1/2 or 3/4 strength, and the nurse would calculate how much water to add to the formula. Although feedings are rarely diluted today due to the increased risk of bacterial contamination, knowing how to dilute an enteral feeding may come in handy. The formula may be used to dilute other liquids as well.

To calculate the amount of water to add to a formula, use the following equation:

$$\text{volume of water to add (mL)} = \frac{\text{total volume of formula on hand (mL)}}{\text{diluted strength}} - \text{total volume of formula on hand (mL)}$$

Note: Dimensional analysis does not work for diluting formulas. You must memorize this formula.

Example 1: A provider orders a formula to be diluted to half strength. The formula comes in a can containing 240 mL. How much water (mL) should the nurse add? Round to the nearest whole number.

1. Set up the dilution equation, using the information given in the question.

$$\text{Volume of water to add (mL)} = \frac{240 \text{ mL}}{\frac{1}{2}} - 240 \text{ mL}$$

2. Divide 240 mL by the fraction ½ to obtain the *total volume* of the feeding. (See Chapter 2 to review dividing fractions.)

$$\frac{240 \text{ mL}}{\frac{1}{2}} = \frac{240}{1} \times \frac{2}{1} = \frac{240 \text{ mL} \times 2}{1 \times 1} = 480 \text{ mL}$$

3. Subtract the amount of formula on hand from the total volume of the feeding to calculate the amount of water to add.

$$\text{Volume of water to add (mL)} = 480 - 240 = 240 \text{ mL}$$

For a half-strength feeding, the total volume will be 480 mL—half composed of formula and half composed of water. See Figure 14-10.

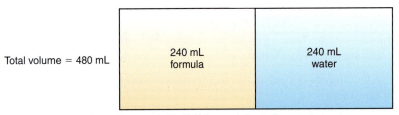

Total volume = 480 mL

240 mL formula

240 mL water

Figure 14-10 Half-Strength Formula

Example 2: A provider orders a formula to be diluted to three-quarters strength. The formula comes in a can containing 240 mL. How much water (mL) should the nurse add? Round to the nearest whole number.

1. Change the fraction 3/4 into a percent. (Sometimes using a percent is less confusing than trying to divide fractions.)

Note: To find the percentage of a number, divide the denominator into the numerator.

$$4)\overline{3.00} \quad \frac{0.75}{}$$

$$\text{Volume of water to add (mL)} = \frac{240 \text{ mL}}{0.75} - 240 \text{ mL}$$

2. Divide 240 mL by 0.75 to calculate the total volume of the feeding.

$$\frac{240 \ mL}{0.75} = 320 \ mL$$

3. Subtract the amount of formula on hand from the total volume of the feeding.

Volume of water to add (mL) = 320 - 240 = 80 mL

For a three-quarters-strength feeding, the total volume will be 320 mL—three-quarters of the total feeding will be composed of formula, and one-quarter composed of water. See Figure 14-11.

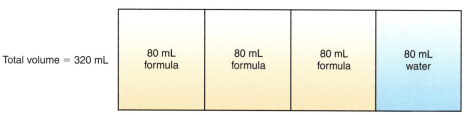

Total volume = 320 mL

| 80 mL formula | 80 mL formula | 80 mL formula | 80 mL water |

Figure 14-11 Three-Quarters-Strength Formula

Example 3: A provider orders a formula to be diluted to two-thirds strength. The formula comes in a can containing 240 mL. How much water (mL) should the nurse add? Round to the nearest whole number.

1. Set up the equation.

Volume of water to add (mL) = $\dfrac{240 \ mL}{\dfrac{2}{3}} - 240 \ mL$

2. Next, divide 240 mL by the fraction 2/3.

$$\frac{240 \ mL}{\dfrac{2}{3}} = \frac{240 \ mL}{1} \times \frac{3}{2} = \frac{240 \ mL \times 3}{1 \times 2} = 360 \ mL$$

3. Subtract the amount of formula on hand from the total volume of the feeding.

Volume of water to add (mL) = 360 - 240 = 120 mL

For a two-thirds-strength feeding, the total volume will be 360 mL—two-thirds composed of formula, and one-third composed of water. See Figure 14-12.

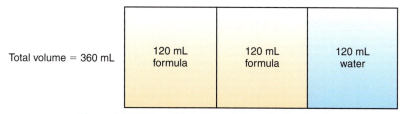

Total volume = 360 mL

| 120 mL formula | 120 mL formula | 120 mL water |

Figure 14-12 Two-Thirds-Strength Formula, Problem 1

Recalculate Example 3 again, this time changing the fraction 2/3 to a decimal:

1. Change the fraction ⅔ into a percent.

Note: To find the percentage of a number, divide the denominator into the numerator:

$$\frac{0.6\overline{6}}{3\overline{)2.00}} = 0.67$$

$$\text{Volume of water to add (mL)} = \frac{240 \text{ mL}}{0.67} - 240 \text{ mL}$$

2. Divide 240 mL by 0.67.

$$\frac{240 \text{ mL}}{0.67} = 358.2 = 358 \text{ mL}$$

3. Subtract the amount of formula on hand from the total volume of the feeding.

$$\text{Volume of water to add (mL)} = 358 - 240 = 118 \text{ mL}$$

See Figure 14-13.

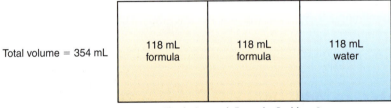

Total volume = 354 mL

| 118 mL formula | 118 mL formula | 118 mL water |

Figure 14-13 Two-Thirds-Strength Formula, Problem 2

Notice that the answer is slightly different when using a fraction such as 2/3 that results in a decimal that is rounded. The more the decimal is rounded (for example, rounding to the nearest tenth instead of the nearest hundredth place), the less precise the answer will be.

Practice Diluting Enteral Feedings

(answers on page 291)

Calculate the amount of water to add to the formula to obtain the feeding strength in the question. Round to the nearest whole number.

1. A provider orders a formula to be diluted to one-third strength; 240 mL of formula are available.

2. A provider orders a formula to be diluted to three-quarters strength; 200 mL of formula are available.

3. A provider orders a formula to be diluted to two-thirds strength; 300 mL of formula are available.

4. A provider orders a formula to be diluted to half strength; 480 mL of formula are available.

5. A provider orders a formula to be diluted to one-quarter strength; 240 mL of formula are available.

Case Study 14–1

Mr. Jasper McManus, date of birth May 7, 1938, is transferred from a long-term-care facility to the medical unit for pneumonia. He has a history of a stroke that has left him with the inability to swallow food and fluids without aspirating. He has chronic renal failure. He has a gastrostomy tube through which he receives all of his nutrition. Mr. McManus's physician has completed the enteral nutrition order shown in Figure 14-14. You are the RN.

1. Calculate the estimated daily calories needed by Mr. McManus, assuming that he has normal calorie requirements (25 cal/kg).
2. Given the flow rate ordered by the physician, will Mr. McManus receive the estimated amount of calories needed each day?
3. When should you withhold a feeding?
4. How often should you check the gastric residual volume?
5. What nursing actions should you take before starting the ordered feeding?
6. List four ways to maintain aseptic technique during feeding administration.

After five days, Dr. Klein discontinues the continuous feedings, and writes an order for Mr. McManus to receive intermittent feedings of 240 mL over 30 minutes 5 times per day, at 0600, 1000, 1400, 1800, and 2200.

7. Calculate the mL/hr flow rate for each of these feedings.
8. How many calories per day will Mr. McManus receive with the new feeding regimen?

Key Points

1. Enteral nutrition provides nutrients for individuals who have a functioning or partially functioning GI tract, but who are unable to swallow or cannot eat adequate amounts of food normally.
2. Enteral nutrition is delivered to the stomach or the small intestine through tubes placed in the nares or placed directly into the stomach or jejunum.
3. The four basic delivery methods for enteral feedings are bolus, continuous, cyclic, and intermittent.
4. Enteral formulas may be delivered via enteral pump or by gravity.
5. An enteral pump should never be used to deliver intravenous fluids.
6. The choice of formula will depend on the specific needs of the patient, and the formula may be polymeric, monomeric, or disease-specific.
7. Closed systems of enteral delivery may hang for up to 48 hours after opening. An open system of delivery may hang for a maximum of 4 to 8 hours, depending upon facility policy.
8. Open system enteral bags and associated equipment must be discarded after 24 hours.
9. Nursing care of a patient receiving enteral nutrition encompasses—
   a. Verifying provider order
   b. Correct labeling of the delivery system (syringe or enteral bag)
   c. Verifying placement of the tubes and checking the insertion site (if PEG or PEJ tube placed)
   d. Maintaining aseptic technique while administering the formula
   e. Preventing aspiration by elevating the head of the bed
   f. Checking gastric residual volume
10. Medications in a liquid form are preferable for feeding tube administration.
11. Medications that cannot be crushed should not be given through an enteral tube.
12. Medications should be given one at a time.
13. A feeding tube should be flushed with sterile water or normal saline before and after instilling each medication.

References

1. Bankhead, R., Boullata, J., Brantley, S., Corkins, M., Guenter, P., Krenitsky, J., Lyman, B., Metheny, N. A., Mueller, C., Robbins, S., & Wessel, J. (2009). A.S.P.E.N. Enteral nutrition practice recommendations. *Journal of Parenteral and Enteral Nutrition, 33*(122), 122–167. doi: 10.1177/0148607108330314

FORMULA

Pt DOB: __5/7/1938__   Weight: __83.6 kg__

☐ Standard _____ cal/mL   ☐ Reduced carbohydrate _____ cal/mL

☐ High protein   ☑ With fiber

☑ Other: _Renal formula 1.8 cal/mL_____

ROUTE AND ACCESS

Route: Access:

☑ Gastric   ☐ Orogastric   ☐ Nasogastric   ☑ Gastrostomy (PEG)

☐ Duodenum   ☐ Nasoduodenal

☐ Jejunum   ☐ Nasojejunal   ☐ Gastrojejunostomy (PEGJ)   ☐ Jejunostomy (PEJ)

METHOD OF ADMINISTRATION

Method: Rate:

☑ Enteral pump   ☑ Initial rate: __48__ mL/hr

                               ☐ Advance by ____ mL/hr every ____ hr to a goal of _____mL/hr.

☐ Gravity-assisted   ☐ Initial rate: _____mL over _____ min _____ times per day.

  (infuse over 30–60 min)   ☐ Advance by ____ mL over _____ min each day to a goal of
                                 _____ mL feeding over _____ min _____ times daily.

☐ Bolus (syringe)   ☐ Initial _____ mL bolus over _____min _____ times daily.

                               ☐ Advance by _____ mL each day to a goal of _____ mL feeding
                                 over _____ min _____ times daily.

GASTRIC RESIDUAL AND FLUSHING

☑ Check residual every _____4_____ hr.

     ☑ If residual greater than _____48_____ mL, hold feeding for ____1____ hours and recheck.

     ☐ If residual greater than 500 mL, hold feeding and notify provider.

☑ Flush tube with __100__ mL sterile water or NS every _____8_____ hours.

OTHER

☑ Observe for abdominal distension, firmness, or discomfort every __4__ hours.

☑ Weigh patient daily.

☑ Strict I&O every 8 hours.

☑ Keep HOB elevated 30 to 45 degrees.

☑ _CBC and electrolytes Mondays, Wednesdays, and Fridays_

☐ _____

Physician's Signature _Amy Klein, MD_____   Date: _4/17/2018_   Time: _0840_____
Noted by:_____ RN   Date: _____   Time:_____

McManus, Jasper A.
DOB: May 7, 1938
MR #: 3910568
Acct #: 37910389769
Physician: A. Klein, MD

**ADULT ENTERAL NUTRITION ORDER FORM
GENERAL HOSPITAL**

Figure 14-14 Enteral Nutrition Order

Chapter Post-Test

(answers in Unit 4)

Multiple Choice

Choose the best answer for each question.

1. A feeding tube placed through the nares into the jejunum is called a:
   a. percutaneous endoscopic jejunostomy tube.
   b. percutaneous endoscopic gastrostomy tube.
   c. nasogastric tube.
   d. nasojejunal tube.

2. The choice of feeding tube placement depends upon all of the following conditions except:
   a. the reason why the patient needs the feeding tube.
   b. the length of time the tube is expected to be used.
   c. the presence of a functioning or partially functioning GI tract.
   d. the gender of the patient.

3. A feeding that is delivered continuously over a period of 8 to 12 hours, often during the night, is called a:
   a. continuous feeding.
   b. bolus feeding.
   c. cyclic feeding.
   d. intermittent feeding.

4. Which feeding most closely mimics natural mealtimes?
   a. continuous feeding
   b. bolus feeding
   c. cyclic feeding
   d. intermittent feeding

5. Which type of tube feeding offers the highest risk of aspiration?
   a. nasogastric tube
   b. nasojejunal tube
   c. percutaneous endoscopic gastrostomy tube
   d. percutaneous endoscopic jejunostomy tube

6. Which formula type is most likely to be ordered for a patient who has a normal functioning GI tract?
   a. monomeric
   b. monosterol
   c. polymeric
   d. polysterol

7. The nurse is preparing to document findings about gastric residual volume. Which of the following statements provides the most accurate information?
   a. "Aspirated large quantity of white gastric residual."
   b. "Aspirated 100 mL white, slightly curdled gastric residual from PEG tube. Contents returned to stomach."
   c. "Aspirated 150 mL greenish brown gastric residual from PEG tube."
   d. "Aspirated small quantity of white, liquid gastric residual. Returned to stomach."

8. How often should the nurse check gastric residual for a critically ill patient receiving continuous feedings?
   a. every 15 minutes
   b. every hour
   c. every 4 hours
   d. every 8 hours

Select all that apply.

9. Enteral nutrition is preferred over intravenous nutrition because:
   a. enteral nutrition stimulates normal GI function.
   b. enteral nutrition provides more carbohydrate, fat, and protein than intravenous nutrition.
   c. enteral nutrition helps maintain intestinal immunity.
   d. enteral nutrition stimulates the release of digestive enzymes.

10. The nurse is preparing to give medications through a feeding tube. Which of the following types of water is the most appropriate to reduce the risk of bacterial contamination?
    a. normal saline (0.9% sodium chloride solution)
    b. distilled water
    c. tap water
    d. sterile water for irrigation

Feeding Calculations

Calculate the daily calorie and protein needs for these patients. Assume the patient requires normal amounts of calories (25 cal/kg/day) and protein (0.8 g/kg/day). Round the final answer to the nearest whole number.

11. Patient weight: 94 kg

12. Patient weight: 58.2 kg

13. Patient weight: 62 kg

14. Patient weight: 88.4 kg

15. Patient weight: 76 kg

Calculate the daily amount of formula (mL/day) needed for these patients. Assume the patient requires normal amounts of calories (25 cal/kg/day) and protein (0.8 g/kg/day). Round the final answer to the nearest whole number.

16. Patient weight: 68 kg. The formula provides 240 calories per 240 mL.

17. Patient weight: 86.5 kg. The formula provides 22 g protein per 240 mL.

18. Patient weight: 61.9 kg. The formula provides 1200 calories per 1 L.

19. Patient weight: 77 kg. The formula provides 60 g protein per 1 L.

20. Patient weight: 93.1 kg. The formula provides 1800 calories per 1000 mL.

Calculate the flow rate (mL/hr) for these feedings. Round the final answer to the nearest whole number.

21. The provider orders a feeding of 720 mL of formula over 12 hours via enteral feeding pump.

22. The provider orders a feeding of 350 mL of formula over 3 hours via enteral feeding pump.

23. The nurse is to administer a 200-mL bolus feeding over 15 minutes using an enteral feeding syringe.

24. The provider orders a 1 L-formula feeding over 18 hours via enteral feeding pump.

25. The provider orders a 400-mL formula feeding over 2 hours via enteral feeding pump.

26. The nurse is to administer a 120-mL bolus feeding over 20 minutes using an enteral feeding syringe.

27. The nurse is to administer a 500-mL feeding over 2.5 hours using an enteral feeding pump.

28. The provider orders a 1000-mL formula feeding over 10 hours via enteral feeding pump.

29. The provider orders a 240-mL formula feeding over 20 minutes using an enteral feeding syringe.

30. The provider orders a 800-mL formula feeding over 3 hours via enteral feeding pump.

Calculate the amount of water to add to the formula to make the diluted feeding strength indicated in the question. Round to the nearest whole number.

31. A provider orders a formula to be diluted to one-quarter-strength; 240 mL of formula are available.

32. A provider orders a formula to be diluted to one-third strength; 480 mL of formula are available.

33. A provider orders a formula to be diluted to half strength; 720 mL of formula are available.

34. A provider orders a formula to be diluted to two-thirds strength; 300 mL of formula are available.

35. A provider orders a formula to be diluted to three-quarters strength; 400 mL of formula are available.

Answers to Practice Questions

Routes of Administration, Delivery Methods, and Types of Formulas

1. b
2. c
3. a
4. a
5. a
6. False
7. True
8. True
9. False
10. True

Open and Closed Feeding Systems, Powdered Formulas, Nursing Care for a Patient on Enteral Nutrition, and Giving Medications Through a Feeding Tube

1. c
2. a
3. d
4. a
5. d
6. c
7. d

Calculating Calorie and Protein Needs for Patients Receiving Enteral Feedings

1. Calorie needs: $\dfrac{cal}{day} = \dfrac{25\ cal}{kg/day} \times 48.3\ kg = 1207.5 = 1208\ \dfrac{cal}{day}$

   Protein needs: $\dfrac{g}{day} = \dfrac{0.8\ g}{kg/day} \times 48.3\ kg = 38.6 = 39\ \dfrac{g}{day}$

2. Calorie needs: $\dfrac{cal}{day} = \dfrac{25\ cal}{kg/day} \times 97\ kg = 2425\ \dfrac{cal}{day}$

   Protein needs: $\dfrac{g}{day} = \dfrac{0.8\ g}{kg/day} \times 97\ kg = 77.6 = 78\ \dfrac{g}{day}$

3. Calorie needs: $\dfrac{cal}{day} = \dfrac{25\ cal}{kg/day} \times 44.5\ kg = 1112.5 = 1113\ \dfrac{cal}{day}$

   Protein needs: $\dfrac{g}{day} = \dfrac{0.8\ g}{kg/day} \times 44.5\ kg = 35.6 = 36\ \dfrac{g}{day}$

4. Calorie needs: $\dfrac{cal}{day} = \dfrac{25\ cal}{kg/day} \times 62\ kg = 1550\ \dfrac{cal}{day}$

   Protein needs: $\dfrac{g}{day} = \dfrac{0.8\ g}{kg/day} \times 62\ kg = 49.6 = 50\ \dfrac{g}{day}$

5. Calorie needs: $\dfrac{cal}{day} = \dfrac{25\ cal}{kg/day} \times 77\ kg = 1925\ \dfrac{cal}{day}$

   Protein needs: $\dfrac{g}{day} = \dfrac{0.8\ g}{kg/day} \times 77\ kg = 61.6 = 62\ \dfrac{g}{day}$

6. Calorie needs: $\dfrac{cal}{day} = \dfrac{25\ cal}{kg/day} \times 94.6\ kg = 2365\ \dfrac{cal}{day}$

   $\dfrac{mL}{day} = \dfrac{240\ mL}{360\ cal} \times \dfrac{2365\ cal}{day} = \dfrac{567,600\ mL}{360\ day} = 1576.6 = 1577\ \dfrac{mL}{day}$

7. Protein needs: $\dfrac{g}{day} = \dfrac{0.8\ g}{kg/day} \times 58.2\ kg = 46.6 = 47\ \dfrac{g}{day}$

   $\dfrac{mL}{day} = \dfrac{240\ mL}{16\ g} \times \dfrac{47\ g}{day} = \dfrac{11,280\ mL}{16\ day} = 705\ \dfrac{mL}{day}$

8. Calorie needs: $\dfrac{cal}{day} = \dfrac{25\ cal}{kg/day} \times 65\ kg = 1625\ \dfrac{cal}{day}$

   $\dfrac{mL}{day} = \dfrac{1000\ ml}{1\ L} \times \dfrac{1.5\ L}{3000\ cal} \times \dfrac{1625\ cal}{day} = \dfrac{2,437,500\ mL}{3000\ day} = 812.5 = 813\ \dfrac{mL}{day}$

9. Protein needs: $\dfrac{g}{day} = \dfrac{0.8\ g}{kg/day} \times 70\ kg = 56\ \dfrac{g}{day}$

   $\dfrac{mL}{day} = \dfrac{1000\ ml}{1\ L} \times \dfrac{1\ L}{50\ g} \times \dfrac{56\ g}{day} = \dfrac{56,000\ mL}{50\ day} = 1120\ \dfrac{mL}{day}$

10. Calorie needs: $\dfrac{cal}{day} = \dfrac{25\ cal}{kg/day} \times 86.1\ kg = 2152.5 = 2153\ \dfrac{cal}{day}$

    $\dfrac{mL}{day} = \dfrac{1000\ ml}{1\ L} \times \dfrac{1\ L}{1000\ cal} \times \dfrac{2153\ cal}{day} = \dfrac{2,153,000\ mL}{1000\ day} = 2153\ \dfrac{mL}{day}$

Calculating Flow Rates for Enteral Feedings

1. $\dfrac{mL}{hr} = \dfrac{480\ mL}{4\ hr} = 120\ \dfrac{mL}{hr}$

2. $\dfrac{mL}{hr} = \dfrac{240\ mL}{30\ min} \times \dfrac{60\ min}{1\ hr} = \dfrac{14,400\ mL}{30\ hr} = 480\ \dfrac{mL}{hr}$

3. $\dfrac{mL}{min} = \dfrac{150\ mL}{20\ min} = 7.5 = 8\ \dfrac{mL}{min}$

4. $\dfrac{mL}{hr} = \dfrac{1000\ ml}{1\ L} \times \dfrac{1.5\ L}{24\ hr} = \dfrac{1500\ mL}{24\ hr} = 62.5 = 63\ \dfrac{mL}{hr}$

5. $\dfrac{mL}{hr} = \dfrac{300\ mL}{2\ hr} = 150\ \dfrac{mL}{hr}$

6. $\dfrac{mL}{hr} = \dfrac{200\ mL}{15\ min} \times \dfrac{60\ min}{1\ hr} = \dfrac{12{,}000\ mL}{15\ hr} = 800\ \dfrac{mL}{hr}$

7. $\dfrac{mL}{min} = \dfrac{240\ mL}{20\ min} = 12\ \dfrac{mL}{min}$

8. $\dfrac{mL}{hr} = \dfrac{1000\ mL}{12\ hr} = 83.3 = 83\ \dfrac{mL}{hr}$

9. $\dfrac{mL}{hr} = \dfrac{720\ mL}{8\ hr} = 90\ \dfrac{mL}{hr}$

10. $\dfrac{mL}{hr} = \dfrac{480\ mL}{40\ min} \times \dfrac{60\ min}{1\ hr} = \dfrac{28{,}800\ mL}{40\ hr} = 720\ \dfrac{mL}{hr}$

Diluting Enteral Feedings

1. $mL\ water = \dfrac{240\ mL}{\frac{1}{3}} - 240\ mL = \dfrac{240\ mL \times 3}{1 \times 1} - 240\ mL$

$= 720\ mL - 240\ mL = 480\ mL$

2. $mL\ water = \dfrac{200\ mL}{\frac{3}{4}} - 200\ mL = \dfrac{200\ mL \times 4}{1 \times 3} - 200\ mL$

$= 267\ mL - 200\ mL = 67\ mL$

3. $mL\ water = \dfrac{300\ mL}{\frac{2}{3}} - 300\ mL = \dfrac{300\ mL \times 3}{1 \times 2} - 300\ mL$

$= 450\ mL - 300\ mL = 150\ mL$

4. $\text{mL water} = \dfrac{480 \text{ mL}}{\frac{1}{2}} - 480 \text{ mL} = \dfrac{480 \text{ mL} \times 2}{1 \times 1} - 480 \text{ mL}$

$= 960 \text{ mL} - 480 \text{ mL} = \textbf{480 mL}$

5. $\text{mL water} = \dfrac{240 \text{ mL}}{\frac{1}{4}} - 240 \text{ mL} = \dfrac{240 \text{ mL} \times 4}{1 \times 1} - 240 \text{ mL}$

$= 960 \text{ mL} - 240 \text{ mL} = \textbf{720 mL}$

■ Answers to Case Study 14–1

1. Estimated daily calories needed: $\left(\dfrac{cal}{day}\right) = \dfrac{25 \text{ cal}}{kg/day} \times 83.6 \text{ kg} = 2090\dfrac{cal}{day}$

2. Calories supplied by formula per day:

$\dfrac{1.8 \text{ cal}}{mL} \times \dfrac{48 \text{ mL}}{hr} \times \dfrac{24 \text{ hr}}{day} = 2073.6 = 2074\dfrac{cal}{day}$

The estimated amount of calories needed by Mr. McManus and the amount of calories that he will receive is close—only 14 mL difference in quantity. However, feedings may be interrupted for periods of time during the day for medication administration or other procedures. Maintaining an accurate daily record of the amount of formula received by Mr. McManus is crucial in determining whether he is getting the calories ordered. In the long run, a stable weight and normal nutrition-related lab values will validate that adequate nutrition was received.

3. You should withhold a feeding if the gastric residual volume is greater than 48 mL. The feeding should be withheld for 1 hour. If the gastric residual volume is less than 48 mL, the feeding may be restarted.

4. Gastric residual volume should be checked every 4 hours.

5. Before beginning the feeding, you should verify the following information:
   a. the physician's order, including the type of formula, route of administration, delivery method, rate of administration, and frequency of feeding
   b. patient identifiers
   c. gastric residual volume
   d. type of tube placed
   e. that the head of the bed is elevated 30 to 45 degrees

6. Maintain aseptic technique by:
   a. washing hands before handling formula and equipment.
   b. wiping the formula container top (if can) or opening with an alcohol swab and allowing it to dry before opening.
   c. wearing gloves.
   d. not allowing the formula to hang longer than dictated by facility policy.

7. Flow rate: $\left(\dfrac{ml}{hr}\right) = \dfrac{240 \text{ mL}}{30 \text{ min}} \times \dfrac{60 \text{ min}}{1 \text{ hr}} = 480\dfrac{mL}{hr}$

8. Calories received: $\left(\dfrac{cal}{day}\right) = \dfrac{1.8 \text{ cal}}{mL} \times \dfrac{240 \text{ mL}}{feeding} \times \dfrac{5 \text{ feeding}}{day} = 2160\dfrac{cal}{day}$

Mr. McManus will receive 2160 cal/day on this new regimen, a slight increase from 2074 calories on the continuous feedings.

Chapter 15
Insulin Administration

Glossary

Algorithm: A set of rules specifying the instructions for accomplishing a task or achieving a goal.

Basal: The minimum level necessary to sustain life.

Endogenous: Derived or produced from inside the human body.

Exogenous: Derived or produced from sources outside the human body.

Hyperglycemia: Abnormally high blood glucose levels.

Hypoglycemia: Abnormally low blood glucose levels.

Insulin analog: An altered form of insulin.

NPH insulin: Neutral protamine Hagedorn insulin.

Particulates: Particles of solids suspended in a liquid.

Preprandial: Before meals (abbreviation: ac).

Postprandial: After meals (abbreviation: pc).

Objectives

After completing this chapter, the learner will be able to—

1. Describe the various types of diabetes.
2. Discuss the onset, peak, and duration of action of rapid-, short-, intermediate-, and long-acting types of insulin preparations.
3. Identify the various types of insulin orders.
4. Explain the three types of subcutaneous insulin delivery systems.
5. Differentiate between various types of insulin syringes.
6. Describe the steps in drawing up insulin from a vial.
7. Identify the components of an intravenous insulin protocol.
8. Describe the steps in mixing NPH and rapid-acting or regular insulin.

Diabetes Mellitus

Diabetes mellitus is a group of metabolic diseases characterized by hyperglycemia that results from impaired pancreatic secretion of insulin and/or defects in the action of insulin inside cells. There are three basic types of diabetes: type 1 diabetes mellitus, type 2 diabetes mellitus, and gestational diabetes. Type 1 diabetes is thought to be caused by an autoimmune process that destroys the beta cells in the pancreas. Persons with type 1 diabetes are unable to produce endogenous insulin, so they must inject exogenous insulin to survive. In type 2 diabetes, the pancreas may still produce some insulin, but the insulin is not used effectively by the body's cells. Gestational diabetes is the presence of diabetes during pregnancy and may be caused by hormonal changes and/or a lack of insulin. Gestational diabetes may disappear after delivery of the baby, although a small percentage of women will continue to have diabetes (usually type 2) after the pregnancy. Other women may develop type 2 diabetes later in life.

Diabetes mellitus is managed with diet (Box 15-1), exercise, and medications—all three of which are equally important in managing blood glucose levels. Medications used to treat diabetes include

■ **Box 15-1 Carbohydrate Counting**

Individuals with diabetes should eat a diet that balances protein, fat, and carbohydrate intake to manage blood glucose levels, cholesterol levels, and body weight. The carbohydrates found in bread, cereal, pasta, and sweets are the substances responsible for increasing blood glucose levels. To manage blood glucose levels, many individuals with diabetes use a method called carbohydrate counting.

Carbohydrate counting requires determining the number of grams of carbohydrates to be eaten during a meal, then injecting a predetermined dose of rapid-acting insulin to metabolize the ingested carbohydrates. Most meals should contain 30 to 60 grams of carbohydrates. An individual using carbohydrate counting should be able to read food labels and accurately calculate the amount of needed insulin.

Table 15-1 Oral and Injected Antidiabetic Medications

Classification of Antidiabetic Drug	Generic (Trade) Names	Method of Delivery	Mechanism of Action
Alpha-glucosidase inhibitors	acarbose (Precose), miglitol (Glyset)	Oral	Delays and reduces carbohydrate absorption in the gastrointestinal tract.
Biguanides	metformin (Glucophage)	Oral	Decreases glucose production in the liver. Decreases intestinal absorption of glucose. Increases sensitivity to insulin.
DPP-4 Enzyme inhibitors	sitagliptin (Januvia), saxagliptin (Onglyza) linagliptin (Tradjenta)	Oral	Stimulates insulin release from beta cells. Reduces glucose production in the liver. Slows gastric emptying time.
Amylin analog	pramlinitide (Symlin)	Injected (subcutaneous)	Controls blood sugar levels after meals.
GLP-1 analog (incretin mimetic)	exenatide (Byetta) liraglutide (Victoza)	Injected (subcutaneous)	Stimulates release of insulin from the pancreas.
Meglitinides	nateglinide (Starlix), repaglinide (Prandin)	Oral	Stimulates release of insulin from the pancreas.
Sulfonylureas	glimepiride (Amaryl), glipizide (Glucotrol), glyburide (Micronase)	Oral	Stimulates release of insulin from the pancreas. Increases sensitivity to insulin.
Thiazolidinediones	pioglitazone (Actos), rosiglitazone (Avandia)	Oral	Increases sensitivity to insulin.

insulin and oral or injected antidiabetic medications. See Table 15-1. This chapter focuses on insulin.

Insulin

Insulin is the hormone responsible for allowing the body to utilize and store glucose. It was discovered in 1921 by Canadian scientists Fredrick Banting and Charles Best. In the early days insulin was produced from beef and porcine (pig) sources. Unfortunately, many people suffered from allergies to insulin or developed tissue damage at injection sites. Now, insulin is produced in the laboratory using recombinant DNA technology. It is typically referred to as "human" insulin because its chemistry closely resembles the insulin produced by humans, not because it comes from humans.

The amount of insulin that an individual with diabetes needs depends on numerous factors: (1) the type of diabetes, (2) the presence of other diseases or illnesses, and (3) the individual's body weight. The total daily dose of insulin to maintain normal or near-normal blood glucose levels varies greatly from person to person.

Types of Insulin

A wide variety of insulin preparations are on the market. Over the years, insulin has been modified to produce other products (called *insulin analogs*) with different onset, peaks, and durations of action. Insulin analogs allow individuals with diabetes to have more freedom in planning meals and activities. Insulin is categorized according to its action: rapid-acting, short-acting, intermediate-acting, and long-acting. Table 15-2 outlines the different types of insulin and the recommended timing for administering subcutaneous dosages.

Nurses need to know the onset, peak, and duration of action for insulin so that adverse reactions may be anticipated and managed (see Box 15-2 for managing hypoglycemia). It is also the responsibility of nurses to teach their patients about insulin and diabetes management principles so patients can manage their disease effectively at home.

Insulin Concentration

Most types of insulin come in a concentration of 100 units per mL (designated on the insulin package label as "U-100"). Only regular (short-acting) insulin comes in two strengths: U-100 and U-500. U-500 regular insulin is more concentrated, providing 500 units of insulin per mL. This highly concentrated insulin is prescribed for individuals who are severely resistant to insulin and require very large doses.

Table 15-2	Insulin Types				
Insulin Preparation	Onset	Peak	Duration of Action	Recommended Timing of Administration	
Rapid-acting					
Insulin aspart (NovoLog)	10–20 minutes	1–3 hours	3–5 hours	5–10 minutes before meals	
Insulin lispro (Humalog)	Within 15 minutes	1 to 1½ hours	3–4 hours	15 minutes before meals or immediately after a meal	
Insulin glulisine (Apidra)	Within 15 minutes	1 hour	2–4 hours	15 minutes before meals or within 20 minutes after starting a meal	
Insulin (human) inhalation powder (Afrezza)	12–15 minutes	50 minutes	3 hours	At the beginning of each meal	
Short-acting					
Regular insulin (Novolin R, Humulin R)	30–60 minutes	2–4 hours	5–7 hours	15–30 minutes before meals	
Intermediate-acting					
NPH insulin/isophane insulin suspension (Novolin N, Humulin N)	1–2 hours	4–12 hours	18–24 hours	30–60 minutes before meals	
Long-acting					
Insulin detemir (Levemir)	3–4 hours	3–14 hours	24 hours	With evening meal or at bedtime	
Insulin glargine (Lantus, Toujeo)	3–4 hours	No peak	24 hours	At same time each day	
Insulin Mixtures					
Insulin lispro protamine suspension/insulin lispro solution (Humalog Mix 75/25, Humalog Mix 50/50)	15–30 minutes	2.8 hours	24 hours	Up to 15 minutes before meals	
Insulin aspart protamine suspension/ insulin aspart solution (NovoLog Mix 70/30)	15 minutes	1–4 hours	18–24 hours	Up to 15 minutes before meals	
NPH/regular insulin mixture (Humulin 70/30, Novolin 70/30)	30 minutes	4–8 hours	24 hours	30–60 minutes before meals	

■ **Box 15-2 Managing Hypoglycemia**

Hypoglycemia is defined as an abnormally low blood glucose level, typically below 70 mg/dL. Symptoms of hypoglycemia include feelings of weakness, shakiness, hunger, and anxiety. Patients may complain of a headache, heart palpitations, blurred vision, and sweating. If not treated promptly, hypoglycemia can lead to loss of consciousness, seizures, and possibly death.

Treatment of hypoglycemia depends on whether the patient is conscious, is able to eat, or has intravenous access.

For a patient with hypoglycemia who is able to eat, provide 15 g of a simple carbohydrate in the form of glucose gel (or tablets), 6 ounces of nondiet soda, or 4 ounces of fruit juice.

For a patient who is unconscious or unable to eat but has intravenous access, administer 25 mL of dextrose 50% intravenously over 1 to 3 minutes.

For a patient who is unconscious or unable to eat and does not have intravenous access, administer 1 mg glucagon by subcutaneous or intramuscular injection. Roll the person onto his or her side after administrating the glucagon, since it can cause vomiting. Obtain intravenous access if possible. Once the person is conscious, provide an oral form of carbohydrate if the person is able to eat.

For each of the scenarios, retest the patient's blood glucose level 15 minutes after providing treatment. Continue the treatment until the blood glucose level is greater than 70 mg/dL. Call the provider for further orders if the patient's blood glucose level remains below 70 mg/dL after two rounds of treatment. If there is more than 1 hour until the next scheduled meal, and the patient is able to eat, provide a snack with carbohydrates and protein, such as milk or crackers and cheese to prevent hypoglycemia from recurring.

Insulin Orders

Insulin may be ordered in a number of ways:

1. on a routine or "fixed" schedule
2. to be given before a meal
3. to be given after a meal
4. as a correction dose
5. using a sliding scale
6. using a combination of methods

Routine Administration (Fixed Schedule)

Intermediate- and long-acting insulin (including mixtures of insulin, such as Humalog Mix 75/25 or NovoLog Mix 70/30) are usually ordered on a routine basis. This means that the patient will receive insulin injections at specific times during the day. This regimen provides a slow release of insulin over a relatively long period (called a basal level), which mimics the body's own natural release of insulin throughout the day.

Examples of routine insulin orders include the following:

• Insulin glargine (Lantus) 20 units, subcut, every evening
• NPH insulin 14 units, subcut, before breakfast
• NPH insulin 25 units, subcut, before evening meal
• NovoLog Mix 70/30, 18 units, subcut, before breakfast and dinner

Pre-Meal Administration of Insulin

Many providers prefer that patients inject rapid- or short-acting insulin just before their meals. These injections provide a burst of insulin that helps metabolize the glucose eaten during the meal. The benefit of this type of dosing is that patients have a little more freedom in planning meal times. The amount of insulin injected depends on the quantity of carbohydrates that the patient plans for the meal. To provide a steady release of insulin between meals, pre-meal insulin regimens are usually combined with routine doses of long-acting insulin administered once or twice per day.

Post-Meal Administration of Insulin

Rapid-acting insulin may occasionally be administered after meals. A patient who is very ill may not be able to eat well. Giving a routine or standard dose of insulin before a meal may cause the individual to experience hypoglycemia. To prevent low blood glucose levels, the provider may order the insulin to be given after meals, based on the amount of food eaten by the patient.

Correction Doses of Insulin

Correction doses of insulin are administered when a patient's blood glucose level is unexpectedly high. In such cases, routine pre-meal doses of insulin are not enough to reduce the patient's blood glucose level to normal. The correction dose of insulin varies depending on the severity of the blood glucose reading and the patient's total daily insulin requirements.

Sliding-Scale Insulin Administration

With a sliding-scale protocol, a patient is administered rapid- or short-acting insulin based upon the blood glucose level drawn prior to meals. A disadvantage of the sliding scale is that it does not account for the carbohydrates that will be consumed in the upcoming meal.

Here is an example of a sliding-scale order:

Administer insulin aspart (Humalog), subcut, before meals, based on the following blood glucose levels:

BG level less than or equal to 110 mg/dL:	*0 units*
BG level between 111 and 130 mg/dL:	*3 units*
BG level between 131 and 150 mg/dL:	*4 units*
BG level between 151 and 200 mg/dL:	*6 units*
BG level over 200 mg/dL:	*Call provider*

Combination of Methods

Effective management of a patient's blood glucose level generally involves a combination of methods. Figure 15-1 provides a sample insulin protocol that demonstrates different methods of insulin management. Each facility should also have a record on which nurses can document blood glucose levels and administered insulin. Some facilities use the medication administration record to accomplish this, while others may use a separate flow sheet (Fig. 15-2).

Practice Insulin Types and Orders

(answers on page 316)

Select the best answer for each question.

1. Which of the following types of diabetes mellitus is characterized by the complete destruction of beta cells in the pancreas?
   a. gestational diabetes
   b. type 1 diabetes
   c. type 2 diabetes
   d. type 3 diabetes

2. Human insulin refers to:
   a. insulin collected from a human pancreas.
   b. insulin collected from a pig's pancreas.
   c. synthetic insulin that closely resembles insulin produced by humans.
   d. insulin collected from the pancreas of a cow.

General Hospital

Date:_____ Time:_____

Diagnosis: ☐ Type 1 Diabetes   ☐ Gestational Diabetes

☐ Type 2 Diabetes   ☐ Hyperglycemia

Place patient ID label here

Subcutaneous Insulin Protocol	**Initials**
☐ **Discontinue all previous insulin orders.**	
Labs: ☐ Electrolytes ☐ Urinalysis (with C&S if indicated) ☐ HbA1C ☐ CBC	

Treat for Hypoglycemia:
  • Call lab for STAT blood glucose level.
  • If conscious and taking PO foods/fluids, provide 8 oz juice or milk and ½ of a meat, cheese, or peanut butter sandwich.
  • If unconscious or NPO, administer 25 mL Dextrose 50%, intravenously STAT. May repeat × 1.
  • Re-check blood glucose in 20 minutes.
  • If blood glucose less than 70 mg/dL × 2, call provider.	

Diet: ☐ NPO   ☐ Enteral Feeding   ☐ TPN   ☐ Carbohydrate Counting:

Calories	**Carbohydrate Units per Meal**
☐ 1200–1500 cal/day	45 grams
☐ 1600–2000 cal/day	60 grams
☐ 2100–2400 cal/day	75 grams
☐ Over 2400 cal/day	90 grams
☐ Gestational	30 grams breakfast, 60 grams lunch, 75 grams dinner

☐ Snack at bedtime (15 grams Carbohydrate)

Fingerstick Blood Glucose Monitoring: ☐ ac and hs   ☐ every 6 hours   ☐ Other: _____

Insulin Regimen

Basal Insulin: ☐ Insulin glargine: _____units every _____

☐ NPH insulin: _____units every _____

☐ Mixture: _____units every _____

☐ Other: _____

Mealtime Insulin: ☐ Insulin aspart   ☐ Other: _____

_____units at breakfast _____units at lunch

_____units at dinner _____units at bedtime

Correction Insulin: Correction insulin (use table here) should be administered with mealtime insulin (if ordered) if blood glucose is over 150 mg/dL. Use ☐ Insulin aspart or ☐ Other: _____

If glucose is:	☐ **Low Dose Regimen**	☐ **Medium Dose Regimen**	☐ **High Dose Regimen**
151–200 mg/dL	1 unit	1 unit	1 unit
201–250 mg/dL	2 units	3 units	4 units
251–300 mg/dL	3 units	5 units	7 units
301–350 mg/dL	4 units	7 units	10 units
351–400 mg/dL	5 units	8 units	12 units
Over 400 mg/dL	6 units and call provider	9 units and call provider	14 units and call provider

Physician's Signature: _____ Date:_____ Time:_____

Nursing Verification

Signature	**Initials**	**Signature**	**Initials**

Figure 15-1 Sample Subcutaneous Insulin Protocol

Date	Time	Blood Glucose (mg/dL)	Insulin Administered			Treatment for Hypoglycemia	Initials
			Type	Amount	Site		

**General Hospital
Subcutaneous Insulin Flow Sheet**

Place patient ID label here

Nursing Verification					
Signature	Init	Signature	Init	Signature	Init

Figure 15-2 Sample Subcutaneous Insulin Flow Sheet

3. Which of the following types of insulin has an approximate onset of 15 minutes, peaks in 1 hour, and has a duration of action of 3 to 4 hours?
   a. regular insulin (Humulin R)
   b. insulin detemir (Levemir)
   c. NPH insulin (Novolin N)
   d. insulin lispro (Humalog)

4. Which of the following types of insulin is long-acting?
   a. insulin aspart (NovoLog)
   b. insulin glargine (Lantus)
   c. NPH insulin (Novolin N)
   d. insulin glulisine (Apidra)

5. A provider writes the following order: "Insulin detemir (Levemir) 13 units, subcut, every evening." This order is an example of which type of insulin order?
   a. sliding-scale order
   b. pre-meal insulin order
   c. routine (fixed schedule) order
   d. correction dose order

Choose True or False for each statement.

6. A correction dose of insulin is administered when a patient's blood glucose level is abnormally low.   True   False

7. U-100 insulin refers to insulin preparations that contain 100 units of insulin per mL.   True   False

Questions 8 through 10 refer to this scenario.

A provider writes the following sliding scale insulin order for a patient:
   Insulin glulisine (Apidra), subcut, before meals, according to the following fingerstick blood glucose (BG) levels:

BG less than 100 mg/dL	0 units
BG 100–120 mg/dL	1 unit
BG 121–150 mg/dL	2 units
BG 151–180 mg/dL	4 units
BG over 180 mg/dL	Call provider

8. The nurse obtains a fingerstick blood glucose level just before breakfast. It is 108 mg/dL. How many units of insulin should the nurse administer to the patient?
   a. 0 units
   b. 1 unit
   c. 2 units
   d. 4 units

9. According to Table 15-2, what is the recommended time to administer the subcutaneous injection of insulin glulisine (Apidra)?
   a. 15 minutes before starting a meal
   b. 30 minutes before starting a meal
   c. Within 20 minutes after starting a meal
   d. Both a and c are correct.

10. At lunchtime, the nurse obtains another fingerstick blood glucose level from the patient. It is now 219 mg/dL. What action should be taken by the nurse?
    a. Administer 2 units of insulin glulisine (Apidra).
    b. Administer 4 units of insulin glulisine (Apidra).
    c. Administer 4 units of insulin glulisine (Apidra), then call the provider.
    d. Call the provider for further orders.

Insulin Delivery Systems

Prior to 2006, insulin could be administered into the body only by way of subcutaneous or intravenous injection. Standard insulin preparations taken orally were destroyed by the digestive system before they could reach the bloodstream, rendering them ineffective in reducing blood glucose levels. In 2006, a powdered form of insulin that could be inhaled was introduced to the U.S. market, but production was discontinued after several years because the drug was expensive, few people were using it, and there was concern that the drug might be linked to lung disease. In 2014, the FDA approved a new inhaled powdered insulin Afrezza. Clinical trials are underway for an oral form of insulin.

Subcutaneous Insulin Delivery Systems

Subcutaneous insulin may be administered periodically or continuously. Insulin that is given periodically is administered with single-use syringes or insulin pen devices. For insulin that is delivered continuously, the patient must use an external insulin pump.

Administering Insulin Using Syringes and Vials

Administering insulin with a syringe and vial requires the full attention of the nurse. It is easy to make errors when drawing up insulin because insulin doses tend to be small, and some different insulin vials look similar. Fortunately, insulin syringes have several unique features that differentiate them from other syringes:

1. Syringe caps of U-100 syringes are orange. Syringe caps of U-500 insulin syringes are green.
2. Calibration markings include mL and units.
3. U-100 syringe sizes vary from 0.3 mL (30 units), 0.5 mL (50 units), and 1 mL (100 units). See Figure 15-3. U-500 syringes are designed to administer up to 250 units. At this time, they only come in one size.
4. U-100 syringes must be used with U-100 insulin. U-500 syringes must be used with U-500 insulin.
5. The needles used with insulin syringes are very fine and short—ranging from 27 to 31 gauge and 3/8 to 5/16 inches in length. Most needles have special coatings that make injections easier and less painful.

Selection of the appropriate syringe and needle depends upon the concentration of insulin to be administered (U-100 versus U-500) and the amount of insulin to be injected.

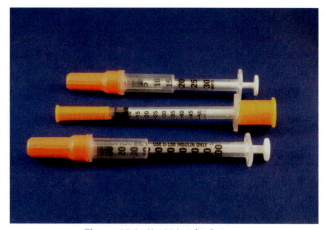

Figure 15-3 U-100 Insulin Syringes

Select the syringe size that corresponds most closely with the amount of insulin being administered. For example, if the patient is to receive 26 units of NPH insulin, select the 0.3-mL/30-unit syringe (or the 0.5-mL/50-unit syringe if a 0.3-mL/30-unit syringe is not available). If the patient is to receive 64 units of insulin, select the 1-mL/100-unit syringe. After selecting the appropriate syringe, draw up the insulin according to facility policy. Box 15-3 provides guidelines for removing insulin from a vial. Always ask another nurse to check the insulin dose for accuracy before administering it.

■ Box 15-3 Guidelines for Removing Insulin From a Vial

1. Select the correct vial of insulin, based on the provider's order.
2. Inspect the insulin for appearance. NPH (neutral protamine Hagedorn) insulin contains zinc chloride and protamine sulfate, which gives NPH its characteristic cloudy appearance. Rapid-acting, long-acting, and regular insulin should be clear, colorless, and without particulates or crystals. Insulin that has been frozen should not be used.
3. Check the manufacturer's expiration date printed on the bottle. Do not use the insulin if the expiration date has passed.
4. If the vial has already been opened, check the date written on the bottle and compare it to the manufacturer's guidelines for the length of time it may be used. If no date has been written on the vial, do not use the insulin—it may be outdated.
5. Select the appropriate syringe size.
6. Compare the concentration of insulin written on the vial to the concentration marking on the syringe. Remember: U-100 insulin must be drawn up with a U-100 syringe and U-500 insulin must be drawn up with a U-500 syringe.
7. Clean the vial's rubber stopper using aseptic technique. Check your facility's policy regarding cleansing of medication vials.
8. Carefully uncap the insulin syringe, being careful to keep the cap clean and the needle shaft and plunger sterile.
9. Draw back air into the syringe in the same amount of the insulin that will be injected. For example, if 35 units of insulin will be injected, draw up approximately 35 units of air. This step prevents a vacuum from forming inside the vial.
10. Insert the needle into the center of the rubber stopper in the vial and inject the air.
11. Turn the vial upside down and draw back the necessary dosage of insulin, being careful to remove any bubbles that have collected inside the syringe.
12. Remove the needle from the vial and carefully recap the needle according to facility policy.
13. Have the dosage drawn double-checked by another nurse.
    Note: This step may be done prior to removing the needle from the vial. Follow your facility's policy.

Administering Insulin Using an Injection Pen

As an alternative to using vials and syringes, injection pens offer patients convenience and portability. The size of a large marking pen, insulin pens contain prefilled cartridges containing up to 315 units of insulin, allowing for days or weeks of use. The pens are reusable, although a new disposable pen needle should be used with each injection.

Injection pens are particularly useful for individuals who have poor eyesight or have difficulty manipulating syringes and vials with their hands. The pens require only dialing-in the insulin dose and administering the injection. Most injection pens have magnified dials for anyone with impaired vision, and the body of the pen is thicker than insulin syringes, making it much easier to handle.

Injection pens from various manufacturers may work slightly differently from one another. Before using an injection pen device, thoroughly read the manufacturer's directions to ensure that the correct dosage of insulin is being administered in the approved manner. Prefilled insulin cartridges are not designed to be opened and mixed together.

Administering Insulin Using an External Insulin Pump

External insulin pumps are pager-sized devices that can be worn on a belt or tucked inside a piece of clothing. Insulin pumps contain rapid- or short-acting insulin in prefilled syringes, which is infused though a very thin tube that is inserted into the subcutaneous tissue of the abdomen. The catheter is inserted through the skin using a very small, fine needle. The needle is then removed, and the catheter is secured to the skin with tape or a transparent dressing. The catheter can stay in place for up to three days. The pump can be disconnected for short periods for bathing or other activities.

Insulin pumps can be programmed to deliver both basal and bolus doses of insulin. Basal doses are injected continuously to provide a small amount of insulin throughout the day and night, whereas bolus doses are delivered around mealtimes. Some insulin pumps can even test blood glucose levels, providing individuals with warnings that blood glucose levels may be out of their target range. Not all individuals are candidates for external insulin pumps, though—they are best suited to individuals who are willing to check their blood sugar frequently and are able to manage the necessary adjustments to their insulin intake.

Intravenous Administration of Insulin

Insulin may be administered intravenously to treat individuals with extremely high blood glucose levels. Most intravenous protocols use regular insulin; however, several of the rapid-acting insulins, such as insulin aspart and insulin glulisine, may also be infused intravenously. The rapid- and short-acting insulins have a relatively fast onset of action, allowing the nurse to adjust, or titrate, the insulin infusion based on the patient's current blood glucose level. Intermediate, long-acting, and mixtures of insulin are not appropriate for intravenous infusions because of their long duration of action, which makes titration of insulin less predictable.

When infusing intravenous insulin, the nurse must frequently check the patient's blood glucose level and titrate the infusion rate until the patient's blood glucose is within a specified target range. The target range is tailored to the patient's medical status. Most healthcare institutions have an intravenous insulin infusion protocol in place (Fig. 15-4) as well as a flow sheet for documentation by nurses (Fig. 15-5). The protocol should include the following information:

- the type of insulin to be infused and directions for dilution (e.g., "Mix 100 units of regular insulin in 100 ml 0.9 sodium chloride solution.")
- the target glucose range
- a procedure (often called an algorithm) for titrating the infusion based on blood glucose levels
- frequency of fingerstick and/or lab blood glucose testing
- procedures for managing abnormally high or low blood glucose levels

Because of the high risk of adverse reactions that occur with intravenous insulin infusions, the nurse needs to clearly understand the protocol before initiating the infusion. A second nurse should verify all calculations or infusion rate changes.

General Hospital

Date:_____   Time:_____

Diagnosis: ☐ Type 1 Diabetes   ☐ Gestational Diabetes

☐ Type 2 Diabetes   ☐ Hyperglycemia

Place patient ID label here

Intravenous Insulin Protocol

☐ Standard intravenous insulin dilution for infusion:
- Mix 100 units human regular insulin in 100 mL 0.9% sodium chloride solution (1unit/1 mL).
- Use an infusion pump. Hang the insulin as a secondary infusion. Start a primary intravenous infusion of 0.9% sodium chloride solution at _____mL/hr.

☐ Begin insulin infusion using the Standard Insulin Infusion Algorithm below.

☐ Target glucose range:_____mg/dL.

☐ Notify provider:
  a. If blood glucose level is less than 70 mg/dL or over 400 mg/dL.
  b. Blood glucose changes greater than 100 mg/dL in one (1) hour.

Standard Insulin Infusion Algorithm

Blood Glucose Level (mg/dL)	Intravenous Infusion Rate (mL/hr)
Less than 100	Turn off infusion
100–119	1
120–149	1.5
150–199	2
200–249	2.5
250–299	3
300–349	4
350–399	6
Greater than 400	7

Bedside Glucose Monitoring

a. Fingerstick blood glucose level every hour until glucose level within target range.
b. After target glucose range reached, fingerstick blood glucose level every two (2) hours × 3 times; if blood glucose remains within the target range, decrease to every four (4) hours.

Treatment of Hypoglycemia (glucose less than 70 mg/dL)

a. Discontinue insulin infusion.
b. Call lab for STAT blood glucose level.
c. Give Dextrose 50% 25 mL intravenously.
d. Recheck blood glucose level in 15 minutes.
e. Repeat Dextrose 50% 25 mL intravenously if blood glucose is less than 70 mg/dL.
f. Repeat fingerstick blood glucose level in 15 minutes.
g. Notify provider.

☐ Other orders:

Physician's Signature: _____ Date:_____Time:_____

Nursing Verification

Signature	Initials	Signature	Initials

Figure 15-4 Sample Intravenous Insulin Protocol

Date	Time	Current Rate (mL/hr)	Blood Glucose (mg/dL)	New Rate (mL/hr)	Next Blood Glucose	Notes	Initials

General Hospital
Intravenous Insulin Flow Sheet

Place patient ID label here

Nursing Verification

Signature	Init	Signature	Init	Signature	Init

Figure 15-5 Sample Intravenous Insulin Flow Sheet

Mixing Insulin

Occasionally, patients may have more than one type of insulin ordered to be given at the same time. To reduce the number of injections given to patients, nurses may be tempted to mix two types of insulin together. However, only a few types of insulin may be mixed in the same syringe (Table 15-3). Mixing insulin in a syringe or contaminating one insulin vial with a different type of insulin may result in the alteration of the onset, peak, and duration of action. There is no

Table 15-3	Insulins That May Be Mixed	
Combinations	**Directions for Mixing**
Insulin glulisine (Apidra) + NPH insulin	Draw insulin glulisine into syringe first.
Insulin lispro (Humalog) + NPH insulin	Draw insulin lispro into syringe first.
Insulin aspart (Novolog) + NPH insulin	Draw insulin aspart into syringe first.
Regular insulin + NPH insulin	Draw regular insulin into syringe first.

rule of thumb as to which types of insulin may be mixed—always refer to the manufacturer's package insert for guidance, and always administer the injection as quickly as possible after mixing. Box 15-4 describes the process of mixing two types of insulin together in one syringe. See Figure 15-6.

■ Box 15-4   Mixing NPH Insulin With Regular or Rapid-Acting Insulin

1. Remove the vials of NPH and the rapid-acting or regular insulin from the storage area.
2. Ensure that the insulin has not expired. Check both the manufacturer's date of expiration and the open date written on the vials. If the vial has not been previously opened, write the date and initial the vial.
3. Inspect the insulin for appearance.
4. Gently mix the NPH insulin before it is drawn into a syringe so that the particles are dispersed evenly. The correct method of mixing NPH is to roll it between the palms of your hands for one minute. Avoid shaking NPH, as shaking creates air bubbles.
5. Cleanse the rubber stoppers of the NPH insulin vial and the rapid-acting or regular insulin vial using two separate alcohol wipes or other antiseptic. (Follow your facility's procedure for the type of antiseptic and amount of time spent cleansing the stopper.)
6. Using the appropriate size insulin syringe, draw up an amount of air approximately equal to the total number of units of insulin to be injected (units of NPH insulin + units of rapid-acting or regular insulin).
7. Inject air into the NPH insulin vial in the amount that you will be drawing up. Withdraw the needle.
8. Inject air into the rapid-acting or regular insulin vial in the amount that you will be drawing up. Do not remove the needle. Turn the vial of insulin upside down and withdraw the amount of insulin ordered, making sure to remove all air bubbles and maintaining the sterility of the needle and plunger. Remove the needle from the vial of rapid-acting or regular insulin. Ensure that the correct number of units have been drawn up.
9. Insert the needle into the bottle of NPH insulin. Slowly draw up the necessary number of units to equal the total number of units to be injected. (For example, if the patient is to receive 12 units of regular insulin and 13 units of NPH, the total number of units to be injected is 25.) Be sure to withdraw only the amount that is needed. If you withdraw more NPH insulin than is needed, do not inject the excess into the vial. You may change the onset, peak, and duration of action of the insulin. Drawing up the NPH slowly will also prevent air bubbles from being introduced into the syringe.
10. Administer the insulin mixture as soon as possible after preparation.

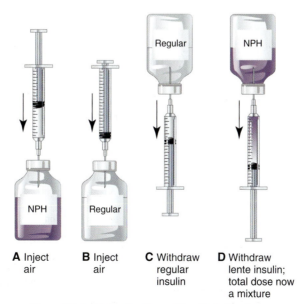

A Inject air   **B** Inject air   **C** Withdraw regular insulin   **D** Withdraw lente insulin; total dose now a mixture

Figure 15-6 Mixing Two Types of Insulin in One Syringe

Practice Insulin Delivery Systems and Mixing Insulin

(answers on page 316)

Choose the best answer for each question.

1. The nurse is to draw up 14 units of insulin lispro (Humalog). Which syringe is the most appropriate to use?
   a. 1-mL tuberculin syringe
   b. 0.3-mL/30-unit insulin syringe
   c. 0.5-mL/50-unit insulin syringe
   d. 1-mL/100-unit insulin syringe

2. The nurse is to draw up 78 units of NPH insulin (Novolin N). Which syringe is the most appropriate to use?
   a. 1-mL tuberculin syringe
   b. 0.3-mL/30-unit insulin syringe
   c. 0.5-mL/50-unit insulin syringe
   d. 1-mL/100-unit insulin syringe

3. The nurse is to draw up 2 units of regular insulin (Humulin R). Which syringe is the most appropriate to use?
   a. 1-mL tuberculin syringe
   b. 0.3-mL/30-unit insulin syringe
   c. 0.5-mL/50-unit insulin syringe
   d. 1-mL/100-unit insulin syringe

4. Which of these items should the nurse check before withdrawing insulin from a vial?
   a. the manufacturer's expiration date
   b. the appearance of the insulin
   c. the date the vial was opened
   d. All of the above

5. Which type of insulin may be given intravenously?
   a. regular insulin (Humulin R)
   b. NPH insulin (Novolin N)
   c. insulin detemir (Levemir)
   d. insulin glargine (Lantus)

On the syringes shown, indicate the correct amount of insulin to be administered.

6. 21 units

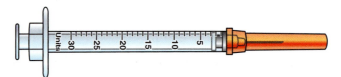

Figure 15-7 0.3-mL/30-Unit Syringe

7. 3 units

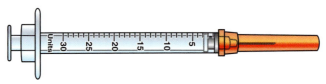

Figure 15-8 0.3-mL/30-Unit Syringe

8. 67 units

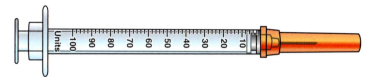

Figure 15-9 1-mL/100-Unit Syringe

Choose True or False for each statement.

9. Injection pen devices are a good choice for individuals who have poor eyesight.   True   False

10. NPH insulin (Novolin N) may be mixed with insulin aspart (NovoLog).   True   False

Read Case Studies 15-1 and 15-2 and answer the questions.

Case Study 15–1

Lilly Reid, a 79-year-old female, is admitted to the medical unit for pneumonia. She has a history of heart disease, hypothyroidism, and type 2 diabetes. Her provider initiates the subcutaneous insulin protocol described in Figure 15-10. You are the RN.

1. *Ms. Reid's blood fingerstick blood glucose levels have been ordered ac and hs. What does this mean? At what times should her blood glucose levels be tested?*

2. *How many grams of carbohydrates is Ms. Reid allowed with each meal? At bedtime?*

3. *What two types of insulin are prescribed for Ms. Reid?*

4. *Is Ms. Reid on the low-dose, medium-dose, or high-dose regimen?*

You are preparing to administer Ms. Reid's lunchtime dose of insulin. Ms. Reid's blood glucose level at 1145 was 208 mg/dL.

5. *How much insulin will you administer? Document your actions on the Subcutaneous Insulin Flow Sheet in Figure 15-11.*

At dinnertime, Ms. Reid's blood glucose level is 263 mg/dL.

6. *How much insulin will you administer? Document your actions on the Subcutaneous Insulin Flow Sheet in Figure 15-11.*

At bedtime, Ms. Reid's blood glucose level is 175 mg/dL.

7. *How much insulin will you administer? Document your actions on the Subcutaneous Insulin Flow Sheet in Figure 15-11.*

GENERAL HOSPITAL

Date: _12/13/2018_ Time: ___0715___

Diagnosis: ☐ Type 1 Diabetes   ☐ Gestational Diabetes

☑ Type 2 Diabetes   ☐ Hyperglycemia

Reid, Lilly R.
DOB: 06/29/1939
MR#: B93017483
Dr. Helen Michel

SUBCUTANEOUS INSULIN PROTOCOL	Initials
☑ **Discontinue all previous insulin orders.**	WM
Labs: ☑ Electrolytes ☑ Urinalysis (with C&S if indicated) ☑ HbA1C ☑ CBC	WM
Treat for Hypoglycemia: • Call lab for STAT blood glucose level. • If conscious and taking PO foods/fluids, provide 8 oz juice or milk and ½ of a meat, cheese, or peanut butter sandwich. • If unconscious or NPO, administer 25 mL Dextrose 50%, intravenously STAT. May repeat × 1. • Re-check blood glucose in 20 minutes. • If blood glucose less than 70 mg/dL × 2, call provider.	WM

Diet: ☐ NPO   ☐ Enteral Feeding   ☐ TPN   ☑ Carbohydrate Counting: — WM

Calories	Carbohydrate Units per Meal
☑ 1200–1500 cal/day	45 grams
☐ 1600–2000 cal/day	60 grams
☐ 2100–2400 cal/day	75 grams
☐ Over 2400 cal/day	90 grams
☐ Gestational	30 grams breakfast, 60 grams lunch, 75 grams dinner

☑ Snack at bedtime (15 grams Carbohydrate)

Fingerstick Blood Glucose Monitoring: ☑ ac and hs   ☐ every 6 hours   ☐ Other: _____   WM

INSULIN REGIMEN

Basal Insulin: ☑ Insulin glargine: ____10____ units every __evening at 2200__   WM

☐ NPH insulin: _____ units every _____

☐ Mixture: _____ units every _____

☐ Other: _____

Mealtime Insulin: ☑ Insulin aspart   ☐ Other: _____

___3___ units at breakfast ___3___ units at lunch

___3___ units at dinner ___0___ units at bedtime

Correction Insulin: Correction insulin (use table here) should be administered with mealtime insulin (if ordered) if blood glucose is over 150 mg/dL. Use ☑ Insulin aspart or ☐ Other: _____

If glucose is:	☑ Low Dose Regimen	☐ Medium Dose Regimen	☐ High Dose Regimen
151–200 mg/dL	1 unit	1 unit	1 unit
201–250 mg/dL	2 units	3 units	4 units
251–300 mg/dL	3 units	5 units	7 units
301–350 mg/dL	4 units	7 units	10 units
351–400 mg/dL	5 units	8 units	12 units
Over 400 mg/dL	6 units and call provider	9 units and call provider	14 units and call provider

PHYSICIAN'S SIGNATURE: _Helen Michel, MD_   Date: _12/13/2018_ Time: _0715_

NURSING VERIFICATION

Signature	Initials	Signature	Initials
W. MANNERING, RN	WM		

Figure 15-10 Subcutaneous Insulin Protocol

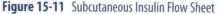

Date	Time	Blood Glucose (mg/dL)	Insulin Administered			Treatment for Hypoglycemia	Initials
			Type	Amount	Site		

General Hospital
Subcutaneous Insulin Flow Sheet

Reid, Lilly R.
DOB: 06/29/1939
MR#: B93017483
Dr. Helen Michel

Nursing Verification					
Signature	Init	Signature	Init	Signature	Init

Figure 15-11 Subcutaneous Insulin Flow Sheet

Case Study 15–2

Gary Smith, a 21-year-old male, has type 1 diabetes. He was diagnosed with the disease when he was 3 years old. Mr. Smith manages his diabetes using an external insulin pump and was doing well up until 2 days ago when his blood glucose levels began rising. Mr. Smith was admitted to the hospital this morning with a severe urinary tract infection. His blood glucose levels are ranging from 280 mg/dL to 350 mg/dL. Mr. Smith's physician places him on the intravenous insulin protocol described in Figure 15-12. You are the RN.

1. What is the blood glucose target range selected for Mr. Smith by his physician?
2. Under what conditions should you notify Mr. Smith's physician?
3. How often should you check Mr. Smith's blood glucose level by fingerstick?

You receive the intravenous insulin bag from the pharmacy and check the bag to ensure that it was mixed as ordered.

4. How many total mL of 0.9% sodium chloride solution should the bag contain?
5. How many total units of insulin should the bag contain?
6. What is the final concentration of insulin in the bag in units/mL?

You prepare to begin the infusion. You make sure that Mr. Smith's intravenous line is working as it should and that the primary solution hanging is 0.9% sodium chloride infusing at 100 mL/hr. You hang the insulin bag as a secondary infusion. Mr. Smith's fingerstick blood glucose level at 1430 is 342 mg/dL.

7. Refer to the standard insulin infusion algorithm on the physician's order sheet. At what rate (mL/hr) should you set the infusion rate for the insulin? Document your answers on the Intravenous Insulin Flow Sheet in Figure 15-13.
8. When should you do the next blood glucose check? Document your answers on the Intravenous Insulin Flow Sheet in Figure 15-13.
9. At 1530, Mr. Smith's blood glucose level is 361 mg/dL. What actions should you take? Document these actions of the Intravenous Insulin Flow Sheet in Figure 15-13. When is the next blood glucose due?

Continued

General Hospital

Date: *10/03/2018*　Time: *1345*

Diagnosis: ☑ Type 1 Diabetes　☐ Gestational Diabetes

　　　　　　☐ Type 2 Diabetes　☐ Hyperglycemia

Smith, Gary L.
DOB: 4/15/1997
MR#: B93017589
Dr. James R. Deleon

Intravenous Insulin Protocol

☑ Standard intravenous insulin dilution for infusion:
- Mix 100 units human regular insulin in 100 mL 0.9% sodium chloride solution (1unit/1 mL).
- Use an infusion pump. Hang insulin as a secondary infusion. Start a primary intravenous infusion of 0.9% sodium chloride at *100* mL/hr.

☑ Begin insulin infusion using the Standard Insulin Infusion Algorithm below.

☑ Target glucose range: *80-110* mg/dL.

☑ Notify provider:
　a. If blood glucose level is less that 70 mg/dL or over 400 mg/dL.
　b. Blood glucose changes greater than 100 mg/dL in one (1) hour.

Standard Insulin Infusion Algorithm

Blood Glucose Level (mg/dL)	Intravenous Infusion Rate (mL/hr)
Less than 100	Turn off infusion
100–119	1
120–149	1.5
150–199	2
200–249	2.5
250–299	3
300–349	4
350–399	6
Greater than 400	7

Bedside Glucose Monitoring

　a. Fingerstick blood glucose level every hour until glucose level within target range.
　b. After target glucose range reached, fingerstick blood glucose level every two (2) hours × 3 times; if blood glucose remains within the target range, decrease to every four (4) hours.

Treatment of Hypoglycemia (glucose less than 70 mg/dL)

　a. Discontinue insulin infusion.
　b. Call lab for STAT blood glucose level.
　c. Give Dextrose 50% 25 mL intravenously.
　d. Recheck blood glucose level in 15 minutes.
　e. Repeat Dextrose 50% 25 mL intravenously if blood glucose is less than 70 mg/dL.
　f. Repeat fingerstick blood glucose level in 15 minutes.
　g. Notify provider.

☐ Other orders:

Physician's Signature: *James Deleon, MD*　Date: *10/03/2018*　Time: *1345*

Nursing Verification

Signature	Initials	Signature	Initials
Andy Rivas, RN	AR		

Figure 15-12 Intravenous Insulin Protocol

General Hospital
Intravenous Insulin Flow Sheet

Smith, Gary L.
DOB: 04/15/1997
MR#: B93017589
Dr. James R. Deleon

Date	Time	Current Rate (mL/hr)	Blood Glucose (mg/dL)	New Rate (mL/hr)	Next Blood Glucose	Notes	Initials

Nursing Verification					
Signature	Init	Signature	Init	Signature	Init

Figure 15-13 Intravenous Insulin Flow Sheet

Case Study 15–2—cont'd

After 12 hours of intravenous insulin, Mr. Smith's blood sugar is within target range and you increase the time between fingersticks as ordered. On 10/04/18 at 0730, Mr. Smith's fingerstick blood glucose level is 56 mg/dL.

10. *What action should you take, based on the blood glucose reading of 56 mg/dL?*

After receiving the first dose of dextrose 50%, 25 mL, Mr. Smith's blood glucose level is 84 mg/dL and he is eating breakfast. The physician discontinues the intravenous insulin protocol and orders blood glucose levels before meals and at bedtimes. He places Mr. Smith on a subcutaneous insulin regimen starting at lunch.

11. *Document the last blood glucose reading and the time of the next blood glucose level on the Intravenous Insulin Flow Sheet in Figure 15-13.*

Key Points

1. Diabetes mellitus is a group of metabolic diseases characterized by hyperglycemia. Diabetes is managed through a combination of medications, diet, and exercise.
2. Insulin is the hormone, produced in the beta cells of the pancreas, that allows the body to use and store glucose.
3. Synthetic insulin is available in rapid-acting, short-acting, intermediate-acting, and long-acting forms.
4. Regular (short-acting) insulin is available in two strengths: 100 units/mL and 500 units/mL.
5. Insulin may be ordered on a routine (fixed) schedule, to be administered either before or after meals, as a correction dose, or on a sliding-scale basis. Most insulin regimens consist of a combination of methods.
6. Insulin may be administered subcutaneously using a syringe and vial, an insulin pen device, or an external insulin pump.
7. Insulin may be administered intravenously. Only regular insulin and several of the rapid-acting types of insulin may be given intravenously. Careful attention is needed when titrating an insulin infusion based on the patient's blood glucose level.
8. NPH insulin may be mixed with rapid-acting and regular insulin. Care must be taken to avoid cross-contaminating the vials of insulin, as this may alter the onset, peak, and duration of action.

Chapter Post-Test

(answers in Unit 4)

Multiple Choice

Select the best answer for each question.

1. Diabetes that is present only during pregnancy is called:
   a. type 1 diabetes.
   b. type 2 diabetes.
   c. borderline diabetes.
   d. gestational diabetes.

2. Diabetes mellitus is managed by:
   a. diet, exercise, and meditation.
   b. diet, exercise, and medication.
   c. medication only.
   d. diet and exercise only.

3. The amount of insulin that an individual needs to maintain normal or near-normal blood glucose levels:
   a. is the same for everybody.
   b. varies, depending on the age of the person.
   c. varies greatly from person to person.
   d. depends upon the individual's body type.

4. Which type of insulin has an onset of 1 to 2 hours, peaks in 4 to 12 hours, and has a duration of action from 18–24 hours?
   a. NPH insulin (Novolin N)
   b. insulin glulisine (Apidra)
   c. insulin detemir (Levemir)
   d. regular insulin (Humulin R)

5. Which insulin has an onset of 3 to 4 hours, does not peak, and has a duration of action of 24 hours?
   a. NPH insulin (Novolin N)
   b. insulin glulisine (Apidra)
   c. regular insulin (Humulin R)
   d. insulin glargine (Lantus)

6. Which insulin should be administered 30 to 60 minutes before meals?
   a. NPH insulin (Novolin N)
   b. regular insulin (Humulin R)
   c. insulin aspart (NovoLog)
   d. insulin lispro (Humalog)

7. Which insulin may be mixed together in the same syringe?
   a. NPH insulin (Novolin N) and insulin detemir (Levemir)
   b. NPH insulin (Novolin N) and regular insulin (Humulin R)
   c. insulin glargine (Lantus) and regular insulin (Humulin R)
   d. insulin aspart (NovoLog) and insulin lispro (Humalog)

8. Which insulin is rapid-acting?
   a. insulin aspart (NovoLog)
   b. insulin glargine (Lantus)
   c. regular insulin (Humulin R)
   d. insulin detemir (Levemir)

9. Which insulin should be injected right before a meal?
   a. insulin glargine (Lantus)
   b. insulin detemir (Levemir)
   c. NPH insulin (Novolin N)
   d. insulin glulisine (Apidra)

Questions 10 through 13 refer to this scenario:

A provider writes this sliding scale insulin order for a patient:

Regular insulin (Humulin R), subcut, before meals, according to the following fingerstick blood glucose (BG) levels:

BG less than or equal to 140 mg/dL	0 units
BG 140–150 mg/dL	1 unit
BG 151–160 mg/dL	2 units
BG 161–170 mg/dL	4 units
BG 171–180 mg/dL	6 units
BG 181–200 mg/dL	8 units
BG over 200 mg/dL	Call provider

10. The nurse obtains a fingerstick blood glucose level just before lunch. It is 196 mg/dL. How many units of insulin should the nurse administer to the patient?
    a. 2 units
    b. 4 units
    c. 6 units
    d. 8 units

11. Just before dinner, the nurse obtains another fingerstick blood glucose level from the patient. It is now 148 mg/dL. Which action should be taken by the nurse?
    a. administer 0 units of insulin
    b. administer 1 unit of insulin
    c. administer 2 units of insulin then call the provider
    d. call the provider for further orders

12. If the nurse administers the regular insulin injection at 1700 (5:00 p.m.), at what time would the nurse expect the insulin to peak?
    a. between 1700 (5 p.m.) and 1900 (6 p.m.)
    b. between 1800 (6 p.m.) and 2000 (8 p.m.)
    c. between 1900 (7 p.m.) and 2100 (9 p.m.)
    d. between 2000 (8 p.m.) and 2200 (10 p.m.)

13. If the nurse administers the regular insulin injection at 1700 (5:00) p.m., at what time would the nurse expect the insulin to lose effectiveness?
    a. between 1900 (7 p.m.) and 2100 (9 p.m.)
    b. between 2000 (8 p.m.) and 2200 (10 p.m.)
    c. between 2100 (9 p.m.) and 2300 (11 p.m.)
    d. between 2200 (10 p.m.) and 2400 (12 a.m.)

14. One characteristic of a U-100 insulin syringe that differentiates it from a standard syringe is:
    a. The cap of the insulin syringe is orange.
    b. An insulin syringe can hold up to 3 mL of solution.
    c. The needles on an insulin syringe may be up to 1½ inches long.
    d. An insulin syringe has the U-250 designation on it.

15. A nurse is preparing to administer an injection of insulin glargine (Lantus) from an unopened vial. The package insert states that insulin glargine may be used for 28 days after it is opened. If the current date is October 3, on which date will this vial of insulin expire (assuming the manufacturer's expiration date has not passed)?
    a. October 29
    b. October 30
    c. October 31
    d. November 1

Insulin Administration

On the syringes shown in Figures 15-14 through 15-21, indicate the correct amount of insulin to be administered.

16. 27 units

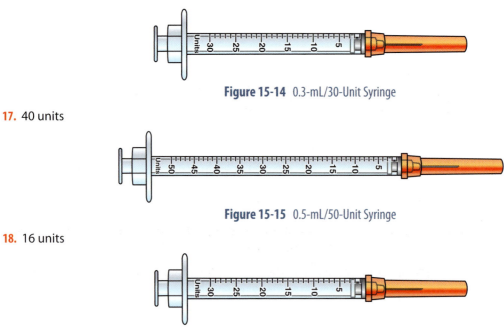

Figure 15-14 0.3-mL/30-Unit Syringe

17. 40 units

Figure 15-15 0.5-mL/50-Unit Syringe

18. 16 units

Figure 15-16 0.3-mL/30-Unit Syringe

19. 88 units

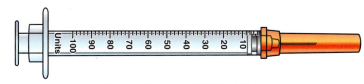

Figure 15-17 1-mL/100-Unit Syringe

20. 9 units

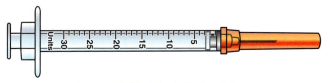

Figure 15-18 0.3-mL/30-Unit Syringe

21. 50 units

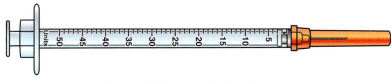

Figure 15-19 0.5-mL/50-Unit Syringe

22. 22 units

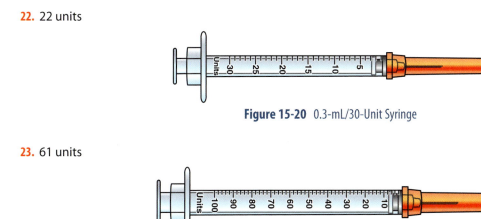

Figure 15-20 0.3-mL/30-Unit Syringe

23. 61 units

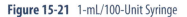

Figure 15-21 1-mL/100-Unit Syringe

True or False

24. External insulin pumps are a good choice for individuals who are able and willing to check their blood glucose levels often, and are able to make adjustments to their insulin intake.   True   False

25. Only the intermediate- and long-acting types of insulin should be used in intravenous infusions.   True   False

Answers to Practice Questions

Insulin Types and Orders

1. b
2. c
3. d
4. b
5. c
6. False
7. True
8. b
9. d
10. d

Insulin Delivery Systems and Mixing Insulin

1. b
2. d
3. b
4. d
5. a
6.

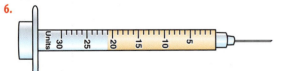

Figure 15-22 0.3-mL/30-Unit Syringe Filled to 21 Units

7.

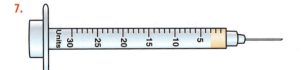

Figure 15-23 0.3-mL/30-Unit Syringe Filled to 3 Units

8.

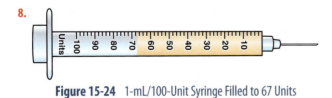

Figure 15-24 1-mL/100-Unit Syringe Filled to 67 Units

9. True
10. True

■ *Answers to Case Study 15–1*

1. *The abbreviation ac means before meals. The abbreviation hs means at bedtime. The actual times that meals are served depends upon a facility's schedule. Generally, blood glucose levels are taken anywhere from 1 hour to immediately before a patient's meal. Check the facility's policy for guidance.*

2. *Ms. Reid is allowed 45 grams of carbohydrates with each meal. She may have a snack at bedtime that contains 15 grams of carbohydrates.*

3. *Ms. Reid's physician prescribed both insulin glargine and insulin aspart. The insulin glargine provides the basal amount of insulin Ms. Reid needs between meals. The insulin aspart provides the short burst of insulin she needs for meals and snacks.*

4. *Ms. Reid was placed on the low-dose regimen. Individuals with type 2 diabetes who are placed on medium- or high-dose regimens have increased resistance to insulin.*

5. *You should administer 3 units of insulin aspart for the mealtime dose, plus 2 units of insulin aspart for the correction dose for a total of 5 units of insulin aspart.*

6. *You should administer 3 units of insulin aspart for the mealtime dose, plus 3 units of insulin aspart for the correction dose for a total of 6 units of insulin aspart.*

7. *You should administer 10 units of insulin glargine at bedtime. The rapid-acting insulin is only ordered for mealtimes, not bedtime.*

All the steps should be documented in the patient's medical record, taking care to note times and the patient's response to the interventions (Fig. 15-25).

Answers to Practice Questions

**General Hospital
Subcutaneous Insulin Flow Sheet**

Reid, Lilly R.
DOB: 06/29/1939
MR#: B93017483
Dr. Helen Michel

Date	Time	Blood Glucose (mg/dL)	Insulin Administered			Treatment for Hypoglycemia	Initials
			Type	**Amount**	**Site**		
12/13/18	1145	208	ASPART	5 UNITS	LEFT ABD.		WM
12/13/18	1700	263	ASPART	6 UNITS	RIGHT ABD.		WM
12/13/18	2200	175	GLARGINE	10 UNITS	LEFT LOWER ABD.		WM

Nursing Verification					
Signature	**Init**	**Signature**	**Init**	**Signature**	**Init**
W. MANNERING, RN	WM				

Figure 15-25 Completed Subcutaneous Insulin Flow Sheet

■ *Answers to Case Study 15–2*

1. *Mr. Smith's physician selected a blood glucose target range of 80–110 mg/dL.*
2. *You should notify Mr. Smith's physician if his blood glucose level is less than 70 mg/dL, over 400 mg/dL, or if Mr. Smith's blood glucose changes greater than 100 mg/dL in 1 hour. The protocol also requires that you notify the physician if Mr. Smith is treated for hypoglycemia.*
3. *You should check Mr. Smith's blood glucose level by fingerstick every hour until his blood glucose level is within target range (80–110 mg/dL), then every 2 hours for 6 hours (every 2 hours × 3 times), then every 4 hours until the protocol is discontinued by the physician.*
4. *The bag should contain 100 mL of 0.9% sodium chloride solution.*
5. *The bag should contain a total of 100 units of regular insulin.*
6. *The final concentration of the bag should be 1 unit/mL $\left(\dfrac{100\ units}{100\ mL} \right)$.*
7. *Based on a fingerstick blood glucose level of 342 mg/dL, you should set the infusion rate for the insulin at 4 mL/hr.*
8. *The next fingerstick blood glucose is due at 1530.*
9. *The infusion rate of insulin should be increased to 6 mL/hr. The next blood glucose level will be due at 1630.*
10. *The protocol states that the following actions should be taken if Mr. Smith's blood glucose level falls below 70 mg/dL:*
    a. *Discontinue the insulin infusion.*
    b. *Call the lab and order a STAT blood glucose level.*
    c. *Administer dextrose 50% (25 mL) by IV push.*
    d. *Recheck Mr. Smith's blood glucose level in 15 minutes. If his blood glucose remains less than 70 mg/dL, repeat the dextrose 50% (25 mL). Notify Mr. Smith's physician.*
11. *Document the blood glucose level of 84 mg/dL on the Intravenous Insulin Flow Sheet, noting the time it was taken. The next blood glucose level will be due before lunch, usually between 1130 and 1200. (Fig. 15-26).*

General Hospital **Subcutaneous Insulin Flow Sheet**					Smith, Gary L. DOB: 04/15/1997 MR#: B93017589 Dr. James R. Deleon		

Date	Time	Current Rate (mL/hr)	Blood Glucose (mg/dL)	New Rate (mL/hr)	Next Blood Glucose	Notes	Initials
10/03/18	1430	0	342	4	1530	Infusion started.	AR
10/03/18	1530	4	361	6	1630	Rate increased.	AR
10/04/18	0730	1	56	0	0745	D50 25mL given intravenously.	DK
10/04/18	0745	0	84	0	1145	intravenous insulin protocol discontinued.	DK

Nursing Verification					
Signature	Init	Signature	Init	Signature	Init
Andy Rivas, RN	AR	D. Klein RN	DK		

Figure 15-26 Completed Intravenous Insulin Flow Sheet

Chapter 16

Heparin Administration

Glossary

Aggregation: Clumping together of red blood cells.
Anticoagulant: A medication that prevents or delays the formation of blood clots.
Bolus or loading dose: A high initial dose of a medication that may be administered at the beginning of a course of treatment.
Embolism: The obstruction of a blood vessel by a foreign object or substance.
Hematoma: A collection of blood caused by a broken blood vessel.
International unit (IU): A designated amount of a substance that is accepted internationally.
Loading dose: Another name for bolus.
Reagent: A substance used to create a chemical reaction for detecting or measuring other substances.
Serum: Plasma; the clear, straw-colored fluid present in blood.
Thromboembolism: The blockage of a blood vessel by a thrombus that has detached and migrated from its site of origin.
Thrombosis: The formation of a blood clot within the vascular system.
Thrombus: A blood clot (plural is "thrombi").
Unfractionated: Not fractionated; whole.

Objectives

After completing this chapter, the learner will be able to—
1. Explain the process of a blood clot formation in a vein.
2. Describe the difference between unfractionated heparin and low molecular weight heparin.
3. Discuss the laboratory tests used to monitor heparin effectiveness.
4. Calculate subcutaneous doses of heparin and low molecular weight heparin.
5. Calculate an intermittent bolus dose of heparin.
6. Calculate the mL/hr flow rate for a continuous infusion of heparin.
7. Calculate the units/hr flow rate for a continuous infusion of heparin.
8. Calculate new flow rates in units/hr and mL/hr for a prescribed change in the dosage of a continuous heparin infusion.

Venous Thrombosis

Venous thrombosis occurs when a blood clot or thrombus forms inside a vein. Composed of red blood cells, platelets, and other clotting factors, thrombi may develop in association with a number of risk factors, such as blood disorders, blood vessel injuries, prolonged immobility, or major surgeries. Venous thrombi can form in both the shallow and deep veins in the body. A clot that forms in a deep vein is called a deep vein thrombosis (DVT) and tends to be more dangerous because pieces of the clot can break off and travel to other parts of the body, known as a thromboembolism. A thromboembolism may lodge in smaller vessels and cause damage to the surrounding tissues. For example, a thromboembolism that lodges in the arteries in the lungs is called a pulmonary embolism (PE), which can be fatal.

A number of medications may be prescribed to treat venous thrombosis or prevent the formation of a thrombus in patients who have risk factors. This chapter focuses specifically on heparin preparations, which require advanced math skills when administered intravenously.

Heparin

Heparin is an anticoagulant derived from bovine (cow) lungs and porcine (pig) intestines. Two types of heparin are used in treating thromboembolic disorders: unfractionated heparin (UH) and low molecular weight heparin (LMWH). The difference between the two substances is related to molecular size. UH is a very large molecule, compared with LMWH. Each type has specific uses, advantages, and disadvantages. Which heparin type is prescribed depends on the thromboembolic disorder being treated.

Subcutaneous Heparin Administration

Both UH and LMWH can be administered subcutaneously. LMWH is almost exclusively given subcutaneously except for enoxaparin, which may be given intravenously under certain circumstances. Heparin cannot be given orally because it is inactivated by stomach acids, and it cannot be administered intramuscularly because of the increased risk of hematoma formation.

UH is supplied in vials (Fig. 16-1 and Fig. 16-2) containing a specific concentration of heparin, such as 10 units/mL, 100 units/mL, 1000 units/mL, 5000 units/mL, 10,000 units/mL, 20,000 units/mL, and 40,000 units/mL. Very low concentrations of UH (10 units/mL and 100 units/mL) are not useful in treating thromboembolic disorders, but are helpful in keeping certain types of intravenous lines from clotting with blood (Fig. 16-3 and Fig. 16-4). This is known as a "heparin lock flush." The concentration and volume instilled into the catheter depends on the catheter's intended use and the recommendations of the manufacturer.

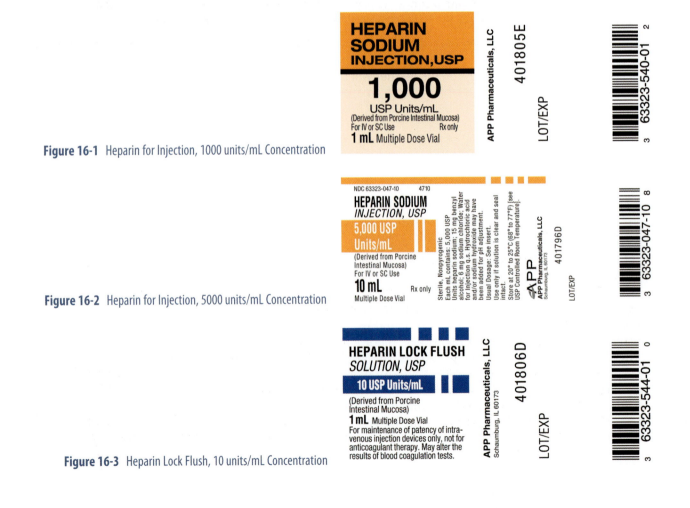

Figure 16-1 Heparin for Injection, 1000 units/mL Concentration

Figure 16-2 Heparin for Injection, 5000 units/mL Concentration

Figure 16-3 Heparin Lock Flush, 10 units/mL Concentration

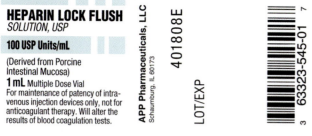

HEPARIN LOCK FLUSH
SOLUTION, USP

100 USP Units/mL

(Derived from Porcine
Intestinal Mucosa)
1 mL Multiple Dose Vial
For maintenance of patency of intravenous injection devices only, not for
anticoagulant therapy. Will alter the
results of blood coagulation tests.

APP Pharmaceuticals, LLC
Schaumburg, IL 60173

401808E

LOT/EXP

63323-545-01

Figure 16-4 Heparin Lock Flush, 100 units/mL Concentration

The highly concentrated solutions (20,000 units/mL and 40,000 units/mL) are added to large volumes of intravenous fluids for continuous infusions. Given subcutaneously, these highly concentrated UH preparations may cause excessive bleeding. Therefore, extreme care must be exercised when preparing UH for administration. It is imperative that the correct concentration be selected. Because of the high risk of adverse drug events associated with heparin, The Joint Commission's National Patient Safety Goal 03.05.01 (2017) was developed that delineates a hospital's responsibilities for the administration of UH and LMWH. See Box 16-1.

LMWH (enoxaparin, dalteparin, and tinzaparin) is supplied in prefilled syringes and multidose vials. The concentration of LMWH varies depending upon the type of LMWH selected and the diagnosis of the patient. Again, the nurse should read the medication label carefully when choosing the syringe or vial.

Calculating Subcutaneous Doses of UH and LMWH

Example 1: A provider orders UH 5000 units subcutaneously every 12 hours. The pharmacy provides a 10-mL vial of UH with a concentration of 5000 units/mL. How many mL's per dose should the nurse draw into the syringe? Round the answer to the nearest hundredth mL.

1. Set up the equation using dimensional analysis. The first set of quantities will be the concentration of the UH.

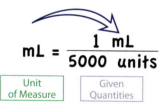

$$mL = \frac{1\ mL}{5000\ units}$$

Unit of Measure   Given Quantities

■ Box 16-1 National Patient Safety Goal 03.05.01

National Patient Safety Goal 03.05.01 was developed by The Joint Commission to decrease the chance of patient injury associated with anticoagulant use in hospitals. Anticoagulation therapy increases a patient's risk for injury because of its complexity of dosing, need for close follow-up monitoring, and inconsistency of patient compliance with treatment. In order to meet accreditation standards, hospitals must have an anticoagulation management program, which includes the following:
- Using prefilled syringes or premixed infusion bags when possible
- Having an approved protocol for the initiation and maintenance of anticoagulation therapy
- Utilizing programmable infusion pumps when heparin is administered continuously through an intravenous line
- Having a written policy that addresses baseline and ongoing laboratory testing for both unfractionated heparin and low molecular weight heparin
- Providing anticoagulation therapy education to prescribers, staff members, patients, and families about the necessity for follow-up testing, diet, potential adverse reactions, possible drug interactions, and issues regarding compliance with treatment

2. Insert the next given quantity—the dosage—to cancel the units in the denominator and solve the equation.

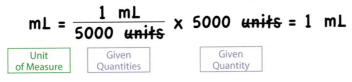

$$mL = \frac{1\ mL}{5000\ \cancel{units}} \times 5000\ \cancel{units} = 1\ mL$$

| Unit of Measure | Given Quantities | Given Quantity |

For Examples 2 and 3, refer to the directions in Example 1.

Example 2: A provider orders UH 8000 units subcutaneously every 8 hours. The pharmacy provides UH in a 1-mL vial with a concentration of 10,000 units/mL. How many mL per dose should the nurse draw into the syringe? Round the answer to nearest hundredth mL.

$$mL = \frac{1\ mL}{10,000\ \cancel{units}} \times 8000\ \cancel{units} = \frac{1\ mL \times 8000}{10,000} = 0.8\ mL$$

Example 3: A provider orders tinzaparin 16,000 IU, subcutaneously once daily. Tinzaparin is supplied in a 2-mL multidose vial containing 20,000 IU/mL. How many mL of tinzaparin per dose should the nurse draw into the syringe? Round the answer to the nearest hundredth mL.

$$mL = \frac{1\ mL}{20,000\ \cancel{IU}} \times 16,000\ \cancel{IU} = \frac{1\ mL \times 16,000}{20,000} = 0.8\ mL$$

Example 4: A provider orders enoxaparin 1 mg/kg subcutaneously every 12 hours. The patient weighs 70 kg. The pharmacy provides enoxaparin in a 3-mL vial containing 300 mg. How many mL of enoxaparin per dose should the nurse draw into the syringe? Round the answer to the nearest hundredth mL.

1. Set up the equation using dimensional analysis. Insert the given quantities related to the concentration of the enoxaparin.

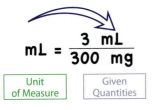

$$mL = \frac{3\ mL}{300\ mg}$$

| Unit of Measure | Given Quantities |

2. Insert the next set of quantities—the prescribed weight-based dosage.

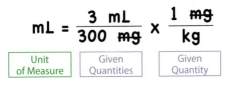

$$mL = \frac{3\ mL}{300\ \cancel{mg}} \times \frac{1\ \cancel{mg}}{kg}$$

| Unit of Measure | Given Quantities | Given Quantity |

3. Insert the last given quantity—the patient's weight—and solve the equation.

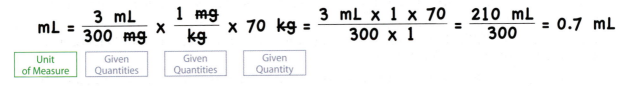

$$mL = \frac{3\ mL}{300\ \cancel{mg}} \times \frac{1\ \cancel{mg}}{\cancel{kg}} \times 70\ \cancel{kg} = \frac{3\ mL \times 1 \times 70}{300 \times 1} = \frac{210\ mL}{300} = 0.7\ mL$$

| Unit of Measure | Given Quantities | Given Quantities | Given Quantity |

For Example 5, refer to the directions in Example 4.

Example 5: A provider orders dalteparin 120 IU/kg subcutaneously once daily. The patient weighs 62.5 kg. The pharmacy provides dalteparin in prefilled syringes with concentrations of 5000 IU/0.2 mL, 7500 IU/0.3 mL, or 10,000 IU/0.4 mL. How many mL's of dalteparin should the nurse administer? Round the answer to the nearest hundredth mL. Which prefilled syringe should the nurse select?

1. Set up the equation using dimensional analysis, inserting the prescribed weight-based dosage of dalteparin as the first set of given quantities.

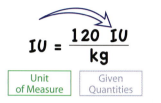

$$IU = \frac{120\ IU}{kg}$$

Unit of Measure	Given Quantities

2. Insert the next given quantity—the patient's weight—and solve the equation.

$$IU = \frac{120\ IU}{kg} \times 62.5\ kg = 120\ IU \times 62.5 = 7500\ IU$$

Unit of Measure	Given Quantities	Given Quantity

3. Select the appropriate prefilled syringe of dalteparin. Since the patient will be receiving 7500 IU of dalteparin, select the prefilled syringe with 7500 IU in 0.3 mL. The nurse should administer the full 0.3 mL of dalteparin.

Practice Calculating Subcutaneous Doses of UH and LMWH

(answers on page 340)

Calculate the volumes (in mL's) of UH or LMWH that the nurse should draw into a syringe. Round the answers to the nearest hundredth mL.

1. A provider orders UH 5000 units, subcutaneously, every 12 hours. The pharmacy provides a 5-mL vial of UH with a concentration of 10,000 units/mL.

2. A provider orders enoxaparin 120 mg, subcutaneously, daily. The pharmacy provides a prefilled syringe with 120 mg in 0.8 mL.

3. A provider orders UH 2500 units, subcutaneously, daily. The pharmacy provides a 5-mL vial of UH with a concentration of 5000 units/mL.

4. A provider orders UH 7500 units, subcutaneously, daily. The pharmacy provides a 5-mL vial of UH with a concentration of 10,000 units/mL.

5. A provider orders tinzaparin 15,000 anti-Xa units, subcutaneously, daily. The pharmacy supplies tinzaparin in a vial containing 20,000 anti-Xa units/mL.

6. A provider orders UH 1000 units, subcutaneously, every 12 hours. The pharmacy provides a 5-mL vial of UH with a concentration of 5000 units/mL.

7. A provider orders UH 2000 units, subcutaneously, every 12 hours. The pharmacy provides a 5-mL vial of UH with a concentration of 5000 units/mL.

8. A provider orders dalteparin 5000 IU subcutaneously, daily. The pharmacy supplies dalteparin in a vial containing 10,000 IU/mL.

9. A provider orders UH 7500 units, subcutaneously, every 12 hours. The pharmacy provides a 5-mL vial of UH with a concentration of 20,000 units/mL.

10. A provider orders UH 3500 units, subcutaneously, every 12 hours. The pharmacy provides a 5-mL vial of UH with a concentration of 5000 units/mL.

Intravenous UH Administration

UH may be administered intravenously as well as subcutaneously. It may be infused intermittently as a bolus dose or continuously as a maintenance solution. A bolus dose of UH is given to increase the blood level of heparin rapidly. It is administered just prior to a continuous infusion or intermittently during a continuous infusion if the patient has not reached an anticoagulated state. Most UH protocols are based on patient weight, so it is vital that the patient be weighed prior to beginning the infusion.

Note: UH is typically referred to as heparin in the clinical setting. From this point on in the chapter, any reference to heparin will be referring to unfractionated heparin (UH), not LMWH.

Calculating Intermittent Bolus Doses of Heparin

Example 1: A provider orders a heparin bolus dose of 80 units/kg intravenously prior to initiating a continuous infusion. The patient weighs 56 kg. The pharmacy provides heparin in a concentration of 5000 units/mL in a 10-mL vial. How many mL's of heparin should the nurse draw up in the syringe? Round the answer to the nearest tenth mL.

1. Set up the equation using dimensional analysis. Insert the given quantities related to the concentration of the heparin.

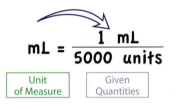

2. Insert the next set of quantities—the prescribed weight-based dosage.

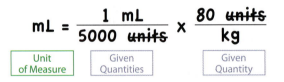

3. Insert the last given quantity—the patient's weight—and solve the equation.

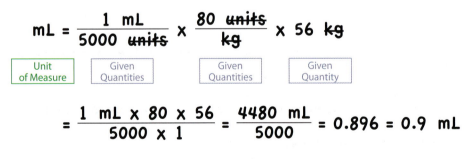

$$= \frac{1 \text{ mL} \times 80 \times 56}{5000 \times 1} = \frac{4480 \text{ mL}}{5000} = 0.896 = 0.9 \text{ mL}$$

Alert! Having to obtain more than one vial of heparin should alert the nurse to double-check the calculation and to have another nurse check the calculation for accuracy.

For Examples 2–5, refer to the directions in Example 1.

Example 2: A provider orders a heparin bolus of 60 units/kg intravenously. The patient weighs 98 kg. The pharmacy provides heparin in a concentration of 10,000 units/mL in a 5-mL vial. How many mL's of heparin should the nurse draw into the syringe? Round the answer to the nearest tenth mL.

$$mL = \frac{1 \text{ mL}}{10,000 \text{ units}} \times \frac{60 \text{ units}}{kg} \times 98 \text{ kg}$$

$$= \frac{1 \text{ mL} \times 60 \times 98}{10,000 \times 1} = \frac{5880 \text{ mL}}{10,000} = 0.588 = 0.6 \text{ mL}$$

Example 3: A provider orders a heparin bolus of 3500 units. The pharmacy provides heparin in a concentration of 1000 units/mL in a 10-mL vial. How many mL of heparin should the nurse draw into the syringe? Round the answer to the nearest tenth mL.

$$mL = \frac{1 \text{ mL}}{1000 \text{ units}} \times 3500 \text{ units} = \frac{1 \text{ mL} \times 3500}{1000} = 3.5 \text{ mL}$$

Example 4: A provider orders a heparin bolus of 7000 units. The pharmacy provides heparin in a concentration of 5000 units/mL in a 10-mL vial. How many mL of heparin should the nurse draw into the syringe? Round the answer to the nearest tenth mL.

$$mL = \frac{1 \text{ mL}}{5000 \text{ units}} \times 7000 \text{ units} = \frac{1 \text{ mL} \times 7000}{5000} = 1.4 \text{ mL}$$

Example 5: A provider orders a heparin bolus of 5000 units. The pharmacy provides heparin in a concentration of 5000 units/mL in a 1-mL vial. How many mL of heparin should the nurse draw into the syringe? Round the answer to the nearest tenth mL.

$$mL = \frac{1 \text{ mL}}{5000 \text{ units}} \times 5000 \text{ units} = \frac{1 \text{ mL} \times 5000}{5000} = 1 \text{ mL}$$

Calculating Continuous Heparin Flow Rates

Every hospital should have a protocol for continuous infusions of heparin. The protocol should specify the following information:

- The laboratory tests needed prior to starting heparin therapy
- The bolus or loading dose of heparin to administer prior to starting the continuous infusion
- The infusion rate
- The type and frequency of laboratory testing during the infusion

In addition, the protocol should provide clear directions for adjusting the heparin dosage if the laboratory test values are outside the expected therapeutic limits. See Figure 16-5.

Heparin is available in commercially premixed solutions of 1000 units in 500 mL 0.9% sodium chloride solution (normal saline), 2000 units in 1000 mL 0.9% sodium chloride solution, 20,000 units in 500 mL 5% dextrose solution, and 25,000 units in 250 mL or 500 mL 5% dextrose solution. To decrease the risk of human error in mixing heparin, many hospital pharmacies prefer to purchase premixed heparin solutions rather than making their own.

Date: _____   Time: _____

Diagnosis:	Allergies:	Patient's Total Body Weight: _____kg
☐ DVT/PE ☐ Cardiovascular		

☐ Draw baseline CBC and aPTT.
☐ Obtain baseline urinalysis.
☐ Administer bolus dose of _____ units heparin intravenously (round to the nearest 100 units).
  ☐ Note: suggested dose for prevention dose (cardiovascular/thrombolytic indications) is 60 units/kg.
  ☐ Note: suggested dose for treatment dose (DVT/PE) is 80 units/kg.
☐ NO LOADING DOSE INDICATED.
☐ Begin heparin infusion at _____ units/hour intravenously (rounded to the nearest 100 units).
  ☐ Note: suggested prevention dose 12–15 units/kg/hour.
  ☐ Note: suggested treatment dose 18 units/kg/hour.
☐ Use standard heparin infusion concentration of 25,000 units in 250 mL D5W.
☐ Use an infusion pump.
☐ Draw aPTT every 6 hours until two aPTTs drawn at least 24 hours apart are within the therapeutic range. Based on the aPTT results, adjust the heparin infusion rate as indicated on the chart below. Record rate of infusion, aPTT results, boluses given, and any adjustments made on the Heparin Flow Sheet.

aPTT Results (seconds)	Bolus Dose	Stop Infusion?	Infusion Rate Change
Under 50	4000 units	NO	Increase rate by 200 units/hr.
50–59	2000 units	NO	Increase rate by 100 units/hr.
60–100	No bolus	NO	No change in rate.
101–110	No bolus	NO	Decrease rate by 100 units/hr.
111–120	No bolus	NO	Decrease rate by 200 units/hr.
121–150	No bolus	Stop infusion for 30 minutes.	Decrease rate by 200 units/hr.
151–199	No bolus	Stop infusion for 60 minutes.	Decrease rate by 200 units/hr.
200	No bolus	Until aPTT is less than 200 seconds.	Redraw aPTT STAT. Draw STAT aPTTs every hour until aPTT less than 100. Then decrease the last infusion rate by 300 units/hr and repeat aPTT in 6 hours. Notify MD.

☐ Draw aPTT, PT, and CBC every morning.
☐ Check all stools for occult blood.
☐ Notify MD for: (1) any signs of bleeding; (2) if unable to obtain blood sample; (3) no intravenous access for greater than 1 hour; (4) if platelet count falls below 100,000.

Patient Identification Sticker	**Intravenous Heparin Administration Protocol** White: Medical Record Pink: Pharmacy Yellow: Nursing

Figure 16-5 Sample Weight-Based IV Heparin Administration Protocol

Heparin must be infused using an intravenous infusion pump. Many intravenous pumps can monitor heparin infusions in mL/hr and units/hr. Nurses need to be able to calculate the flow rate of heparin in both mL/hr and units/hr to verify that the flow rate is correct. Most facilities utilize some type of heparin flow sheet for nursing staff to keep track of changes in heparin infusions (Fig. 16-6). The flow sheet may be embedded within the electronic health record, but the information entered is similar to a paper document.

Date	Time	Current Rate	aPTT	Adjustment to Be Made		New Rate	NEXT aPTT	Initials
				Bolus	**Rate Change**			

Patient Identification Sticker

Intravenous Heparin Flow Sheet

Figure 16-6 Sample IV Heparin Flow Record

Calculating mL/hr Flow Rates

Example 1: A provider orders a continuous heparin infusion to begin at 15 units/kg/hr. The patient weighs 82 kg. The pharmacy supplies heparin in a premixed bag of 25,000 units in 250 mL 5% dextrose solution. Calculate the mL/hr flow rate. Round the answer to the nearest tenth mL.

    1. Set up the equation using dimensional analysis. Insert the given quantities—the volume of IV fluid and amount of heparin in the IV fluid.

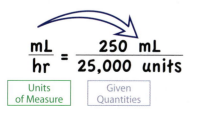

$$\frac{mL}{hr} = \frac{250\ mL}{25{,}000\ units}$$

Units of Measure   Given Quantities

2. Insert the next set of given quantities—the flow rate of the infusion.

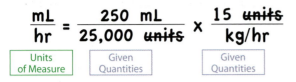

$$\underbrace{\frac{mL}{hr}}_{\substack{\text{Units} \\ \text{of Measure}}} = \underbrace{\frac{250 \ mL}{25,000 \ \cancel{units}}}_{\substack{\text{Given} \\ \text{Quantities}}} \times \underbrace{\frac{15 \ \cancel{units}}{kg/hr}}_{\substack{\text{Given} \\ \text{Quantities}}}$$

3. Insert the last given quantity—the weight of the patient—and solve the equation.

$$\underbrace{\frac{mL}{hr}}_{\substack{\text{Units} \\ \text{of Measure}}} = \underbrace{\frac{250 \ mL}{25,000 \ \cancel{units}}}_{\substack{\text{Given} \\ \text{Quantities}}} \times \underbrace{\frac{15 \ \cancel{units}}{\cancel{kg}/hr}}_{\substack{\text{Given} \\ \text{Quantities}}} \times \underbrace{82 \ \cancel{kg}}_{\substack{\text{Given} \\ \text{Quantity}}}$$

$$= \frac{250 \ mL \times 15 \times 82}{25,000 \ hr} = \frac{307,500 \ mL}{25,000 \ hr} = 12.3 \ \frac{mL}{hr}$$

For Examples 2–5, refer to the directions in Example 1.

Example 2: A provider orders a continuous heparin infusion to begin at 18 units/kg/hr. The patient weighs 73.4 kg. The pharmacy supplies heparin in a premixed bag of 25,000 units in 500 mL 5% dextrose solution. Calculate the mL/hr flow rate. Round the answer to the nearest tenth mL.

$$\frac{mL}{hr} = \frac{500 \ mL}{25,000 \ \cancel{units}} \times \frac{18 \ \cancel{units}}{\cancel{kg}/hr} \times 73.4 \ \cancel{kg}$$

$$= \frac{500 \ mL \times 18 \times 73.4}{25,000 \ hr} = 26.4 \ \frac{mL}{hr}$$

Example 3: A provider orders a continuous heparin infusion to begin at 14 units/kg/hr. The patient weighs 69.3 kg. The pharmacy supplies heparin in a premixed bag of 20,000 units in 500 mL 5% dextrose solution. Calculate the mL/hr flow rate. Round the answer to the nearest tenth mL.

$$\frac{mL}{hr} = \frac{500 \ mL}{20,000 \ \cancel{units}} \times \frac{14 \ \cancel{units}}{\cancel{kg}/hr} \times 69.3 \ \cancel{kg}$$

$$= \frac{500 \ mL \times 14 \times 69.3}{20,000 \ hr} = 24.3 \ \frac{mL}{hr}$$

Example 4: A provider orders a continuous heparin infusion to begin at 8 units/kg/hr. The patient weighs 45 kg. The pharmacy supplies heparin in a premixed bag of 20,000 units in 500 mL 5% dextrose solution. Calculate the mL/hr flow rate. Round the answer to the nearest tenth mL.

$$\frac{mL}{hr} = \frac{500 \ mL}{20,000 \ \cancel{units}} \times \frac{8 \ \cancel{units}}{\cancel{kg}/hr} \times 45 \ \cancel{kg} = \frac{500 \ mL \times 8 \times 45}{20,000 \ hr} = 9 \ \frac{mL}{hr}$$

If the patient's weight is in pounds instead of kilograms, an extra step must be inserted into the equation to convert pounds to kilograms. The conversion can be done before the equation is started, or it can be inserted into the equation, as shown in Example 5.

Example 5: A provider orders a continuous heparin infusion to begin at 16 units/kg/hr. The patient weighs 154 lb. The pharmacy supplies heparin in a premixed bag of 25,000 units in 250 mL 5% dextrose solution. Calculate the mL/hr flow rate. Round the answer to the nearest tenth mL.

$$\frac{mL}{hr} = \frac{250\ mL}{25{,}000\ \cancel{units}} \times \frac{16\ \cancel{units}}{kg/hr} \times \frac{1\ \cancel{kg}}{2.2\ \cancel{lb}} \times 154\ \cancel{lb}$$

$$= \frac{250\ mL \times 16 \times 1 \times 154}{25{,}000\ hr \times 2.2} = 11.2\ \frac{mL}{hr}$$

Calculating units/hr Flow Rates

Nurses need to be able to calculate the units/hr flow rate for IV heparin as well as the mL/hr flow rate. To calculate those flow rates, two pieces of information are necessary: the current mL/hr flow rate and the concentration of heparin in the intravenous bag.

Example 1: A nurse is verifying the dosage of a heparin infusion. The intravenous pump is infusing at 9.7 mL/hr. The intravenous bag hanging has 40,000 units of heparin in 500 mL 5% dextrose solution. Calculate the units/hr flow rate. Round the answer to the nearest whole unit.

1. Set up the equation using dimensional analysis. The first set of given quantities is the concentration of heparin in the bag.

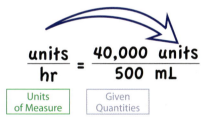

$$\frac{units}{hr} = \frac{40{,}000\ units}{500\ mL}$$

Units of Measure   Given Quantities

2. Insert the next set of given quantities—the flow rate—and solve the equation

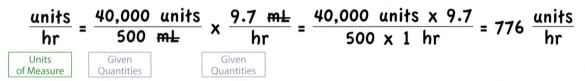

$$\frac{units}{hr} = \frac{40{,}000\ units}{500\ \cancel{mL}} \times \frac{9.7\ \cancel{mL}}{hr} = \frac{40{,}000\ units \times 9.7}{500 \times 1\ hr} = 776\ \frac{units}{hr}$$

Units of Measure   Given Quantities   Given Quantities

For Examples 2–5, refer to the directions in Example 1.

Example 2: An intravenous pump is infusing heparin at a flow rate of 11.3 mL/hr. The intravenous bag hanging has 25,000 units of heparin in 500 mL 5% dextrose solution. Calculate the units/hr flow rate. Round the answer to the nearest whole unit.

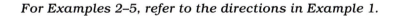

$$\frac{units}{hr} = \frac{25{,}000\ units}{500\ \cancel{mL}} \times \frac{11.3\ \cancel{mL}}{hr} = \frac{25{,}000\ units \times 11.3}{500 \times 1\ hr} = 565\ \frac{units}{hr}$$

Example 3: An intravenous pump is infusing heparin at a flow rate of 8.2 mL/hr. The intravenous bag hanging has a concentration of 1000 units/mL. Calculate the units/hr flow rate, rounding to the nearest whole unit.

> **Note:** In this example the concentration of heparin is given, not the number of units in a specific volume of solution. The equation remains the same.

$$\frac{units}{hr} = \frac{1000\ units}{1\ mL} \times \frac{8.2\ mL}{hr} = \frac{1000\ units \times 8.2}{1 \times 1\ hr} = 820\ \frac{units}{hr}$$

Example 4: An intravenous pump is infusing heparin at a flow rate of 13 mL/hr. The intravenous bag hanging has 25,000 units of heparin in 500 mL 5% dextrose solution. Calculate the units/hr flow rate. Round the answer to the nearest whole unit.

$$\frac{units}{hr} = \frac{25,000\ units}{500\ mL} \times \frac{13\ mL}{hr} = \frac{25,000\ units \times 13}{500 \times 1\ hr} = 650\ \frac{units}{hr}$$

Example 5: An intravenous pump is infusing heparin at a flow rate of 4.9 mL/hr. The intravenous bag hanging has a concentration of 200 units/mL. Calculate the units/hr flow rate. Round the answer to the nearest whole unit.

$$\frac{units}{hr} = \frac{200\ units}{1\ mL} \times \frac{4.9\ mL}{hr} = \frac{200\ units \times 4.9}{1 \times 1\ hr} = 980\ \frac{units}{hr}$$

Adjusting Heparin Flow Rates

Continuous heparin flow rates may need to be adjusted frequently at the beginning of therapy, depending on the patient's laboratory test results. Before changing the flow rate, determine whether the IV pump is infusing heparin in units/hr or mL/hr.

Adjusting units/hr Flow Rates

Increasing or decreasing a heparin flow rate when the pump is infusing in units/hr requires adding or subtracting the prescribed dosage change to the current flow rate.

Example 1: A patient has a continuous heparin infusion running at 800 units/hr. According to the hospital's heparin protocol, the infusion should be increased by 100 units/hr. The intravenous pump should be programmed to what new flow rate in units/hr?
   Add the prescribed change in dosage (100 units/hr) to the current flow rate (800 units/hr).

```
Current flow rate:        800 units/hr
Prescribed increase:    + 100 units/hr
New flow rate:            900 units/hr
```

Example 2: A patient has a continuous heparin infusion running at 623 units/hr. According to the hospital's heparin protocol, the heparin infusion should be decreased by 200 units/hr. The intravenous pump should be programmed to what new flow rate in units/hr?
   In this example, the flow rate needs to be decreased. Subtract the prescribed decrease of 200 units/hr from the current flow rate.

```
Current flow rate:        623 units/hr
Prescribed decrease:    - 200 units/hr
New flow rate:            423 units/hr
```

Alert!   Changes in heparin flow rates should always be double-checked with another RN.

Adjusting mL/hr Flow Rates

Changing the heparin dose when the intravenous pump is infusing in mL/hr requires additional information. The necessary data to collect includes the following:

- The concentration of heparin in the bag (units/mL)
- The current flow rate of heparin (mL/hr or units/hr)
- The prescribed increase of heparin (usually designated in units/hr)

Example 3:   A patient has a continuous heparin infusion running at 12.3 mL/hr. According to the hospital's heparin protocol, the heparin infusion should be increased by 200 units/hr. The current heparin bag hanging contains 25,000 units in 500 mL 5% dextrose. The intravenous pump should be programmed to what new flow rate in mL/hr? Round the answer to the nearest tenth mL.

    1. Calculate the mL/hr flow rate change needed to increase the current unit/hr flow rate by 200 units/hr.

$$\frac{mL}{hr}\ rate\ increase = \frac{500\ mL}{25,000\ \cancel{units}} \times \frac{200\ \cancel{units}}{1\ hr}$$

$$= \frac{500\ mL \times 200}{25,000 \times 1\ hr} = 4\ \frac{mL}{hr}\ rate\ increase$$

    2. Add the prescribed rate increase to the current flow rate.

```
Current flow rate:      12.3 mL/hr
Prescribed increase:  + 4.0 mL/hr
New flow rate:          16.3 mL/hr
```

Example 4:   A patient has a continuous heparin infusion running at 9.6 mL/hr. According to the hospital's heparin protocol, the heparin infusion should be decreased by 100 units/hr. The current heparin bag hanging contains 40,000 units in 500 mL 5% dextrose. The intravenous pump should be programmed to what new flow rate in mL/h? Round the answer to the nearest tenth mL.

    1. Calculate the mL/hr flow rate change needed to decrease the current unit/hr flow rate by 100 units/hr.

$$\frac{mL}{hr}\ rate\ decrease = \frac{500\ mL}{40,000\ \cancel{units}} \times \frac{100\ \cancel{units}}{1\ hr}$$

$$= \frac{500\ mL \times 100}{40,000 \times 1\ hr} = 1.3\ \frac{mL}{hr}\ rate\ decrease$$

    2. Subtract the prescribed rate decrease from the current flow rate.

```
Current flow rate:     9.6 mL/hr
Prescribed decrease: - 1.3 mL/hr
New flow rate:         8.3 mL/hr
```

Practice Calculating IV Heparin Boluses and Flow Rates

(answers on page 341)

Calculate the volume (in mLs) of UH or LMWH to be drawn up in the syringe for these boluses. Round the answers to the nearest tenth mL.

1. A provider orders a heparin bolus of 4500 units, intravenously. The pharmacy provides heparin in a concentration of 1000 units/mL.

2. A provider orders a heparin bolus of 70 units/kg, intravenously, prior to initiating a continuous infusion. The patient weighs 58.7 kg. The pharmacy provides heparin in a concentration of 10,000 units/mL in a 5-mL vial.

Calculate the mL/hr flow rate for these weight-based heparin infusions. Round the answers to the nearest tenth mL.

3. A provider orders a continuous heparin infusion to begin at 17 units/kg/hr. The patient weighs 93.8 kg. The pharmacy supplies heparin in a premixed bag of 25,000 units in 500 mL 5% dextrose solution.

4. A provider orders a continuous heparin infusion to begin at 12 units/kg/hr. The patient weighs 62 kg. The pharmacy supplies heparin in a premixed bag of 25,000 units in 250 mL 5% dextrose solution.

Calculate the new units/hr flow rates for these continuous heparin infusions. Round the answers to the nearest whole number.

5. An intravenous pump is infusing 15.6 mL/hr. The intravenous bag hanging has 40,000 units of heparin in 500 mL 5% dextrose.

6. An intravenous pump is infusing heparin at a rate of 9.5 mL/hr. The intravenous bag hanging has a concentration of 100 units/mL.

Calculate the new units/hr flow rates for these heparin infusion changes. Round the answers to the nearest whole number.

7. A patient has a continuous heparin infusion running at 1112 units/hr. According to the hospital's heparin protocol, the heparin infusion should be decreased by 100 units/hr.

8. A patient has a continuous heparin infusion running at 1250 units/hr. According to the hospital's heparin protocol, the heparin infusion should be increased by 200 units/hr.

Calculate the new mL/hr flow rates for these heparin infusion changes. Round the answers to the nearest tenth mL.

9. A patient has a continuous heparin infusion running at 17.3 mL/hr. According to the hospital's heparin protocol, the heparin infusion should be decreased by 200 units/hr. The current heparin bag hanging contains 25,000 units in 500 mL 5% dextrose.

10. A patient has a continuous heparin infusion running at 14.4 mL/hr. According to the hospital's heparin protocol, the heparin infusion should be increased by 100 units/hr. The current heparin bag hanging contains 40,000 units in 500 mL 5% dextrose.

Monitoring UH and LMWH Effectiveness

Both UH and LMWH may cause serious side effects, such as bleeding. Patients receiving these medications should be closely monitored.

Unfractionated Heparin

The effectiveness of UH can be monitored using one of two laboratory tests: the activated partial thromboplastin time (aPTT), and the heparin anti-factor Xa assay. The aPTT measures the time it takes for a clot to form after chemical reagents are added to the blood sample obtained from the patient. Normal aPTT values range from 25 to 39 seconds; they vary from laboratory to laboratory depending on the type of reagent used to test the blood sample. Since the purpose of heparin therapy is to extend a patient's clotting ability, providers generally want the aPTT value to be prolonged, typically between 1.5 to 2.5 times the normal value.

Alert! If a patient's aPTT is prolonged far beyond the therapeutic range desired by the provider, a drug called protamine sulfate may be ordered. Protamine sulfate is the antidote to heparin and is administered intravenously. Before giving protamine sulfate, assess the patient for allergies to fish (proteins from fish are used to make protamine). Watch the patient closely, as bleeding is a possibility with high aPTT levels.

The heparin anti-factor Xa assay measures the concentration of heparin in a patient's blood. The heparin anti-factor Xa test is not commonly utilized for routine monitoring of heparin effectiveness since it is expensive compared to the aPTT and the test takes longer to complete.

Low Molecular Weight Heparin

Patients who receive LMWH do not need routine laboratory monitoring. However, pregnant women and patients who are obese or who have impaired kidney function should be monitored using the heparin anti-factor Xa assay (Hirsh, Bauer, Donati, Gould, Samama, & Weitz, 2008).

Read Case Study 16-1 and answers the questions.

Case Study 16–1

Read the case study and answer the questions.

Ali Hall, a 58-year-old female with a pulmonary embolism, is admitted to the intensive care unit where you are the RN. Her physician initiates the IV Heparin Administration Protocol. See Figure 16-7.

1. *Double-check the calculations made by the physician for the bolus and infusion doses of heparin. Pay close attention to the rounding instructions of the IV Heparin Administration Protocol.*
   a. *Has the bolus dose been calculated correctly?   Yes   No*
   b. *Has the continuous infusion flow rate (units/hr) been calculated correctly?   Yes   No*
2. *When should the aPTT be drawn during Ms. Hall's treatment with heparin?*
   a. _____
   b. _____
   c. _____
3. *Ms. Hall's baseline aPTT results are faxed from the laboratory. Her aPTT is 19 seconds. You prepare to administer the heparin bolus. You select a vial of heparin that contains 10,000 units/mL from the automated medication dispensing cabinet. How much heparin will you draw up in the syringe? Round to the nearest hundredth mL. _____ mL*
4. *You administer the heparin bolus at 1420 (2:20 p.m.). Record the heparin bolus administered on the IV Heparin Flow Record (Fig. 16-8).*
5. *You prepare to begin the continuous infusion at 1435 (2:35 p.m.). If you program the intravenous pump to deliver the heparin in mL/hr, at what flow rate should the pump be set? (**Tip:** The heparin concentration is prescribed on the IV Heparin Administration Protocol sheet.) _____ mL/hr*
6. *If you program the pump to deliver the heparin in units/hr, at what rate should the pump be set? _____ units/hr*
7. *Record the necessary data on the IV Heparin Flow Record in Figure 16-8. Include the date, time, current rate in mL/hr, aPTT results, and the time the next aPTT is due.*
8. *At 2055 (8:55 p.m.), the laboratory technician draws the patient's aPTT. The report faxed to the unit 10 minutes later states that the aPTT level is now 46 seconds. Given the patient's aPTT level, what nursing action is indicated based on the IV Heparin Administration Protocol?*

Continued

Case Study 16–1—cont'd

9. Calculate these flow rates and volume.
   a. If a heparin bolus is indicated, what volume (in mL's) of heparin should the nurse draw up in the syringe? The pharmacy supplied heparin in a vial containing 5000 units/mL. Round to the nearest hundredth mL.
   b. Calculate the new flow rates:
      units/hr rate: _____
      mL/hr rate: _____

10. Record the necessary data on the IV Heparin Flow Record in Figure 16-8.

11. The nurse reprograms the pump according to the new calculations at 2105 (9:05 p.m.). Another aPTT is drawn 6 hours later, at 0300 (3:00 a.m.). This time the aPTT is 106 seconds. Given the patient's aPTT level, what nursing action is indicated based on the IV Heparin Administration Protocol?

12. Calculate these flow rates and volume:
    a. If a heparin bolus is indicated, what volume (in mL's) of heparin should you draw up in the syringe? The pharmacy supplied heparin in a vial containing 5000 units/mL. Round to the nearest hundredth mL
    b. Calculate the new flow rates:
       units/hr rate: _____
       mL/hr rate: _____

13. Record the necessary data on the IV Heparin Flow Record in Figure 16-8.

14. The third aPTT is drawn at 0910 (9:10 a.m.), 6 hours after the last aPTT was drawn and 18 hours after the heparin infusion was started. The aPTT is 92 seconds. Given the patient's aPTT level, what nursing action is indicated based on the IV Heparin Administration Protocol?

15. Calculate these flow rates and volume:
    a. If a heparin bolus is indicated, what volume (in mL's) of heparin should you draw up in the syringe? The pharmacy supplied heparin in a vial containing 5000 units/mL. Round to the nearest hundredth mL.
    b. Calculate the new flow rates:
       units/hr rate: _____
       mL/hr rate: _____

16. Record the necessary data on the IV Heparin Flow Record in Figure 16-8.

Key Points

1. Nurses need to have a solid understanding of the action of heparin, the indications for its use, and the potential for adverse reactions. They must have the ability to quickly and accurately calculate heparin flow rates to ensure that the correct dosage is being administered.

2. Venous thrombosis is the formation of a blood clot in a vein. These blood clots have the potential to break away and travel to other parts of the body, such as the heart and lungs, and cause extensive damage and even death.

3. Heparin is an anticoagulant that is used to prevent and treat venous thrombosis. There are two types of heparin: unfractionated heparin (UH) and low molecular weight heparin (LMWH).

4. UH can be administered subcutaneously or intravenously. As an intravenous medication, it can be delivered in a bolus or as a continuous infusion. Many hospitals use weight-based heparin protocols to manage continuous heparin infusions. Heparin protocols should have clear directions on initiating and managing a continuous infusion.

5. Changes in heparin flow rates should always be checked by another nurse.

6. The effectiveness of UH anticoagulation is usually monitored using the activated partial thromboplastin time (aPTT). In some cases, effectiveness may be monitored using the heparin anti-factor Xa assay instead of the aPTT.

7. LMWH is typically administered by subcutaneous injection. Patients receiving LMWH do not need laboratory monitoring; however, patients who are pregnant, who are obese, or who have kidney disease may be monitored using the heparin anti-factor Xa assay.

Date: _09/13/2018_   Time: _1420_

Diagnosis: ☑ DVT/PE ☐ Cardiovascular	Allergies: *Penicillin*	Patient's Total Body Weight: _69.9_ kg

☑ Draw baseline CBC and aPTT.
☑ Obtain baseline urinalysis.
☑ Administer bolus dose of __5600__ units heparin intravenously (round to the nearest 100 units).
   ☐ Note: suggested dose for prevention dose (cardiovascular/thrombolytic indications) is 60 units/kg.
   ☑ Note: suggested dose for treatment dose (DVT/PE) is 80 units/kg.
   NO LOADING DOSE INDICATED.
☑ Begin heparin infusion at _1300_ units/hour intravenously (rounded to the nearest 100 units).
   ☐ Note: suggested prevention dose 12–15 units/kg/hour.
   ☑ Note: suggested treatment dose 18 units/kg/hour.
☑ Use standard heparin infusion concentration of 25,000 units in 250 mL D_5W.
☑ Use an infusion pump.
☑ Draw aPTT every 6 hours until two aPTTs drawn at least 24 hours apart are within the therapeutic range. Based on the aPTT results, adjust the heparin infusion rate as indicated on the chart below. Record rate of infusion, aPTT results boluses given, and any adjustments made on the Heparin Flow Sheet.

aPTT Results (seconds)	Bolus Dose	Stop Infusion?	Infusion Rate Change
Under 50	4000 units	NO	Increase rate by 200 units/hr.
50–59	2000 units	NO	Increase rate by 100 units/hr.
60–100	No bolus	NO	No change in rate.
101–110	No bolus	NO	Decrease rate by 100 units/hr.
111–120	No bolus	NO	Decrease rate by 200 units/hr.
121–150	No bolus	Stop infusion for 30 minutes.	Decrease rate by 200 units/hr.
151–199	No bolus	Stop infusion for 60 minutes.	Decrease rate by 200 units/hr.
200	No bolus	Until aPTT is less than 200 seconds.	Redraw aPTT STAT. Draw STAT aPTTs every hour until aPTT less than 100. Then decrease the last infusion rate by 300 units/hr and repeat aPTT in 6 hours. Notify MD.

☑ Draw aPTT, PT, and CBC every morning.
☑ Check all stools for occult blood.
☑ Notify MD for: (1) any signs of bleeding; (2) if unable to obtain blood sample; (3) no intravenous access for greater than 1 hour; (4) if platelet count falls below 100,000.

Patient Identification Sticker
 	
   Ali Hall
   DOB: 03/15/1960
   MR: 19873489139
   ACCT: 294-29878987
	Intravenous Heparin Administration Protocol
	General Hospital
	
	White: Medical Record Pink: Pharmacy Yellow: Nursing

Figure 16-7 IV Heparin Administration Protocol

Date	Time	Current Rate	aPTT	Adjustment to Be Made		New Rate (mL/hr)	NEXT aPTT	Initials
				Bolus	Rate Change			

Patient Identification Sticker

Ali Hall
DOB: 03/15/1960
MR: 19873489139
ACCT: 294-29878987

**Intravenous Heparin Flow Sheet
General Hospital**

White: Medical Record Pink: Pharmacy Yellow: Nursing

Figure 16-8 IV Heparin Flow Record

References

1. Hirsh, J., Bauer, K. A., Donati, M. B., Gould, M., Samama, M. M., & Weitz, J. I. (2008). Parenteral anticoagulants. *Chest*, 133, 141S–159S. doi:10.1378/chest.08-0689

2. The Joint Commission. (2017). *Accreditation Program: Hospital. Chapter: National Patient Safety Goals*. National Patient Safety Goals Manual. Retrieved from http://www.jointcommission.org

Chapter Post-Test   *(answers in Unit 4)*

Multiple Choice

Select the best answer for each question.

1. A potential serious side effect of heparin includes:
   a. bleeding.
   b. nausea.
   c. constipation.
   d. stuffy nose.

2. According to The Joint Commission's Patient Safety Goal 03.05.01 (2011), a hospital's responsibilities for the administration of heparin includes:
   a. having the hospital's nurses mix all infusion bags of heparin.
   b. using prefilled syringes and infusion bags when available.
   c. having a written policy that addresses baseline and ongoing laboratory testing.
   d. both b and c.

3. Which of the following lab tests monitors unfractionated heparin (UH) effectiveness?
   a. international normalized ratio (INR)
   b. activated partial thromboplastin time (aPTT)
   c. white blood cell count (WBC)
   d. blood urea nitrogen (BUN)

True or False

4. The heparin anti-factor Xa assay measures serum heparin concentration.   True   False

5. It is always a good idea to have another nurse check heparin dosage calculations.   True   False

Calculations

Calculate the volume (in mL) of UH or LMWH to be drawn into the syringe for subcutaneous injection. Round the answer to the nearest hundredth mL.

6. A provider orders heparin 4000 units subcutaneously, every 12 hours. The pharmacy supplies heparin in a 1-mL vial containing 5000 units/mL.

7. A provider orders heparin 6500 units, subcutaneously, every 12 hours. The pharmacy provides a 5-mL vial of heparin with a concentration of 10,000 units/mL.

8. A provider orders enoxaparin 1 mg/kg subcutaneously every 12 hours. The patient weighs 72.8 kg. The pharmacy provides enoxaparin in a 3-mL vial containing 300 mg/mL.

9. A provider orders dalteparin 10,000 IU, subcutaneously, daily. The pharmacy supplies dalteparin in a vial containing 25,000 IU/mL.

Calculate the volume (in mL) of heparin to be administered for these boluses. Round the answer to the nearest tenth mL.

10. A provider orders a heparin bolus of 80 units/kg, intravenously. The patient weighs 84.2 kg. The pharmacy provides heparin in a concentration of 5000 units/mL.

11. A provider orders a heparin bolus of 60 units/kg. The patient weighs 61.4 kg. The pharmacy supplies heparin in a vial containing 1000 units/mL.

12. A provider orders a heparin bolus of 6000 units, intravenously. The pharmacy provides heparin in a vial containing 10,000 units/mL.

13. A provider orders a heparin bolus of 7500 units intravenously. The pharmacy supplies heparin in a vial containing 5000 units/mL.

Calculate the mL/hr flow rate for these weight-based heparin infusions. Round the answer to the nearest tenth mL.

14. A provider orders a continuous heparin infusion to begin at 15 units/kg/hr. The patient weighs 93.8 kg. The pharmacy supplies heparin in a premixed bag of 40,000 units in 500 mL 5% dextrose solution.

15. A provider orders a continuous heparin infusion to begin at 12 units/kg/hr. The patient weighs 79 kg. The pharmacy supplies heparin in a premixed bag of 25,000 units in 250 mL 5% dextrose solution.

16. A provider orders a continuous heparin infusion to begin at 18 units/kg/hr. The patient weighs 46.4 kg. The pharmacy supplies heparin in a premixed bag of 25,000 units in 500 mL 5% dextrose solution.

17. A provider orders a continuous heparin infusion to begin at 14 units/kg/hr. The patient weighs 71 kg. The pharmacy supplies heparin in a premixed bag of 40,000 units in 500 mL 5% dextrose solution.

Calculate the new mL/hr flow rate for these heparin infusion changes. Round the answer to the nearest tenth mL.

18. A patient has a continuous heparin infusion running at 1100 units/hr. The patient's aPTT is too high, so the flow rate is to be decreased by 100 units/hr. The infusion bag currently hanging has 25,000 units of heparin in 250 mL 5% dextrose solution.

19. A patient has a continuous heparin infusion running at 885 units/hr. The patient's aPTT is too low, so the flow rate is to be increased by 200 units/hr. The infusion bag currently hanging has 40,000 units of heparin in 500 mL 5% dextrose solution.

20. A patient has a continuous heparin infusion running at 900 units/hr. The patient's aPTT is too high, so the flow rate is to be decreased by 50 units/hr. The infusion bag currently hanging has 20,000 units of heparin in 250 mL 5% dextrose solution.

21. A patient has a continuous heparin infusion running at 750 units/hr. The patient's aPTT is too high, so the flow rate is to be decreased by 200 units/hr. The infusion bag currently hanging has 25,000 units of heparin in 500 mL 5% dextrose solution.

Calculate the new units/hr flow rate for these heparin infusion changes. Round the answer to the nearest whole number.

22. A patient has a continuous heparin infusion running at 13.5 mL/hr. The infusion bag currently hanging has 40,000 units in 500 mL 5% dextrose solution. According to the hospital's heparin protocol, the heparin infusion should be increased by 200 units/hr.

23. A patient has a continuous heparin infusion running at 9.7 mL/hr. The infusion bag currently hanging has 25,000 units in 500 mL 5% dextrose solution. According to the hospital's heparin protocol, the heparin infusion should be decreased by 200 units/hr.

24. A patient has a continuous heparin infusion running at 10.1 mL/hr. The infusion bag hanging has 25,000 units in 250 mL 5% dextrose solution. According to the hospital's heparin protocol, the heparin infusion should be decreased by 200 units/hr.

25. A patient has a continuous heparin infusion running at 8.9 mL/hr. The infusion bag hanging has 40,000 units in 500 mL 5% dextrose solution. According to the hospital's heparin protocol, the heparin infusion should be increased by 100 units/hr.

Answers to Practice Questions

Calculating Subcutaneous Doses of Heparin and LMWH

1. $mL = \dfrac{1\ mL}{10{,}000\ \cancel{units}} \times 5000\ \cancel{units} = \dfrac{1\ mL \times 5000}{10{,}000} = 0.5\ mL$

2. $mL = \dfrac{0.8\ mL}{120\ \cancel{mg}} \times 120\ \cancel{mg} = \dfrac{1\ mL \times 120}{120} = 0.8\ mL$

3. $mL = \dfrac{1\ mL}{5000\ \cancel{units}} \times 2500\ \cancel{units} = \dfrac{1\ mL \times 2500}{5000} = 0.5\ mL$

4. $mL = \dfrac{1\ mL}{10{,}000\ \cancel{units}} \times 7500\ \cancel{units} = \dfrac{1\ mL \times 7500}{10{,}000} = 0.75\ mL$

5. $mL = \dfrac{1\ mL}{20{,}000\ \cancel{IU}} \times 15{,}000\ \cancel{IU} = \dfrac{1\ mL \times 15{,}000}{20{,}000} = 0.75\ mL$

6. $mL = \dfrac{1\ mL}{5000\ \cancel{units}} \times 1000\ \cancel{units} = \dfrac{1\ mL \times 1000}{5000} = 0.2\ mL$

7. $mL = \dfrac{1\ mL}{5000\ \cancel{units}} \times 2000\ \cancel{units} = \dfrac{1\ mL \times 2000}{5000} = 0.4\ mL$

8. $mL = \dfrac{1\ mL}{10{,}000\ \cancel{units}} \times 5000\ \cancel{units} = \dfrac{1\ mL \times 5000}{10{,}000} = 0.5\ mL$

9. $mL = \dfrac{1\ mL}{20{,}000\ \cancel{units}} \times 7500\ \cancel{units} = \dfrac{1\ mL \times 7500}{20{,}000} = 0.38\ mL$

10. $mL = \dfrac{1\ mL}{5000\ \cancel{units}} \times 3500\ \cancel{units} = \dfrac{1\ mL \times 3500}{5000} = 0.7\ mL$

IV Heparin Boluses and Flow Rates

1. $mL = \dfrac{1\ mL}{5000\ \text{units}} \times 4500\ \text{units} = \dfrac{1\ mL \times 4500}{5000} = 4.5\ mL$

2. $mL = \dfrac{1\ mL}{10{,}000\ \text{units}} \times \dfrac{70\ \text{units}}{1\ kg/hr} \times 58.7\ \text{kg} = \dfrac{70\ mL \times 58.7}{10{,}000} = 0.4\ mL$

3. $\dfrac{mL}{hr} = \dfrac{500\ mL}{25{,}000\ \text{units}} \times \dfrac{17\ \text{units}}{kg/hr} \times 93.8\ \text{kg} = \dfrac{500\ mL \times 17 \times 93.8}{25{,}000\ hr} = 31.9\ \dfrac{mL}{hr}$

4. $\dfrac{mL}{hr} = \dfrac{250\ mL}{25{,}000\ \text{units}} \times \dfrac{12\ \text{units}}{kg/hr} \times 62\ \text{kg} = \dfrac{250\ mL \times 12 \times 62}{25{,}000\ hr} = 7.4\ \dfrac{mL}{hr}$

5. $\dfrac{units}{hr} = \dfrac{40{,}000\ units}{500\ \text{mL}} \times \dfrac{15.6\ \text{mL}}{hr} = \dfrac{40{,}000\ units \times 15.6}{500\ hr} = 1248\ \dfrac{units}{hr}$

6. $\dfrac{units}{hr} = \dfrac{100\ units}{1\ \text{mL}} \times \dfrac{9.5\ \text{mL}}{hr} = \dfrac{100\ units \times 9.5}{1\ hr} = 950\ \dfrac{units}{hr}$

7.
Current flow rate:	1112 units/hr
Prescribed decrease:	− 100 units/hr
New flow rate:	1012 units/hr

8.
Current flow rate:	1250 units/hr
Prescribed increase:	+ 200 units/hr
New flow rate:	1450 units/hr

9. Rate decrease $\dfrac{mL}{hr} = \dfrac{500\ mL}{25{,}000\ \text{units}} \times \dfrac{200\ \text{units}}{hr} = \dfrac{500\ mL \times 200}{25{,}000\ hr} = 4\ \dfrac{mL}{hr}$

Current flow rate:	17.3 mL/hr
Prescribed decrease:	− 4.0 mL/hr
New flow rate:	13.3 mL/hr

10. Rate increase $\dfrac{mL}{hr} = \dfrac{500\ mL}{40{,}000\ \text{units}} \times \dfrac{100\ \text{units}}{hr} = \dfrac{500\ mL \times 100}{40{,}000\ hr} = 1.3\ \dfrac{mL}{hr}$

Current flow rate:	14.4 mL/hr
Prescribed increase:	+ 1.3 mL/hr
New flow rate:	15.7 mL/hr

■ *Answers to Case Study 16–1*

1. *Physician's bolus and infusion rates:*
   a. *According to the IV Heparin Administration Protocol, the suggested bolus dose of heparin is 80 units/kg. Ms. Hall's weight is 69.9 kg.*

   $$\text{Bolus dose (units)} = \frac{80 \text{ units}}{\text{kg}} \times 69.9 \text{ kg} = 5592 \text{ units}$$

   The protocol directs the provider to round the dosage to the nearest 100 units. The calculated dose is 5592, which is closer to 5600 than 5500. The ordered dose of 5600 units is correct.
   b. *The suggested infusion rate of heparin is 18 units/kg/hr.*

   $$\text{Infusion rate} \left(\frac{\text{units}}{\text{hr}} \right) = \frac{18 \text{ units}}{\text{kg/hr}} \times 69.9 \text{ kg} = 1258.2 = 1300 \frac{\text{units}}{\text{hr}}$$

   The infusion rate of heparin should be rounded to the nearest 100 units. In this case, 1258 units/hr is rounded up to 1300 units/hr (1258 is closer to 1300 than 1200). The flow rate has been calculated correctly.
2. *Frequency of the aPTT:*
   a. *Before the heparin infusion is begun (baseline level)*
   b. *Every 6 hours until two aPTT's drawn at least 24 hours apart are within the therapeutic range (60 to 100 seconds)*
   c. *Every morning*
3. *Bolus dose:*

   $$\text{Bolus dose (mL)} = \frac{1 \text{ mL}}{10,000 \text{ units}} \times 5600 \text{ units} = 0.56 \text{ mL}$$

4. *Heparin Flow Record (See Figure 16-9):*
5. $$\frac{\text{mL}}{\text{hr}} = \frac{250 \text{ mL}}{25,000 \text{ units}} \times \frac{1300 \text{ units}}{1 \text{ hr}} = \frac{250 \text{ mL} \times 1300}{25,000 \times 1 \text{ hr}} = 13 \frac{\text{mL}}{\text{hr}}$$

6. *Units/hr flow rate for continuous infusion:*
   The pump will be set for 1300 units/hr, as calculated in answer 1b.
7. *Heparin Flow Record (See Figure 16-10):*
8. *The heparin infusion should be adjusted according to the chart on the IV Heparin Administration Protocol. Ms. Hall's aPTT value of 46 seconds falls in the "Under 50" range. The actions taken by the nurse will include giving a bolus dose of 4000 units and increasing the rate by 200 units/hr.*

Date	Time	Current Rate	aPTT	Adjustment to Be Made		New Rate (mL/hr)	NEXT aPTT	Initials
				Bolus	Rate Change			
09/13/18	1420	NA	19 sec	5600 units	NA	NA		N.N., RN

Figure 16-9 IV Heparin Flow Record

Date	Time	Current Rate	aPTT	Adjustment to Be Made		New Rate (mL/hr)	NEXT aPTT	Initials
				Bolus	Rate Change			
09/13/18	1420	NA	19 sec	5600 units	NA	NA		N.N., RN
09/13/18	1435	13 mL/hr		NA	NA	NA	2055	N.N., RN

Figure 16-10 IV Heparin Flow Record

■ *Answers to Case Study 16–1—cont'd*

9. *Calculate the following:*
Heparin bolus:
a. *Bolus dose* (mL) $= \dfrac{1\ mL}{5000\ \text{units}} \times 4000\ \text{units} = 0.8\ mL$

b. *Calculate the new flow rates:*
units/hr rate increase:

Current infusion rate:	1300 units/hr
Rate increase:	+ 200 units/hr
New infusion rate:	1500 units/hr

mL/hr rate increase:

$$\frac{mL}{hr} = \frac{250\ mL}{25{,}000\ \text{units}} \times \frac{200\ \text{units}}{1\ hr} = \frac{250\ mL \times 200}{25{,}000 \times 1\ hr} = 2\frac{mL}{hr}$$

Current infusion rate:	13 mL/hr
Rate increase:	+ 2 mL/hr
New infusion rate:	15 mL/hr

10. *IV Heparin Flow Record (See Figure 16-11):*

11. *Nursing actions:*
Ms. Hall's aPTT value of 106 seconds falls in the range of "101–110." The action taken by the nurse will be to decrease the infusion rate by 100 units/hr.

12. *Calculate the following:*
a. *No bolus will be administered.*
b. *units/hr rate decrease:*

Current infusion rate:	1500 units/hr
Rate decrease:	− 100 units/hr
New infusion rate:	1400 units/hr

mL/hr rate decrease:

$$\frac{mL}{hr} = \frac{250\ mL}{25{,}000\ \text{units}} \times \frac{100\ \text{units}}{1\ hr} = \frac{250\ mL \times 100}{25{,}000 \times 1\ hr} = 1\frac{mL}{hr}$$

Current infusion rate:	15 mL/hr
Rate decrease:	− 1 mL/hr
New infusion rate:	14 mL/hr

13. *IV Heparin Flow Record (See Figure 16-12):*

14. *The aPTT of 92 seconds falls within the therapeutic range of "60–100" according to the heparin flow chart. This would be considered the first aPTT to be in therapeutic range. No bolus or change in infusion rate is necessary at this time. aPTT levels should be drawn every 6 hours until at least two aPTT levels drawn at least 24 hours apart are within therapeutic range.*

15. a. *No heparin bolus is indicated.*
b. *No change in flow rates is required at this time.*

16. *IV Heparin Flow Record (See Figure 16-13):*

Date	Time	Current Rate	aPTT	Adjustment to Be Made		New Rate (mL/hr)	NEXT aPTT	Initials
				Bolus	Rate Change			
09/13/18	1420	NA	19 sec	5600 units	NA	NA		N.N., RN
09/13/18	1435	13 mL/hr		NA	NA	NA	2055	N.N., RN
09/13/18	2105	13 mL/HR	46 sec	4000 units	↑ 2 mL	15 mL/HR	0300	V.S., RN

Figure 16-11 IV Heparin Flow Record

Date	Time	Current Rate	aPTT	Adjustment to Be Made		New Rate (mL/hr)	NEXT aPTT	Initials
				Bolus	Rate Change			
09/13/18	1420	NA	19 sec	5600 units	NA	NA		N.N., RN
09/13/18	1435	13 mL/hr		NA	NA	NA	2055	N.N., RN
09/13/18	2105	13 mL/HR	46 sec	4000 units	↑ 2 mL	15 mL/HR	0300	V.S., RN
09/14/18	0310	15 mL/HR	106 sec	NA	↓ 1 mL	14 mL/HR	0910	V.S., RN

Figure 16-12 IV Heparin Flow Record

Date	Time	Current Rate	aPTT	Adjustment to Be Made		New Rate (mL/hr)	NEXT aPTT	Initials
				Bolus	Rate Change			
09/13/18	1420	NA	19 sec	5600 units	NA	NA		N.N., RN
09/13/18	1435	13 mL/hr		NA	NA	NA	2055	N.N., RN
09/13/18	2105	13 mL/HR	46 sec	4000 units	↑ 2 mL	15 mL/HR	0300	V.S., RN
09/14/18	0310	15 mL/HR	106 sec	NA	↓ 1 mL	14 mL/HR	0910	V.S., RN
09/14/18	0930	14 mL/hr	92 sec	NA	NA	14 mL/hr	1510	J.J., RN

Figure 16-13 IV Heparin Flow Record

Chapter 17
Critical Care Dosage Calculations

⚬ Glossary

Critical care: Care received by clients whose illnesses or injuries are life-threatening; also known as intensive care.
Microdrip tubing: IV tubing with a drop factor of 60 drops/mL.
Titrate: To increase or decrease the dose of a medication in small increments to reach a target dose or to elicit a required response.

Objectives

After completing this chapter, the learner will be able to—
1. Calculate mL/hr infusion rates from mg/min or mcg/min dosages.
2. Calculate mL/hr infusion rates from mg/kg/min or mcg/kg/min dosages.
3. Calculate mg/min and mcg/min dosages from mL/hr infusion rates.
4. Titrate dosages according to patient response.
5. Describe the purpose of an IV drip protocol.

Critical Care

Critical care is a nursing specialty that focuses on the care of patients who require close monitoring and frequent or complex interventions to maintain health or prevent death. Patients in critical care units are medically unstable and require intensive medical and nursing care, including medications to keep body functions intact. Critical care medications include those that improve oxygenation, maintain blood pressure, correct an abnormal heartbeat, or dissolve clots in the arteries in the heart. Such medications are potentially dangerous and must be titrated until the desired response is exhibited by the patient or until the upper threshold dose (the dose at which the drug may become toxic) has been reached. For example, a patient who has an irregular heartbeat may be started on a medication at a low or moderate dose that is then increased in small increments over several hours until the patient's heartbeat becomes regular, or the upper limit of the prescribed dosage has been reached. See Figure 17-1.

Critical care drugs administered intravenously should be infused using a programmable infusion pump that allows the nurse to enter the name, dosage, and concentration of the medication. If one is not available, the medication may be infused using microdrip tubing (60 gtt/mL calibration) and a volume control set (a safety device that can limit the amount of fluid available for infusion) as a last resort. However, manual infusion of critical care medications should be initiated only under the most dire of circumstances.

Administering routine IV fluids and IV piggyback medications involves computing a flow rate in either mL/hr (using an electronic infusion device) or gtt/min (manual gravity control) (see Chapter 13). However, when administering high-risk drugs, the nurse may be required to infuse

Date	Physicians' Orders
11/21/18	Diltiazem 0.25 mg/kg loading dose intravenously over 5 minutes, then start a diltiazem infusion
1000	at 5–15 mg/hr until patient converts to normal sinus rhythm.
	——————— Mary Jones, MD

Sarah Dillon
MR 00382991
Account A9184028
Dr. Mary Jones, MD
DOB: 04/08/1935

Figure 17-1 Sample Provider Order

a medication based on drug weight (such as mg, mcg, mEq, or units) per time unit (min or hr), instead of the usual mL/hr flow rate.

Smart infusion pumps have made weight-based IV therapy simpler: The patient's weight, medication dosage, amount of diluent, and desired length of time for the infusion can be programmed into the pump, and the pump will infuse the solution at the correct rate. The drug can be titrated up or down by small increments using the keypad on the pump. However, even with smart technology, the nurse is still responsible for verifying that the correct dosage of medication is infusing.

Calculating mL/hr Infusion Rates From mg/min and mcg/min Dosages

Example 1: A provider orders disopyramide (Norpace) to be infused at a rate of 0.4 mg/min. The pharmacy supplies the medication in an IV bag containing 250 mg in 500 mL D₅W. Calculate the desired infusion rate in mL/hr. Round the answer to the nearest tenth mL.

1. Set up the equation using dimensional analysis and insert the first set of given quantities—the amount of medication contained in the IV bag.

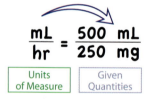

$$\frac{mL}{hr} = \frac{500\ mL}{250\ mg}$$

Units of Measure | Given Quantities

2. Insert the next given quantities—the desired infusion rate.

$$\frac{mL}{hr} = \frac{500\ mL}{250\ mg} \times \frac{0.4\ mg}{1\ min}$$

Units of Measure | Given Quantities | Given Quantities

3. Insert the conversion factor for time as the last set of quantities.

$$\frac{mL}{hr} = \frac{500\ mL}{250\ mg} \times \frac{0.4\ mg}{1\ min} \times \frac{60\ min}{1\ hr}$$

Units of Measure | Given Quantities | Given Quantities | Conversion Factor (Time)

4. Solve the equation.

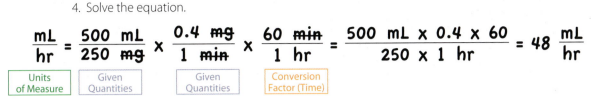

To infuse the disopyramide (Norpace) at a rate of 0.4 mg/min, the nurse should set the pump at 48 mL/hr.

Example 2: A provider orders isoproterenol (Isuprel) to be infused at a rate of 4 mcg/min. The pharmacy supplies the medication in an IV bag containing 1 mg in 250 mL of 0.9% sodium chloride solution (normal saline). What is the desired infusion rate in mL/hr? Round the answer to the nearest tenth mL.

1. Set up the example using dimensional analysis and insert the first set of given quantities—the concentration of isoproterenol (Isuprel) in the solution.

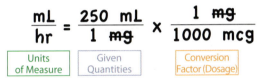

2. Insert the next set of given quantities. In this example, a conversion factor is required to convert mg to mcg.

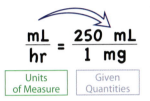

3. Insert the dosage of isoproterenol (Isuprel) as the next set of given quantities.

4. Insert the conversion factor for time to convert minutes into hours.

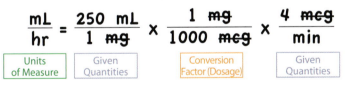

5. Solve the equation.

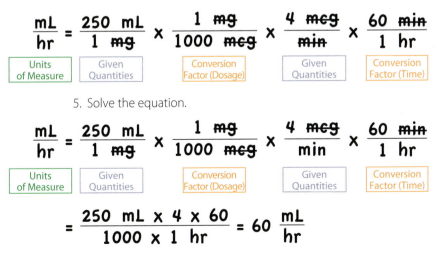

To infuse isoproterenol (Isuprel) at 4 mcg/min, the nurse should set the pump at a rate of 60 mL/hr.

Practice Calculating mL/hr Infusion Rates From mg/min and mcg/min Dosages

(answers on page 364)

Calculate the mL/hr infusion rates for these medication orders. Round the answers to the nearest tenth mL.

1. A provider orders norepinephrine (Levophed) 8 mcg/min IV. The IV bag contains 4 mg norepinephrine (Levophed) in 250 mL D$_5$W.

2. A provider orders amiodarone (Cordarone) 1 mg/min IV. The IV bag contains 900 mg amiodarone (Cordarone) in 500 mL D$_5$W.

3. A provider orders epinephrine 1.5 mcg/min IV. The IV bag contains 1 mg epinephrine in 250 mL NS.

4. A provider orders phenylephrine (Neo-Synephrine) 100 mcg/min IV. The IV bag contains 50 mg phenylephrine (Neo-Synephrine) in 500 mL NS.

5. A provider orders isoproterenol (Isuprel) 5 mcg/min IV. The IV bag contains 1 mg isoproterenol (Isuprel) in 250 mL D$_5$W.

6. A provider orders procainamide (Pronestyl) 2 mg/min IV. The IV bag contains 1 g procainamide (Pronestyl) in 250 mL NS.

7. A provider orders eptifibatide (Integrilin) 160 mcg/min IV. The IV bag contains 75 mg eptifibatide (Integrilin) in 100 mL solution.

8. A provider orders nitroprusside (Nitropress) 225 mcg/min IV. The IV bag contains 100 mg nitroprusside (Nitropress) in 250 mL D$_5$W.

9. A provider orders abciximab (Reopro) 11 mcg/min IV. The IV bag contains 7.2 mg abciximab (Reopro) in 250 mL NS.

10. A provider orders inamrinone (Inocor) 384 mcg/min IV. The IV bag contains 500 mg inamrinone (Inocor) in 200 mL NS.

Calculating mL/hr Infusion Rates From mg/kg/min and mcg/kg/min Dosages

Some critical care medications need to be titrated based on the patient's weight.

Example 1: A provider orders methylprednisolone (Solu-Medrol) 0.05 mg/kg/min for a patient who weighs 67 kg. The infusion bag contains 200 mg methylprednisolone (Solu-Medrol) in 100 mL D$_5$W. Calculate the mL/hr infusion rate. Round the answer to the nearest tenth mL.

1. Set up the equation, inserting the first set of given quantities—the concentration of the solution.

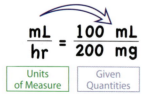

$$\frac{mL}{hr} = \frac{100 \ mL}{200 \ mg}$$

Units of Measure | Given Quantities

2. Insert the second set of given quantities—the weight-based dosage of methylprednisolone (Solu-Medrol).

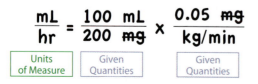

$$\frac{mL}{hr} = \frac{100 \ mL}{200 \ \cancel{mg}} \times \frac{0.05 \ \cancel{mg}}{kg/min}$$

Units of Measure | Given Quantities | Given Quantities

3. Insert the conversion factor that changes minutes into hours.

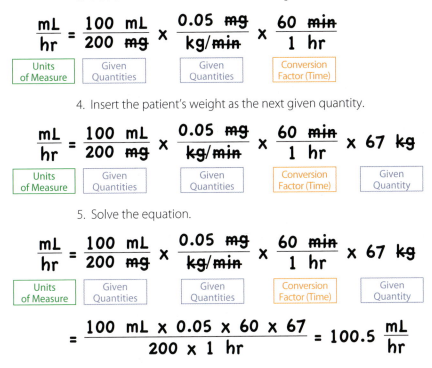

$$\frac{mL}{hr} = \frac{100 \ mL}{200 \ \cancel{mg}} \times \frac{0.05 \ \cancel{mg}}{kg/\cancel{min}} \times \frac{60 \ \cancel{min}}{1 \ hr}$$

| Units of Measure | Given Quantities | Given Quantities | Conversion Factor (Time) |

4. Insert the patient's weight as the next given quantity.

$$\frac{mL}{hr} = \frac{100 \ mL}{200 \ \cancel{mg}} \times \frac{0.05 \ \cancel{mg}}{\cancel{kg}/\cancel{min}} \times \frac{60 \ \cancel{min}}{1 \ hr} \times 67 \ \cancel{kg}$$

| Units of Measure | Given Quantities | Given Quantities | Conversion Factor (Time) | Given Quantity |

5. Solve the equation.

$$\frac{mL}{hr} = \frac{100 \ mL}{200 \ \cancel{mg}} \times \frac{0.05 \ \cancel{mg}}{\cancel{kg}/\cancel{min}} \times \frac{60 \ \cancel{min}}{1 \ hr} \times 67 \ \cancel{kg}$$

| Units of Measure | Given Quantities | Given Quantities | Conversion Factor (Time) | Given Quantity |

$$= \frac{100 \ mL \times 0.05 \times 60 \times 67}{200 \times 1 \ hr} = 100.5 \ \frac{mL}{hr}$$

To infuse methylprednisolone (Solu-Medrol) at 0.05 mg/kg/min, the nurse will set the pump at a rate of 100.5 mL/hr.

Example 2:   A provider orders inamrinone (Inocor) 5 mcg/kg/min as a maintenance IV for a patient who weighs 75 kg. Inamrinone (Inocor) is provided by the pharmacy in bags containing 500 mg in 200 mL 0.9% sodium chloride solution. Calculate the mL/hr infusion rate. Round the answer to the nearest tenth mL.

1. Set up the equation, inserting the first set of given quantities—the concentration of medication in the bag of fluid.

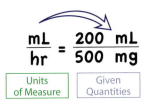

$$\frac{mL}{hr} = \frac{200 \ mL}{500 \ mg}$$

| Units of Measure | Given Quantities |

2. Insert the next set of given quantities. In this case, it must be a conversion factor to change mg into mcg.

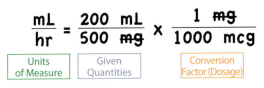

$$\frac{mL}{hr} = \frac{200 \ mL}{500 \ \cancel{mg}} \times \frac{1 \ \cancel{mg}}{1000 \ mcg}$$

| Units of Measure | Given Quantities | Conversion Factor (Dosage) |

3. Insert the weight-based dosage of inamrinone (Inocor) as the next set of given quantities.

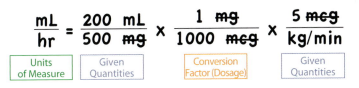

$$\frac{mL}{hr} = \frac{200 \ mL}{500 \ \cancel{mg}} \times \frac{1 \ \cancel{mg}}{1000 \ \cancel{mcg}} \times \frac{5 \ \cancel{mcg}}{kg/min}$$

| Units of Measure | Given Quantities | Conversion Factor (Dosage) | Given Quantities |

4. Insert the conversion factor to convert minutes to hours.

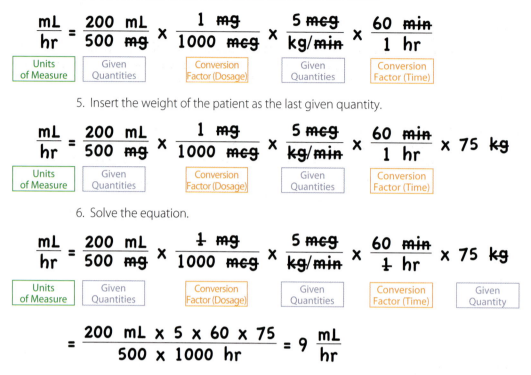

5. Insert the weight of the patient as the last given quantity.

6. Solve the equation.

$$= \frac{200 \text{ mL} \times 5 \times 60 \times 75}{500 \times 1000 \text{ hr}} = 9 \frac{\text{mL}}{\text{hr}}$$

Practice Calculating mL/hr Infusion Rates From mg/kg/min and mcg/kg/min Dosages

(answers on page 365)

Calculate the mL/hr infusion rates from these weight-based dosages. Round the answers to the nearest tenth mL.

1. A provider orders abciximab (Reopro) 0.125 mcg/kg/min IV. The IV bag contains 5.85 mg abciximab (Reopro) in 250 mL NS. The patient weighs 65 kg.

2. A provider orders nitroprusside (Nitropress) 4.5 mcg/kg/min IV. The IV bag contains 50 mg nitroprusside (Nitropress) in 250 mL D₅W. The patient weighs 72 kg.

3. A provider orders inamrinone (Inocor) 0.01 mg/kg/min IV. The IV bag contains 500 mg inamrinone (Inocor) in 200 mL solution. The patient weighs 80 kg.

4. A provider orders milrinone (Primacor) 0.375 mcg/kg/min IV. The IV bag contains 20 mg milrinone (Primacor) in 80 mL NS. The patient weighs 92 kg.

5. A provider orders dobutamine 2.5 mcg/kg/min IV. The IV bag contains 500 mg dobutamine in 250 mL NS. The patient weighs 78 kg.

6. A provider orders dopamine 9.7 mcg/kg/min IV. The IV bag contains 400 mg dopamine in 250 mL D₅W. The patient weighs 56 kg.

7. A provider orders esmolol (Brevibloc) 0.05 mg/kg/min IV for 4 minutes. The IV bag contains 2.5 g esmolol (Brevibloc) in 250 mL D₅W. The patient weighs 63 kg.

8. A provider orders fenoldopam (Corlopam) 0.25 mcg/kg/min IV. The IV bag contains 10 mg fenoldopam (Corlopam) in 250 mL D₅W. The patient weighs 71 kg.

9. A provider orders nesiritide (Natrecor) 0.01 mcg/kg/min IV. The IV bag contains 1.5 mg nesiritide (Natrecor) in 250 mL solution. The patient weighs 84 kg.

10. A provider orders tirofiban (Aggrastat) 0.4 mcg/kg/min IV. The IV bag contains 12.5 mg tirofiban (Aggrastat) in 250 mL solution. The patient weighs 69 kg.

Calculating mg/min and mcg/min Dosages From mL/hr Infusion Rates

The nurse must be able to verify that the correct dose of medication is infusing, especially if a programmable IV pump is not being used. This can be done by gathering the following information: the mL/hr infusion rate, the amount of medication in the IV bag, and the original volume of fluid in the bag.

Example 1:   A nurse walks into a patient's room and sees an IV infusion of lidocaine infusing at a rate of 15 mL/hr. The IV bag contains 500 mg lidocaine in 500 mL 0.9% sodium chloride solution. Calculate the mg/min dosage that is infusing. Round the answer to the nearest hundredth mg.

1. Set up the equation using dimensional analysis. Insert the first set of given quantities relating the dosage of lidocaine to the total volume of fluid in the bag.

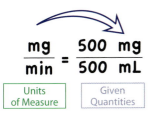

$$\frac{mg}{min} = \frac{500 \ mg}{500 \ mL}$$

Units of Measure   Given Quantities

2. Insert the next set of given quantities—the flow rate of the IV.

$$\frac{mg}{min} = \frac{500 \ mg}{500 \ mL} \times \frac{15 \ mL}{1 \ hr}$$

Units of Measure   Given Quantities   Given Quantities

3. Insert a conversion factor to convert hours into minutes.

$$\frac{mg}{min} = \frac{500 \ mg}{500 \ mL} \times \frac{15 \ mL}{1 \ hr} \times \frac{1 \ hr}{60 \ min}$$

Units of Measure   Given Quantities   Given Quantities   Conversion Factor (Time)

4. Solve the equation.

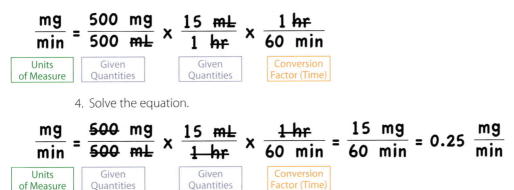

$$\frac{mg}{min} = \frac{500 \ mg}{500 \ mL} \times \frac{15 \ mL}{1 \ hr} \times \frac{1 \ hr}{60 \ min} = \frac{15 \ mg}{60 \ min} = 0.25 \ \frac{mg}{min}$$

Units of Measure   Given Quantities   Given Quantities   Conversion Factor (Time)

The nurse calculates that the infusion, which is running at 15 mL/hr, is providing the patient with lidocaine 0.25 mg/min. To verify that this dosage is in the range specified by the provider, the nurse should refer to the provider's written order. If the dosage is out of the prescribed range, the nurse should notify the provider for additional orders and follow facility protocol for error reporting.

Example 2: A nurse wants to verify the mcg/min dosage of an infusion of drotrecogin alfa (Xigris) running at 9.1 mL/hr. The IV bag contains 20 mg drotrecogin alfa (Xigris) in 100 mL 0.9% sodium chloride solution. What is the mcg/min dosage? Round the answer to the nearest tenth.

1. Set up the equation using dimensional analysis. The first set of given quantities in the equation is the factor converting mg to mcg.

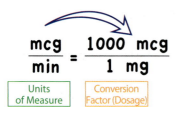

$$\frac{\text{mcg}}{\text{min}} = \frac{1000 \text{ mcg}}{1 \text{ mg}}$$

| Units of Measure | Conversion Factor (Dosage) |

2. Insert the second set of given quantities relating the dosage of drotrecogin alfa (Xigris) in the bag to the total volume of fluid in the bag.

$$\frac{\text{mcg}}{\text{min}} = \frac{1000 \text{ mcg}}{1 \text{ mg}} \times \frac{20 \text{ mg}}{100 \text{ mL}}$$

| Units of Measure | Conversion Factor (Dosage) | Given Quantities |

3. Insert the flow rate of the IV as the next set of given quantities.

$$\frac{\text{mcg}}{\text{min}} = \frac{1000 \text{ mcg}}{1 \text{ mg}} \times \frac{20 \text{ mg}}{100 \text{ mL}} \times \frac{9.1 \text{ mL}}{1 \text{ hr}}$$

| Units of Measure | Conversion Factor (Dosage) | Given Quantities | Given Quantities |

4. Insert the conversion factor for time to convert hours into minutes.

$$\frac{\text{mcg}}{\text{min}} = \frac{1000 \text{ mcg}}{1 \text{ mg}} \times \frac{20 \text{ mg}}{100 \text{ mL}} \times \frac{9.1 \text{ mL}}{1 \text{ hr}} \times \frac{1 \text{ hr}}{60 \text{ min}}$$

| Units of Measure | Conversion Factor (Dosage) | Given Quantities | Given Quantities | Conversion Factor (Time) |

5. Solve the equation.

$$\frac{\text{mcg}}{\text{min}} = \frac{1000 \text{ mcg}}{1 \text{ mg}} \times \frac{20 \text{ mg}}{100 \text{ mL}} \times \frac{9.1 \text{ mL}}{1 \text{ hr}} \times \frac{1 \text{ hr}}{60 \text{ min}}$$

| Units of Measure | Conversion Factor (Dosage) | Given Quantities | Given Quantities | Conversion Factor (Time) |

$$= \frac{1000 \text{ mcg} \times 20 \times 9.1}{1 \times 100 \times 60 \text{ min}} = 30.33 = 30.3 \frac{\text{mcg}}{\text{min}}$$

Practice Calculating mg/min and mcg/min Dosages From mL/hr Infusion Rates

(answers on page 366)

Calculate the mg/min dosage from the mL/hr flow rate of the IV. Round the answers to the nearest tenth mg/min.

1. An IV of ibutilide (Corvert) is infusing at 300 mL/hr. The IV bag contains 1 mg ibutilide (Corvert) in 50 mL D_5W. Calculate the mg/min dosage.

2. An IV of immune globulin is infusing at 60 mL/hr. The IV bag contains 5 g immune globulin in 100 mL solution. Calculate the mg/min dosage.

3. An IV of lidocaine is infusing at 45 mL/hr. The IV bag contains 2 g lidocaine in 500 mL solution. Calculate the mg/min dosage.

4. An IV of magnesium sulfate is infusing at 56 mL/hr. The IV bag contains 2 g magnesium sulfate in 100 mL D_5W. Calculate the mg/min dosage.

5. An IV of tirofiban (Aggrastat) is infusing at 25 mL/hr. The IV bag contains 200 mg tirofiban (Aggrastat) in 250 mL of solution. Calculate the mg/min dosage.

Calculate the mcg/min dosage from the mL/hr flow rate of the IV. Round the answers to the nearest tenth mcg/min.

6. An IV of octreotide (Sandostatin) is infusing at 20 mL/hr. The IV bag contains 1.2 mg octreotide (Sandostatin) in 250 mL solution. Calculate the mcg/min dosage.

7. An IV of epinephrine is infusing at 37 mL/hr. The IV bag contains 1 mg epinephrine in 250 mL NS. Calculate the mcg/min dosage.

8. An IV of nesiritide (Natrecor) is infusing at 9 mL/hr. The IV bag contains 1.5 mg nesiritide (Natrecor) in 250 mL D_5W. Calculate the mcg/min dosage.

9. An IV of infliximab (Remicade) is infusing at 30 mL/hr. The IV bag contains 300 mg infliximab (Remicade) in 250 mL NS. Calculate the mcg/min dosage.

10. An IV of milrinone (Primacor) is infusing at 7.3 mL/hr. The IV bag contains 20 mg milrinone (Primacor) in 100 mL D_5W. Calculate the mcg/min dosage.

Titrating Dosages According to Patient Response

High-risk medications are adjusted, or titrated, up or down according to a patient's physiological response to the drug. For example, the drug dopamine can be infused to help maintain blood pressure when a person is in shock. The nurse's responsibility when infusing dopamine is to obtain frequent blood pressure readings and adjust the dose of dopamine up or down. An order for dopamine may prescribe a predetermined range within which the nurse can increase or decrease the dose. If the patient isn't responding to the dopamine within the dosage range, new orders must be obtained. An adverse drug reaction may occur if the upper limit of the prescribed range is exceeded.

Example 1: A provider writes an order to start a dopamine drip at 5 mcg/kg/min IV. The dopamine drip is to be titrated in 5 mcg/kg/min increments up to 20 mcg/kg/min to maintain the patient's blood pressure within the range ordered by the provider. The patient weighs 66 kg. The pharmacy supplies the medication in premixed infusion bags containing 400 mg dopamine in 250 mL D_5W. Calculate the mL/hr flow rate range (the beginning flow rate and the maximum flow rate) for the dopamine drip. Round the answer to the nearest tenth mL.

1. Set up the equation to find the beginning flow rate in mL/hr using dimensional analysis. The beginning flow rate should deliver 5 mcg/kg/hr.

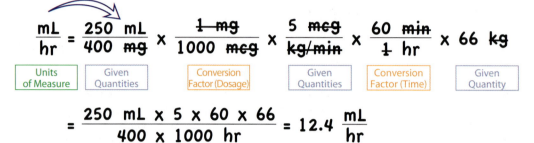

$$= \frac{250 \text{ mL} \times 5 \times 60 \times 66}{400 \times 1000 \text{ hr}} = 12.4 \frac{\text{mL}}{\text{hr}}$$

To infuse dopamine at 5 mcg/kg/min for this patient, the pump must be set at 12.4 mL/hr.

2. Now calculate the upper limit of the dopamine infusion in mL/hr. The upper limit is reached at 20 mcg/kg/min.

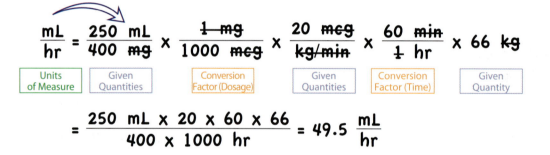

$$= \frac{250 \text{ mL} \times 20 \times 60 \times 66}{400 \times 1000 \text{ hr}} = 49.5 \frac{\text{mL}}{\text{hr}}$$

The flow rate for the maximum dosage of dopamine is 49.5 mL/hr. This flow rate should not be exceeded without contacting the provider.

In summary, the mL/hr flow rate range for this dopamine drip is 12.4 to 49.5 mL/hr based on the prescribed dosage of 5 to 20 mcg/kg/min.

Example 2: A provider orders a nitroglycerin IV drip to titrate between 5 and 15 mcg/min based on the patient's blood pressure. The pharmacy supplies an infusion bag containing 25 mg nitroglycerin in 250 mL D_5W. Calculate the mL/hr flow rate range for the nitroglycerin infusion. Round the answer to the nearest tenth mL.

1. Set up the equation to find the beginning flow rate in mL/hr. The initial flow rate is set to deliver 5 mcg/min.

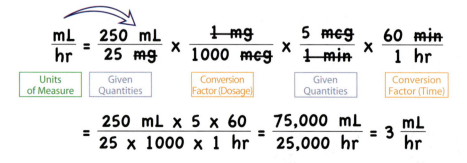

$$= \frac{250 \text{ mL} \times 5 \times 60}{25 \times 1000 \times 1 \text{ hr}} = \frac{75,000 \text{ mL}}{25,000 \text{ hr}} = 3 \frac{\text{mL}}{\text{hr}}$$

2. Calculate the mL/hr flow rate for the maximum dosage (15 mcg/min).

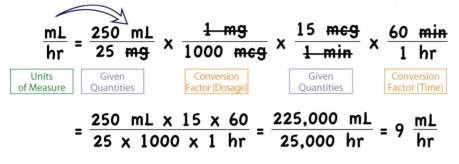

The mL/hr flow rate range for titrating the nitroglycerin drip is from 3 to 9 mL/hr (based on a dosage range of 5 to 15 mcg/min). Any flow rate exceeding 9 mL/hr must be prescribed by the provider.

Example 3:   A nurse is assuming care for a patient on a nitroglycerin drip. The nurse wants to verify that the mL/hr flow rate has been correctly calculated by the previous nurse. The nitroglycerin drip is currently running at 7.7 mL/hr. The nurse reads the label of the bag and notes that it contains 25 mg nitroglycerin in 250 mL D_5W. Calculate the mcg/min dosage that is currently infusing. Round the answer to the nearest tenth mL. Determine whether the dosage infusing is within the prescribed range of 5 to 15 mcg/min.

1. Set up the equation to solve for mcg/min. The first set of given quantities is the conversion factor to convert mg to mcg.

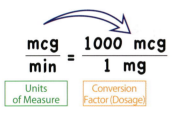

2. Enter the next set of given quantities—the amount of medication in the IV bag (25 mg in 250 mL).

$$\frac{mcg}{min} = \frac{1000 \ mcg}{1 \ mg} \times \frac{25 \ mg}{250 \ mL}$$

| Units of Measure | Conversion Factor (Dosage) | Given Quantities |

3. Enter the next set of given quantities—the mL/hr infusion rate of the IV (7.7 mL/hr).

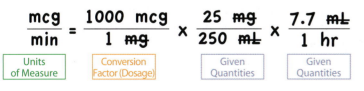

4. Enter the last conversion factor to change hours into minutes (60 min/hr) and solve the equation.

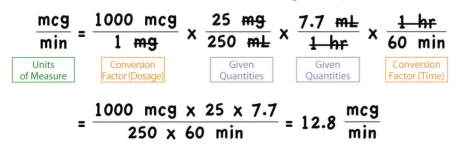

$$= \frac{1000 \ mcg \times 25 \times 7.7}{250 \times 60 \ min} = 12.8 \ \frac{mcg}{min}$$

The patient is receiving 12.8 mcg/min of nitroglycerin when the flow rate is 7.7 mL/hr. The dosage of nitroglycerin the patient is receiving is within the prescribed range of 5 to 15 mcg/min.

Example 4: A patient is receiving a nitroprusside (Nitropress) IV drip. The prescribed range of nitroprusside (Nitropress) that the patient may receive is 0.5 to 8 mcg/kg/min. The patient weighs 68.3 kg. The IV bag contains 50 mg nitroprusside (Nitropress) in 500 mL D_5W. The IV is currently infusing at 24.4 mL/hr. Calculate the mcg/min dosage that is currently infusing, rounding the final answer to the nearest tenth. Determine if the dosage is within the prescribed range of 0.5 to 8 mcg/kg/min.

1. Set up the equation to solve for mcg/min. Insert the first set of quantities—the conversion factor to convert mg to mcg.

$$\frac{mcg}{min} = \frac{1000\ mcg}{1\ mg}$$

Units of Measure | Conversion Factor (Dosage)

2. Enter the next set of given quantities—the amount of medication in the IV bag.

$$\frac{mcg}{min} = \frac{1000\ mcg}{1\ mg} \times \frac{50\ mg}{500\ mL}$$

Units of Measure | Conversion Factor (Dosage) | Given Quantities

3. Enter the next set of given quantities.

$$\frac{mcg}{min} = \frac{1000\ mcg}{1\ mg} \times \frac{50\ mg}{500\ mL} \times \frac{24.4\ mL}{1\ hr}$$

Units of Measure | Conversion Factor (Dosage) | Given Quantities | Given Quantities

4. Enter the last conversion factor to change hours into minutes and solve the equation.

$$\frac{mcg}{min} = \frac{1000\ mcg}{1\ mg} \times \frac{50\ mg}{500\ mL} \times \frac{24.4\ mL}{1\ hr} \times \frac{1\ hr}{60\ min}$$

Units of Measure | Conversion Factor (Dosage) | Given Quantities | Given Quantities | Conversion Factor (Time)

$$= \frac{1000\ mcg \times 50 \times 24.4}{500 \times 60\ min} = 40.7\ \frac{mcg}{min}$$

The patient is receiving 40.7 mcg/min of nitroprusside (Nitropress) when the flow rate is 24.4 mL/hr. However, the dosage range of nitroprusside is based on patient weight, so the appropriate dosage range must be calculated before evaluating whether the patient is receiving a dose within the correct range.

5. Calculate the prescribed dosage range:
   a. Calculate the beginning mcg/min dosage.

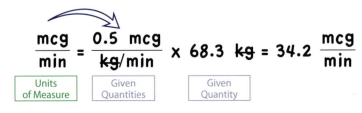

$$\frac{mcg}{min} = \frac{0.5\ mcg}{kg/min} \times 68.3\ kg = 34.2\ \frac{mcg}{min}$$

Units of Measure | Given Quantities | Given Quantity

b. Calculate the maximum mcg/min dosage.

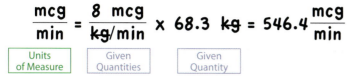

$$\frac{mcg}{min} = \frac{8\ mcg}{kg/min} \times 68.3\ kg = 546.4\ \frac{mcg}{min}$$

Units of Measure   Given Quantities   Given Quantity

The prescribed dosage range of nitroprusside (Nitropress) for this patient is 34.2 to 546.4 mcg/min based on the patient's weight. The current dosage of nitroprusside (Nitropress) that is infusing is 40.7 mcg/min, which is within the prescribed range. If the current dosage had been less than 34.2 mcg/min or greater than 546.4 mcg/min, the nurse would have needed to notify the provider to request new orders.

Practice Titrating Dosages According to Patient Response

(answers on page 367)

Calculate the mL/hr flow rate range for these IV drips. Round the answer to the nearest tenth.

1. A provider orders an argatroban IV drip to begin at 2 mcg/kg/min. The maximum dose is 10 mcg/kg/min. The patient weighs 88 kg. The IV bag contains 250 mg argatroban in 250 mL D_5W.

2. A provider orders a cisatracurium (Nimbex) IV drip to begin at 3 mcg/kg/min. The maximum dose is 10 mcg/kg/min. The patient weighs 74.5 kg. The IV bag contains 250 mg cisatracurium (Nimbex) in 250 mL D_5W.

3. A provider orders a procainamide (Pronestyl) IV drip to begin at 1 mg/min. The maximum dose is 6 mg/min. The IV bag contains 1 g procainamide (Pronestyl) in 250 mL D_5W.

4. A provider orders a norepinephrine IV drip to begin at 2 mcg/min. The maximum dose is 4 mcg/min. The IV bag contains 4 mg norepinephrine in 250 mL D_5W.

5. A provider orders a dobutamine IV drip to begin at 2.5 mcg/kg/min. The maximum dose is 10 mcg/kg/min. The patient weighs 66.3 kg. The IV bag contains 500 mg dobutamine in 250 mL D_5W.

Calculate the mcg/min dosage currently infusing for these IV drips. Indicate whether the dosage is within the prescribed range. Round the answer to the nearest tenth.

6. A diltiazem (Cardizem) IV drip is infusing at 9.8 mL/hr. The IV bag contains 100 mg diltiazem (Cardizem) in 100 mL D_5W. The prescribed dosage range is 84 to 167mcg/min.

7. A conivaptan (Vaprisol) IV drip is infusing at 14 mL/hr. The IV bag contains 20 mg conivaptan (Vaprisol) in 250 mL D_5W. The prescribed dosage range is 13.8 to 26.7 mcg/min.

8. An esmolol (Brevibloc) IV drip is infusing at 48 mL/hr. The IV bag contains 500 mg esmolol (Brevibloc) in 250 mL NS. The prescribed dosage range is 10 to 50 mcg/kg/min. The patient weighs 80 kg.

9. An isoproterenol (Isuprel) IV drip is infusing at 90 mL/hr. The IV bag contains 1 mg isoproterenol (Isuprel) in 250 mL D_5W. The prescribed dosage range is 0.5 to 5 mcg/min.

10. A phenylephrine (Neo-Synephrine) IV drip is infusing at 2.8 mL/hr. The IV bag contains 100 mg phenylephrine (Neo-Synephrine) in 100 mL NS. The prescribed dosage range is 40 to 60 mcg/min.

IV Infusion Protocols for High-Risk Medications

IV infusion protocols are standardized sets of orders that are initiated by a provider when a patient is admitted with a specific disorder, such as an irregular heartbeat, low blood pressure, or chest pain. Nurses should become familiar with the protocols for high-risk medications to ensure patient safety. An example of a diltiazem protocol for an irregular heart beat is shown in Figure 17-2.

Intravenous Diltiazem (Cardizem) Protocol

☐ Place patient on a cardiac monitor. Monitor continually while diltiazem (Cardizem) drip being administered.

☐ Administer intravenous diltiazem (Cardizem) bolus: 0.25 mg/kg over 3 minutes.
Patient weight _____ kg × 0.25 mg = IV bolus of _____ mg.

☐ Immediately after the bolus, begin a continuous infusion of diltiazem (Cardizem) (mixed as 100 mg diltiazem in 100 mL D_5W to equal 1 mg/mL).

☐ May titrate the infusion rate to a maximum of 15 mg/hr if an atrial arrhythmia exists and the heart rate is greater than 100 beats/min.

☐ Monitor BP every 5 minutes for 30 minutes, then every 15 minutes for 3 hours, then every 2 hours.

☐ Call MD for orders to administer a second bolus if the following are present:
 • Heart rate greater than 80% of pre-treatment level 15 minutes after the first bolus.
 • Systolic blood pressure is within 90% of pre-treatment level.

☐ Discontinue infusion and call MD for:
 • A heart rate less than 60 beats/min.
 • A pause of greater than 2 seconds.
 • A second or third degree AV block.
 • A systolic BP below 90 mm Hg.

_____ Date: _____ Time: _____
Provider's Signature

_____ Date: _____ Time: _____
RN Noted

Faxed to Pharmacy by: _____
Date: _____ Time: _____

Patient Label

Intravenous Diltiazem (Cardizem) Protocol

Figure 17-2 Sample Diltiazem (Cardizem) Infusion Protocol

Read Case Study 17-1 and answer the questions.

Case Study 17–1

Harold Bell is admitted to the critical care unit where you are the RN; he has a very slow heartbeat and low blood pressure. His physician places him on the dopamine protocol (see Fig. 17-3). Mr. Bell weighs 82.7 kg. Answer these questions based on the standing orders in the protocol.

1. *Before beginning the dopamine infusion, you must ensure that Mr. Bell is placed on a*
   _____ monitor.
2. *Calculate the beginning mcg/min dose of dopamine, rounding to the nearest whole number.*
3. *Calculate the beginning mL/hr flow rate, rounding to the nearest tenth mL.*

Ten minutes after the dopamine infusion was initiated, Mr. Bell's blood pressure is still low. You increase the rate by 1 mcg/kg/min.

4. *Calculate the new mcg/min dose of dopamine, rounding to the nearest whole number.*
5. *Calculate the new mL/hr flow rate. Round the answer to the nearest tenth mL.*
6. *What is the maximum mcg/min dose that you can give Mr. Bell c without contacting the provider?*
7. *What other monitoring must be done while Mr. Bell is on the dopamine drip?*

Key Points

1. Medications prescribed in critical care are potentially dangerous.
2. Critical care medications should be infused using an electronic infusion device.
3. If the electronic infusion device cannot be programmed for specific drugs, the nurse must calculate the mL/hr flow rate based on the prescribed dosage, the amount of medication in the IV bag, the amount of solution in the IV bag, and the weight of the patient if the dosage is weight-based.
4. Many critical care medications must be titrated incrementally according to the patient's response.
5. Nurses must be able to verify that a drug is being infused at the right dosage and the right flow rate. If an infusion rate exceeds the prescribed limits, the nurse must contact the provider for new orders.

Intravenous Dopamine Protocol
General Hospital

General:

☑ Patient must be on a cardiac monitor while on dopamine.
☑ Dopamine must be administered using an electronic infusion pump.
☐ Central line placement is preferred for a dopamine infusion.

Mixture:

☐ Use the following mixture (check one):
  ☑ Dopamine 400 mg in 500 mL D_5W = 0.8 mg/mL
  ☐ Dopamine 800 mg in 500 mL D_5W = 1.6 mg/mL
  ☐ Dopamine 800 mg in 250 mL D_5W = 3.2 mg/mL

Dosage:

☑ Patient's weight _____82.7_____ kg
☐ Begin the infusion at (choose one):
  ☑ 2 mcg/kg/min = wt (kg) _____ × 2 mcg/kg/min = _____ mcg/min
  ☐ _____ mcg/kg/min = wt (kg) _____ × _____ mcg/kg/min = _____ mcg/min

Titration:

☑ Increase the dose by 1 mcg/kg/min every 5 to 10 minutes until:
  ☑ Systolic BP greater than ___110___ mm Hg
  ☑ Heart rate greater than ___60___ bpm
  ☐ Other: _____
☑ Do not exceed 20 mcg/kg/min dose without notifying provider.
☑ Begin downward titration per provider's order.

Other:

☑ Insert Foley catheter if one not already present.
☑ Concurrent intravenous fluids:
  ☑ NS ___125___ mL/hr   ☐ LR at _____ mL/hr
  ☐ D_5W at _____ mL/hr   ☐ Other: _____

Monitoring:

☑ Monitor Intake & Output hourly.
☑ Monitor blood pressure and pulse every 5 to 10 minutes while titrating dose.
☑ If blood pressure and pulse have been stabilized for at least 1 hour, may monitor hourly.
☑ Obtain temperature and respiratory rate every 2 to 4 hours.
☑ Monitor intravenous site hourly. If the dopamine has infiltrated around the access site, contact provider for orders to treat.

Intravenous Dopamine Protocol

Harold M. Bell
Acct #: 83991856
MR #: A972058
DOB: 08/15/1948
Provider: M. Jones, MN

Figure 17-3 Dopamine Protocol

Chapter Post-Test   *(answers in Unit 4)*

Calculations

Calculate the mL/hr infusion rates for these medication orders. Round the answers to the nearest tenth mL.

1. A provider orders nitroprusside (Nitropress) 175 mcg/min IV. The IV bag contains 50 mg nitroprusside (Nitropress) in 250 mL D$_5$W.

2. A provider orders isoproterenol (Isuprel) 8 mcg/min IV. The IV bag contains 2 mg isoproterenol (Isuprel) in 500 mL D$_5$W.

3. A provider orders norepinephrine (Levophed) 6 mcg/min IV. The IV bag contains 4 mg norepinephrine (Levophed) in 250 mL D$_5$W.

4. A provider orders amiodarone (Cordarone) 2 mg/min. The IV bag contains 900 mg amiodarone (Cordarone) in 500 mL D$_5$W.

5. A provider orders phenylephrine (Neo-Synephrine) 75 mcg/min IV. The IV bag contains 10 mg phenylephrine (Neo-Synephrine) in 100 mL NS.

6. A provider orders eptifibatide (Integrilin) 140 mcg/min IV. The IV bag contains 150 mg eptifibatide (Integrilin) in 200 mL solution.

7. A provider orders abciximab (Reopro) 9 mcg/min IV. The IV bag contains 10 mg abciximab (Reopro) in 250 mL NS.

8. A provider orders procainamide (Pronestyl) 1 mg/min IV. The IV bag contains 2 g procainamide (Pronestyl) in 500 mL NS.

9. A provider orders inamrinone (Inocor) 300 mcg/min IV. The IV bag contains 250 mg inamrinone (Inocor) in 100 mL NS.

10. A provider orders epinephrine 1.5 mcg/min IV. The IV bag contains 2 mg epinephrine in 500 mL NS.

Calculate the mL/hr infusion rates from these weight-based dosages. Round the answers to the nearest tenth mL.

11. A provider orders dopamine 7.6 mcg/kg/min IV. The IV bag contains 400 mg dopamine in 250 mL. The patient weighs 94 kg.

12. A provider orders esmolol (Brevibloc) 0.1 mg/kg/min IV. The IV bag contains 2 g esmolol (Brevibloc) in 100 mL D$_5$W. The patient weighs 64 kg.

13. A provider orders dobutamine 1 mcg/kg/min IV. The IV bag contains 500 mg dobutamine in 250 mL NS. The patient weighs 65 kg.

14. A provider orders abciximab (Reopro) 0.1 mcg/kg/min IV. The IV bag contains 4 mg abciximab (Reopro) in 200 mL NS. The patient weighs 51 kg.

15. A provider orders nitroprusside (Nitropress) 3 mcg/kg/min IV. The IV bag contains 50 mg nitroprusside (Nitropress) in 250 mL D$_5$W. The patient weighs 85 kg.

16. A provider orders inamrinone (Inocor) 0.015 mg/kg/min. The IV bag contains 1 g inamrinone (Inocor) in 500 mL solution. The patient weighs 68 kg.

17. A provider orders milrinone (Primacor) 0.175 mcg/kg/min IV. The IV bag contains 40 mg milrinone (Primacor) in 100 mL NS. The patient weighs 76 kg.

18. A provider orders fenoldopam (Corlopam) 0.3 mcg/kg/min. The IV bag contains 20 mg fenoldopam (Corlopam) in 250 mL D_5W. The patient weighs 82 kg.

19. A provider orders nesiritide (Natrecor) 0.015 mcg/kg/min IV. The IV bag contains 1.5 mg nesiritide (Natrecor) in 250 mL solution. The patient weighs 59 kg.

20. A provider orders tirofiban (Aggrastat) 0.3 mcg/kg/min IV. The IV bag contains 25 mg tirofiban (Aggrastat) in 500 mL solution. The patient weighs 77 kg.

Calculate the mg/min dosage from the mL/hr flow rate of the IV. Round the answers to the nearest tenth mg.

21. An IV of magnesium sulfate is infusing at 64 mL/hr. The IV bag contains 4 g magnesium sulfate in 250 mL D_5W. Calculate the mg/min dosage.

22. An IV of ibutilide (Corvert) is infusing at 150 mL/hr. The IV bag contains 10 mg ibutilide (Corvert) in 100 mL D_5W. Calculate the mg/min dosage.

23. An IV of immune globulin is infusing at 80 mL/hr. The IV bag contains 5 g immune globulin in 250 mL solution. Calculate the mg/min dosage.

24. An IV of lidocaine is infusing at 30 mL/hr. The IV bag contains 1 g lidocaine in 250 mL solution. Calculate the mg/min dosage.

25. An IV of labetalol is infusing at 30 mL/hr. The IV bag contains 200 mg labetalol in 160 mL D_5W. Calculate the mg/min dosage.

Calculate the mcg/min dosage from the mL/hr flow rate of the IV. Round the answers to the nearest tenth mcg.

26. An IV of octreotide (Sandostatin) is infusing at 22 mL/hr. The IV bag contains 2 mg octreotide (Sandostatin) in 250 mL solution. Calculate the mcg/min dosage.

27. An IV of tirofiban (Aggrastat) is infusing at 12.6 mL/hr. The IV bag contains 25 mg tirofiban (Aggrastat) in 250 mL of solution. Calculate the mcg/min dosage.

28. An IV of infliximab (Remicade) is infusing at 32 mL/hr. The IV bag contains 250 mg infliximab (Remicade) in 250 mL NS. Calculate the mcg/min dosage.

29. An IV of milrinone (Primacor) is infusing at 5.9 mL/hr. The IV bag contains 40 mg milrinone (Primacor) in 250 mL D_5W. Calculate the mcg/min dosage.

30. An IV of epinephrine is infusing at 25.8 mL/hr. The IV bag contains 2 mg of epinephrine in 200 mL NS. Calculate the mcg/min dosage.

Calculate the mL/hr flow rate range for these IV infusions. Round the answers to the nearest tenth mL.

31. A provider orders a procainamide (Pronestyl) IV drip to begin at 1.5 mg/min. The maximum dose is 6 mg/min. The IV bag contains 2 g procainamide (Pronestyl) in 500 mL D_5W.

32. A provider orders a norepinephrine (Levophed) IV drip to begin at 3 mcg/min. The maximum dose is 4 mcg/min. The IV bag contains 4 mg norepinephrine (Levophed) in 200 mL D_5W.

33. A provider orders an argatroban IV drip to begin at 2.5 mcg/kg/min. The maximum dose is 10 mcg/kg/min. The patient weighs 54 kg. The IV bag contains 250 mg argatroban in 250 mL D_5W.

34. A provider orders a dobutamine IV drip to begin at 2 mcg/kg/min. The maximum dose is 10 mcg/kg/min. The patient weighs 70.3 kg. The IV bag contains 250 mg dobutamine in 250 mL D_5W.

35. A provider orders a cisatracurium (Nimbex) IV drip to begin at 3 mcg/kg/min. The maximum dose is 10 mcg/kg/min. The patient weighs 83.8 kg. The IV bag contains 125 mg cisatracurium (Nimbex) in 100 mL D$_5$W.

Calculate the mcg/min dosage that is currently infusing for these IV drips. Indicate whether the dosage is within the prescribed range. Round the answers to the nearest tenth mcg.

36. A conivaptan (Vaprisol) IV drip is infusing at 12 mL/hr. The IV bag contains 20 mg conivaptan (Vaprisol) in 200 mL D$_5$W. The prescribed dosage range is 13.8 to 26.7 mcg/min.

37. An isoproterenol (Isuprel) IV drip is infusing at 75 mL/hr. The IV bag contains 2 mg isoproterenol (Isuprel) in 250 mL D$_5$W. The prescribed dosage range is 0.5 to 5 mcg/min.

38. A diltiazem (Cardizem) IV drip is infusing at 20 mL/hr. The IV bag contains 100 mg of diltiazem (Cardizem) in 250 mL D$_5$W. The prescribed dosage range is 84 to 167 mcg/min.

39. A phenylephrine (Neo-Synephrine) IV drip is infusing at 4 mL/hr. The IV bag contains 100 mg phenylephrine (Neo-Synephrine) in 100 mL NS. The prescribed dosage range is 40 to 80 mcg/min.

40. An esmolol (Brevibloc) IV drip is infusing at 42 mL/hr. The IV bag contains 2 g esmolol (Brevibloc) in 200 mL NS. The prescribed dosage range is 50 to 200 mcg/kg/min. The patient weighs 74 kg.

Answers to Practice Questions

Calculating mL/hr Infusion Rates From mg/min and mcg/min Dosages

1. $\dfrac{mL}{hr} = \dfrac{250\ mL}{4\ \cancel{mg}} \times \dfrac{1\ \cancel{mg}}{1000\ \cancel{mcg}} \times \dfrac{8\ \cancel{mcg}}{1\ \cancel{min}} \times \dfrac{60\ \cancel{min}}{1\ hr} = \dfrac{250\ mL \times 8 \times 60}{4 \times 1000 \times 1\ hr} = 30\ \dfrac{mL}{hr}$

2. $\dfrac{mL}{hr} = \dfrac{500\ mL}{900\ \cancel{mg}} \times \dfrac{1\ \cancel{mg}}{1\ \cancel{min}} \times \dfrac{60\ \cancel{min}}{1\ hr} = \dfrac{500\ mL \times 60}{900 \times 1\ hr} = 33.3\ \dfrac{mL}{hr}$

3. $\dfrac{mL}{hr} = \dfrac{250\ mL}{1\ \cancel{mg}} \times \dfrac{1\ \cancel{mg}}{1000\ \cancel{mcg}} \times \dfrac{1.5\ \cancel{mcg}}{1\ \cancel{min}} \times \dfrac{60\ \cancel{min}}{1\ hr} = \dfrac{250\ mL \times 1.5 \times 60}{1000 \times 1 \times 1\ hr} = 22.5\ \dfrac{mL}{hr}$

4. $\dfrac{mL}{hr} = \dfrac{500\ mL}{50\ \cancel{mg}} \times \dfrac{1\ \cancel{mg}}{1000\ \cancel{mcg}} \times \dfrac{100\ \cancel{mcg}}{1\ \cancel{min}} \times \dfrac{60\ \cancel{min}}{1\ hr} = \dfrac{500\ mL \times 100 \times 60}{50 \times 1000 \times 1\ hr} = 60\ \dfrac{mL}{hr}$

5. $\dfrac{mL}{hr} = \dfrac{250\ mL}{1\ \cancel{mg}} \times \dfrac{1\ \cancel{mg}}{1000\ \cancel{mcg}} \times \dfrac{5\ \cancel{mcg}}{1\ \cancel{min}} \times \dfrac{60\ \cancel{min}}{1\ hr} = \dfrac{250\ mL \times 5 \times 60}{1000 \times 1 \times 1\ hr} = 75\ \dfrac{mL}{hr}$

6. $\dfrac{mL}{hr} = \dfrac{250\ mL}{1\ \cancel{g}} \times \dfrac{1\ \cancel{g}}{1000\ \cancel{mg}} \times \dfrac{2\ \cancel{mg}}{1\ \cancel{min}} \times \dfrac{60\ \cancel{min}}{1\ hr} = \dfrac{250\ mL \times 2 \times 60}{1000 \times 1 \times 1\ hr} = 30\ \dfrac{mL}{hr}$

7. $\dfrac{mL}{hr} = \dfrac{100\ mL}{75\ \cancel{mg}} \times \dfrac{1\ \cancel{mg}}{1000\ \cancel{mcg}} \times \dfrac{160\ \cancel{mcg}}{1\ \cancel{min}} \times \dfrac{60\ \cancel{min}}{1\ hr} = \dfrac{100\ mL \times 160 \times 60}{75 \times 1000 \times 1\ hr} = 12.8\ \dfrac{mL}{hr}$

8. $\dfrac{mL}{hr} = \dfrac{250\ mL}{100\ \cancel{mg}} \times \dfrac{1\ \cancel{mg}}{1000\ \cancel{mcg}} \times \dfrac{225\ \cancel{mcg}}{1\ \cancel{min}} \times \dfrac{60\ \cancel{min}}{1\ hr} = \dfrac{250\ mL \times 225 \times 60}{100 \times 1000 \times 1\ hr} = 33.8\ \dfrac{mL}{hr}$

9. $\dfrac{mL}{hr} = \dfrac{250\ mL}{7.2\ \cancel{mg}} \times \dfrac{1\ \cancel{mg}}{1000\ \cancel{mcg}} \times \dfrac{11\ \cancel{mcg}}{1\ \cancel{min}} \times \dfrac{60\ \cancel{min}}{1\ hr} = \dfrac{250\ mL \times 11 \times 60}{7.2 \times 1000 \times 1\ hr} = 22.9\ \dfrac{mL}{hr}$

10. $\dfrac{mL}{hr} = \dfrac{200\ mL}{500\ \cancel{mg}} \times \dfrac{1\ \cancel{mg}}{1000\ \cancel{mcg}} \times \dfrac{384\ \cancel{mcg}}{1\ \cancel{min}} \times \dfrac{60\ \cancel{min}}{1\ hr} = \dfrac{200\ mL \times 384 \times 60}{500 \times 1000 \times 1\ hr} = 9.2\ \dfrac{mL}{hr}$

Calculating mL/hr Infusion Rates From mg/kg/min and mcg/kg/min Dosages

1. $\dfrac{mL}{hr} = \dfrac{250\ mL}{5.85\ \cancel{mg}} \times \dfrac{1\ \cancel{mg}}{1000\ \cancel{mcg}} \times \dfrac{0.125\ \cancel{mcg}}{kg/min} \times \dfrac{60\ \cancel{min}}{1\ hr} \times 65\ \cancel{kg}$

$= \dfrac{250\ mL \times 0.125 \times 60 \times 65}{5.85 \times 1000\ hr} = 20.8\ \dfrac{mL}{hr}$

2. $\dfrac{mL}{hr} = \dfrac{250\ mL}{50\ \cancel{mg}} \times \dfrac{1\ \cancel{mg}}{1000\ \cancel{mcg}} \times \dfrac{4.5\ \cancel{mcg}}{kg/min} \times \dfrac{60\ \cancel{min}}{1\ hr} \times 72\ \cancel{kg}$

$= \dfrac{250\ mL \times 4.5 \times 60 \times 72}{50 \times 1000\ hr} = 97.2\ \dfrac{mL}{hr}$

3. $\dfrac{mL}{hr} = \dfrac{200\ mL}{500\ \cancel{mg}} \times \dfrac{0.01\ \cancel{mg}}{kg/min} \times \dfrac{60\ \cancel{min}}{1\ hr} \times 80\ \cancel{kg}$

$= \dfrac{200\ mL \times 0.01 \times 60 \times 80}{500 \times 1\ hr} = 19.2\ \dfrac{mL}{hr}$

4. $\dfrac{mL}{hr} = \dfrac{80\ mL}{20\ \cancel{mg}} \times \dfrac{1\ \cancel{mg}}{1000\ \cancel{mcg}} \times \dfrac{0.375\ \cancel{mcg}}{kg/min} \times \dfrac{60\ \cancel{min}}{1\ hr} \times 92\ \cancel{kg}$

$= \dfrac{80\ mL \times 0.375 \times 60 \times 92}{20 \times 1000\ hr} = 8.3\ \dfrac{mL}{hr}$

5. $\dfrac{mL}{hr} = \dfrac{250\ mL}{500\ \cancel{mg}} \times \dfrac{1\ \cancel{mg}}{1000\ \cancel{mcg}} \times \dfrac{2.5\ \cancel{mcg}}{kg/min} \times \dfrac{60\ \cancel{min}}{1\ hr} \times 78\ \cancel{kg}$

$= \dfrac{250\ mL \times 2.5 \times 60 \times 78}{500 \times 1000\ hr} = 5.9\ \dfrac{mL}{hr}$

6. $\dfrac{mL}{hr} = \dfrac{250\ mL}{400\ \cancel{mg}} \times \dfrac{1\ \cancel{mg}}{1000\ \cancel{mcg}} \times \dfrac{9.7\ \cancel{mcg}}{kg/min} \times \dfrac{60\ \cancel{min}}{1\ hr} \times 56\ \cancel{kg}$

$= \dfrac{250\ mL \times 9.7 \times 60 \times 56}{400 \times 1000\ hr} = 20.4\ \dfrac{mL}{hr}$

7. $\dfrac{mL}{hr} = \dfrac{250\ mL}{2.5\ \cancel{g}} \times \dfrac{1\ \cancel{g}}{1000\ \cancel{mg}} \times \dfrac{0.05\ \cancel{mg}}{kg/min} \times \dfrac{60\ \cancel{min}}{1\ hr} \times 63\ \cancel{kg}$

$= \dfrac{250\ mL \times 0.05 \times 60 \times 63}{2.5 \times 1000\ hr} = 18.9\ \dfrac{mL}{hr}$

Answers to Practice Questions

8. $\dfrac{mL}{hr} = \dfrac{250 \ mL}{10 \ \cancel{mg}} \times \dfrac{1 \ \cancel{mg}}{1000 \ \cancel{mcg}} \times \dfrac{0.25 \ \cancel{mcg}}{\cancel{kg}/\cancel{min}} \times \dfrac{60 \ \cancel{min}}{1 \ hr} \times 71 \ \cancel{kg}$

$= \dfrac{250 \ mL \times 0.25 \times 60 \times 71}{10 \times 1000 \ hr} = 26.6 \ \dfrac{mL}{hr}$

9. $\dfrac{mL}{hr} = \dfrac{250 \ mL}{1.5 \ \cancel{mg}} \times \dfrac{1 \ \cancel{mg}}{1000 \ \cancel{mcg}} \times \dfrac{0.01 \ \cancel{mcg}}{\cancel{kg}/\cancel{min}} \times \dfrac{60 \ \cancel{min}}{1 \ hr} \times 84 \ \cancel{kg}$

$= \dfrac{250 \ mL \times 0.01 \times 60 \times 84}{1.5 \times 1000 \ hr} = 8.4 \ \dfrac{mL}{hr}$

10. $\dfrac{mL}{hr} = \dfrac{250 \ mL}{12.5 \ \cancel{mg}} \times \dfrac{1 \ \cancel{mg}}{1000 \ \cancel{mcg}} \times \dfrac{0.4 \ \cancel{mcg}}{\cancel{kg}/\cancel{min}} \times \dfrac{60 \ \cancel{min}}{1 \ hr} \times 69 \ \cancel{kg}$

$= \dfrac{250 \ mL \times 0.4 \times 60 \times 69}{12.5 \times 1000 \ hr} = 33.1 \ \dfrac{mL}{hr}$

Calculating mg/min and mcg/min Dosages From mL/hr Infusion Rates

1. $\dfrac{mg}{min} = \dfrac{1 \ \cancel{mg}}{50 \ \cancel{mL}} \times \dfrac{300 \ \cancel{mL}}{1 \ \cancel{hr}} \times \dfrac{1 \ \cancel{hr}}{60 \ min} = \dfrac{1 \ mg \times 300}{50 \times 60 \ min} = 0.1 \ \dfrac{mg}{min}$

2. $\dfrac{mg}{min} = \dfrac{1000 \ mg}{1 \ \cancel{g}} \times \dfrac{5 \ \cancel{g}}{100 \ \cancel{mL}} \times \dfrac{60 \ \cancel{mL}}{1 \ \cancel{hr}} \times \dfrac{1 \ \cancel{hr}}{60 \ min} = \dfrac{1000 \ mg \times 5 \times 60}{1 \times 100 \times 60 \ min} = 50 \ \dfrac{mg}{min}$

3. $\dfrac{mg}{min} = \dfrac{1000 \ mg}{1 \ \cancel{g}} \times \dfrac{2 \ \cancel{g}}{500 \ \cancel{mL}} \times \dfrac{45 \ \cancel{mL}}{1 \ \cancel{hr}} \times \dfrac{1 \ \cancel{hr}}{60 \ min} = \dfrac{1000 \ mg \times 2 \times 45}{1 \times 500 \times 60 \ min} = 3 \ \dfrac{mg}{min}$

4. $\dfrac{mg}{min} = \dfrac{1000 \ mg}{1 \ \cancel{g}} \times \dfrac{2 \ \cancel{g}}{100 \ \cancel{mL}} \times \dfrac{56 \ \cancel{mL}}{1 \ \cancel{hr}} \times \dfrac{1 \ \cancel{hr}}{60 \ min} = \dfrac{1000 \ mg \times 2 \times 56}{1 \times 100 \times 60 \ min} = 18.7 \ \dfrac{mg}{min}$

5. $\dfrac{mg}{min} = \dfrac{200 \ \cancel{mg}}{250 \ \cancel{mL}} \times \dfrac{25 \ \cancel{mL}}{1 \ \cancel{hr}} \times \dfrac{1 \ \cancel{hr}}{60 \ min} = \dfrac{1000 \ mcg \times 200 \times 25}{1 \times 250 \times 60 \ min} = 0.3 \ \dfrac{mg}{min}$

6. $\dfrac{mcg}{min} = \dfrac{1000 \ mcg}{1 \ \cancel{mg}} \times \dfrac{1.2 \ \cancel{mg}}{250 \ \cancel{mL}} \times \dfrac{20 \ \cancel{mL}}{1 \ \cancel{hr}} \times \dfrac{1 \ \cancel{hr}}{60 \ min}$

$= \dfrac{1000 \ mcg \times 1.2 \times 20}{1 \times 250 \times 60 \ min} = 1.6 \ \dfrac{mcg}{min}$

7. $\dfrac{mcg}{min} = \dfrac{1000 \ mcg}{1 \ \cancel{mg}} \times \dfrac{1 \ \cancel{mg}}{250 \ \cancel{mL}} \times \dfrac{37 \ \cancel{mL}}{1 \ \cancel{hr}} \times \dfrac{1 \ \cancel{hr}}{60 \ min} = \dfrac{1000 \ mcg \times 1 \times 37}{1 \times 250 \times 60 \ min} = 2.5 \ \dfrac{mcg}{min}$

8. $\dfrac{mcg}{min} = \dfrac{1000\ mcg}{1\ mg} \times \dfrac{1.5\ mg}{250\ mL} \times \dfrac{9\ mL}{1\ hr} \times \dfrac{1\ hr}{60\ min}$

$= \dfrac{1000\ mcg \times 1.5 \times 9}{1 \times 250 \times 60\ min} = \dfrac{13,500\ mcg}{15,000\ min} = 0.9\ \dfrac{mcg}{min}$

9. $\dfrac{mcg}{min} = \dfrac{1000\ mcg}{1\ mg} \times \dfrac{300\ mg}{250\ mL} \times \dfrac{30\ mL}{1\ hr} \times \dfrac{1\ hr}{60\ min}$

$= \dfrac{1000\ mcg \times 300 \times 30}{1 \times 250 \times 60\ min} = 600\ \dfrac{mcg}{min}$

10. $\dfrac{mcg}{min} = \dfrac{1000\ mcg}{1\ mg} \times \dfrac{20\ mg}{100\ mL} \times \dfrac{7.3\ mL}{1\ hr} \times \dfrac{1\ hr}{60\ min}$

$= \dfrac{1000\ mcg \times 20 \times 7.3}{1 \times 100 \times 60\ min} = 24.3\ \dfrac{mcg}{min}$

Titrating Dosages According to Patient Response

1. Beginning rate:

$\dfrac{mL}{hr} = \dfrac{250\ mL}{250\ mg} \times \dfrac{1\ mg}{1000\ mcg} \times \dfrac{2\ mcg}{kg/min} \times \dfrac{60\ min}{1\ hr} \times 88\ kg$

$= \dfrac{250\ mL \times 2 \times 60 \times 88}{250 \times 1000 \times 1\ hr} = 10.6\ \dfrac{mL}{hr}$

Maximum rate:

$\dfrac{mL}{hr} = \dfrac{250\ mL}{250\ mg} \times \dfrac{1\ mg}{1000\ mcg} \times \dfrac{10\ mcg}{kg/min} \times \dfrac{60\ min}{1\ hr} \times 88\ kg$

$= \dfrac{250\ mL \times 10 \times 60 \times 88}{250 \times 1000 \times 1\ hr} = 52.8\ \dfrac{mL}{hr}$

The flow rate range for the prescribed dosage range of 2 to 10 mcg/kg/min is 10.6 to 52.8 mL/hr.

2. Beginning rate:

$\dfrac{mL}{hr} = \dfrac{250\ mL}{250\ mg} \times \dfrac{1\ mg}{1000\ mcg} \times \dfrac{3\ mcg}{kg/min} \times \dfrac{60\ min}{1\ hr} \times 74.5\ kg$

$= \dfrac{250\ mL \times 3 \times 60 \times 74.5}{250 \times 1000 \times 1\ hr} = 13.4\ \dfrac{mL}{hr}$

Maximum rate:

$\dfrac{mL}{hr} = \dfrac{250\ mL}{250\ mg} \times \dfrac{1\ mg}{1000\ mcg} \times \dfrac{10\ mcg}{kg/min} \times \dfrac{60\ min}{1\ hr} \times 74.5\ kg$

$= \dfrac{250\ mL \times 10 \times 60 \times 74.5}{250 \times 1000 \times 1\ hr} = 44.7\ \dfrac{mL}{hr}$

The flow rate range for the prescribed dosage range of 3 to 10 mcg/kg/min is 13.4 to 44.7 mL/hr.

Answers to Practice Questions

3. **Beginning rate:**

$$\frac{mL}{hr} = \frac{250\ mL}{1\ g} \times \frac{1\ g}{1000\ mg} \times \frac{1\ mg}{1\ min} \times \frac{60\ min}{1\ hr} = \frac{250\ mL \times 60}{1000 \times 1\ hr} = 15\ \frac{mL}{hr}$$

Maximum rate:

$$\frac{mL}{hr} = \frac{250\ mL}{1\ g} \times \frac{1\ g}{1000\ mg} \times \frac{6\ mg}{1\ min} \times \frac{60\ min}{1\ hr} = \frac{250\ mL \times 6 \times 60}{1000 \times 1\ hr} = 90\ \frac{mL}{hr}$$

The flow rate range for the prescribed dosage range of 1 to 6 mg/min is 15 to 90 mL/hr.

4. **Beginning rate:**

$$\frac{mL}{hr} = \frac{250\ mL}{4\ mg} \times \frac{1\ mg}{1000\ mcg} \times \frac{2\ mcg}{1\ min} \times \frac{60\ min}{1\ hr} = \frac{250\ mL \times 2 \times 60}{4 \times 1000 \times 1\ hr} = 7.5\ \frac{mL}{hr}$$

Maximum rate:

$$\frac{mL}{hr} = \frac{250\ mL}{4\ mg} \times \frac{1\ mg}{1000\ mcg} \times \frac{4\ mcg}{1\ min} \times \frac{60\ min}{1\ hr} = \frac{250\ mL \times 4 \times 60}{4 \times 1000 \times 1\ hr} = 15\ \frac{mL}{hr}$$

The flow rate range for the prescribed dosage range of 2 to 4 mcg/min is 7.5 to 15 mL/hr.

5. **Beginning rate:**

$$\frac{mL}{hr} = \frac{250\ mL}{500\ mg} \times \frac{1\ mg}{1000\ mcg} \times \frac{2.5\ mcg}{kg/min} \times \frac{60\ min}{1\ hr} \times 66.3\ kg$$

$$= \frac{250\ mL \times 2.5 \times 60 \times 66.3}{500 \times 1000 \times 1\ hr} = 5\ \frac{mL}{hr}$$

Maximum rate:

$$\frac{mL}{hr} = \frac{250\ mL}{500\ mg} \times \frac{1\ mg}{1000\ mcg} \times \frac{10\ mcg}{kg/min} \times \frac{60\ min}{1\ hr} \times 66.3\ kg$$

$$= \frac{250\ mL \times 10 \times 60 \times 66.3}{500 \times 1000 \times 1\ hr} = 19.9\ \frac{mL}{hr}$$

The flow rate range for the prescribed dosage range of 2.5 to 10 mcg/kg/min is 5 to 19.9 mL/hr.

6. **Current dosage infusing:**

$$\frac{mcg}{min} = \frac{1000\ mcg}{1\ mg} \times \frac{100\ mg}{100\ mL} \times \frac{9.8\ mL}{1\ hr} \times \frac{1\ hr}{60\ min} = \frac{1000\ mcg \times 9.8}{60\ min} = 163.3\ \frac{mcg}{min}$$

The prescribed dosage range of diltiazem is 84 to 167 mcg/min. The current dosage of diltiazem infusing is 163.3 mcg/min, which is within the prescribed range.

7. Current dosage infusing:

$$\frac{mcg}{min} = \frac{1000\ mcg}{1\ \cancel{mg}} \times \frac{20\ \cancel{mg}}{250\ \cancel{mL}} \times \frac{14\ \cancel{mL}}{1\ \cancel{hr}} \times \frac{1\ \cancel{hr}}{60\ min}$$

$$= \frac{1000\ mcg \times 20 \times 14}{1 \times 250 \times 60\ min} = 18.7\ \frac{mcg}{min}$$

The prescribed dosage range of conivaptan is 13.8 to 26.7 mcg/min. The current dosage of conivaptan infusing is 18.7 mcg/min, which is within the prescribed range.

8. Current dosage infusing:

$$\frac{mcg}{min} = \frac{1000\ mcg}{1\ \cancel{mg}} \times \frac{500\ \cancel{mg}}{250\ \cancel{mL}} \times \frac{48\ \cancel{mL}}{1\ \cancel{hr}} \times \frac{1\ \cancel{hr}}{60\ min}$$

$$= \frac{1000\ mcg \times 500 \times 48}{1 \times 1 \times 250 \times 60\ min} = 1600\ \frac{mcg}{min}$$

Prescribed dosage range of esmolol:

Lower limit:

$$\frac{mcg}{min} = \frac{10\ mcg}{\cancel{kg}/min} \times 80\ \cancel{kg} = 800\ \frac{mcg}{min}$$

Upper limit:

$$\frac{mcg}{min} = \frac{50\ mcg}{\cancel{kg}/min} \times 80\ \cancel{kg} = 4000\ \frac{mcg}{min}$$

The current dosage of esmolol infusing is 1600 mcg/min, which is within the prescribed range of 800 to 4000 mcg/min.

9. Current dosage infusing:

$$\frac{mcg}{min} = \frac{1000\ mcg}{1\ \cancel{mg}} \times \frac{1\ \cancel{mg}}{250\ \cancel{mL}} \times \frac{90\ \cancel{mL}}{1\ \cancel{hr}} \times \frac{1\ \cancel{hr}}{60\ min}$$

$$= \frac{1000\ mcg \times 90}{250 \times 60\ min} = \frac{90,000\ mcg}{15,000\ min} = 6\ \frac{mcg}{min}$$

The current dosage of isoproterenol infusing is 6 mcg/min, which is over the prescribed range of 0.5 to 5 mcg/min. The nurse should contact the provider for new orders.

10. Current dosage infusing:

$$\frac{mcg}{min} = \frac{1000\ mcg}{1\ \cancel{mg}} \times \frac{100\ \cancel{mg}}{100\ \cancel{mL}} \times \frac{2.8\ \cancel{mL}}{1\ \cancel{hr}} \times \frac{1\ \cancel{hr}}{60\ min}$$

$$= \frac{1000\ mcg \times 2.8}{1 \times 60\ min} = \frac{2800\ mcg}{60\ min} = 46.7\ \frac{mcg}{min}$$

The current dosage of phenylephrine infusing is 46.7 mcg/min, which is within the prescribed range of 40 to 60 mcg/min.

■ *Answers to Case Study 17–1*

1. *cardiac monitor*

2. $\dfrac{2 \text{ mcg}}{\text{kg/min}} \times 82.7 \text{ kg} = 165\dfrac{\text{mcg}}{\text{min}}$

3. $\dfrac{500 \text{ mL}}{400 \text{ mg}} \times \dfrac{1 \text{ mg}}{1000 \text{ mcg}} \times \dfrac{165 \text{ mcg}}{1 \text{ min}} \times \dfrac{60 \text{ min}}{1 \text{ hr}} = 12.4\dfrac{\text{mL}}{\text{hr}}$

4. *The dosage was increased by 83 mcg/min:*

$\dfrac{1 \text{ mcg}}{\text{kg/min}} \times 82.7 \text{ kg} = 83\dfrac{\text{mcg}}{\text{min}}$

The old dosage of 165 mcg/min + the dosage increase of 83 mcg/min = the new dosage of 248 mcg/min.

5. $\dfrac{500 \text{ mL}}{400 \text{ mg}} \times \dfrac{1 \text{ mg}}{1000 \text{ mcg}} \times \dfrac{248 \text{ mcg}}{1 \text{ min}} \times \dfrac{60 \text{ min}}{1 \text{ hr}} = 18.6\dfrac{\text{mL}}{\text{hr}}$

6. $\dfrac{20 \text{ mcg}}{\text{kg/min}} \times 82.7 \text{ kg} = 1654\dfrac{\text{mcg}}{\text{min}}$

7. *Other monitoring includes blood pressure and pulse every 5 to 10 minutes while the dose is being titrated, then every hour after the blood pressure and pulse have stabilized for at least 1 hour; other vital signs every 2 to 4 hours; hourly intake and output; and hourly IV site checks.*

Chapter 18

Lifespan Considerations in Dosage Calculation

☊ Glossary

Absorption: The process by which a medication moves from its site of administration into the blood.

Burette: A chamber used to ensure precise measurement of small amounts of IV fluids; part of a volume control set.

Comorbid: Coexisting with another unrelated disease process; for example, having diabetes, high blood pressure, depression, and chronic kidney disease at the same time.

Distribution: The transportation of medications throughout the body after having been absorbed.

Excretion: The removal of medications from the body through the kidney, lungs, GI tract, or glands.

Free drug: Medication that is not bound to plasma proteins in the blood.

Infiltration: Fluid or medication that leaks from the blood vessel into the surrounding tissues.

Intake and output: The measurement of all fluid intake and output during a 24-hour period.

Metabolism: The process by which a medication is changed by the body.

PSI: Abbreviation for pounds per square inch; a measure of pressure.

Polypharmacy: The use of many medications.

Volume control set: A device that contains a burette; designed to hold a small volume of IV solution from a larger container to avoid accidental fluid overload.

Objectives

After completing this chapter, the learner will be able to—
1. Describe general considerations when administering medications to children, pregnant or lactating women, and aging adults.
2. Calculate drug dosages for children based on body weight.
3. Calculate drug dosages for children based on body surface area.
4. Describe two methods of safe IV administration in children.
5. Calculate daily fluid maintenance needs for children.

General Considerations for Children

The continuous growth and development of a child's body greatly affects how medications are absorbed, distributed, metabolized, and excreted. Before 2000, few reliable resources about prescribing and administering appropriate medication dosages for children existed. However, in 2002, Congress passed the Best Pharmaceuticals for Children Act. The law established a process for studying medications used in the pediatric population. In 2003, the Pediatric Research Equity Act amended the federal Food, Drug, and Cosmetic Act to authorize the FDA to require pharmaceutical companies to conduct pediatric studies of drugs if the drug might be used for children. These laws have improved product labeling, identification of adverse drug events, and the development of new formulations specific to the pediatric population. In July 2016, the FDA reported to Congress that over 600 drugs had pediatric labeling, and inclusion of children in clinical drug studies were becoming a regular part of drug development by manufacturers.

Until all medication used by children can be studied to determine the appropriate doses, providers should calculate drug dosages and nurses should verify the accuracy of prescribed dosages. All dosage calculations should be double-checked by another nurse or pharmacist before administration.

Calculating Dosages for Infants and Children Using Body Weight

Using body weight to prescribe medications for infants and children allows for rapid dosage calculation; however, body weight is not proportional to the serum drug concentration nor does it take into account age-related variances in absorption, distribution, metabolism, or excretion (Table 18-1). Calculating dosage based on body weight is covered in Chapter 11. More examples and questions are provided here for additional practice.

Example 1: A provider orders ondansetron (Zofran) 0.15 mg/kg, IV, 30 minutes prior to chemotherapy. The patient weighs 36 kg. Calculate the dosage (mg) of ondansetron (Zofran) to be administered. Round the answer to the nearest tenth mg.

1. Set up the equation using dimensional analysis, inserting the given quantities for the dosage.

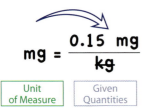

$$mg = \frac{0.15 \ mg}{kg}$$

Unit of Measure | Given Quantities

2. Enter the given quantity for the patient's weight.

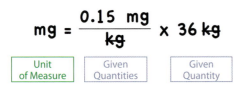

$$mg = \frac{0.15 \ mg}{kg} \times 36 \ kg$$

Unit of Measure | Given Quantities | Given Quantity

Table 18-1	**Alterations in Organ Function Related to Young Age**	
Organ	**Alterations Related to Age**	**Effect on Medication Absorption, Distribution, Metabolism, or Excretion**
Body	High water content relative to fat content.	Increased dilution of water-soluble drugs, leading to decreased serum drug level. Increased serum drug level of fat-soluble drugs.
Gastrointestinal	Increased pH of stomach secretions (alkaline) (infants 2 months or younger). Slowed gastric emptying time.	Altered absorption. Increased or prolonged absorption due to medications taking longer to leave the stomach.
Kidneys	Immature kidney function.	Slowed excretion.
Liver	Immature liver that produces small amounts of plasma proteins. Immature liver enzyme system.	Increased level of free drug in serum. Slowed metabolism.
Muscles	Underdeveloped musculature.	Altered absorption and distribution of drugs given by IM route.
Skin	Thin skin.	Increased absorption of topically applied drugs.
Brain	Immature blood-brain barrier.	Altered central nervous system function.

3. Solve the equation.

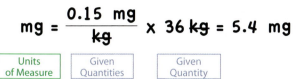

$$mg = \frac{0.15 \text{ mg}}{\text{kg}} \times 36 \text{ kg} = 5.4 \text{ mg}$$

| Units of Measure | Given Quantities | Given Quantity |

The patient should receive 5.4 mg ondansetron (Zofran).

Example 2:   The pharmacy supplies ondansetron (Zofran) in vials containing 2 mg/mL. Using the dosage (mg) calculated in Example 1, calculate the volume (mL) of medication to be administered per dose. Round the answer to the nearest tenth mL.

1. Set up the equation, inserting the given quantities for drug concentration.

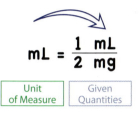

$$mL = \frac{1 \text{ mL}}{2 \text{ mg}}$$

| Unit of Measure | Given Quantities |

2. Insert the next given quantity—the dosage of medication determined in Example 1.

$$mL = \frac{1 \text{ mL}}{2 \text{ mg}} \times 5.4 \text{ mg}$$

| Unit of Measure | Given Quantities | Given Quantity |

3. Solve the equation.

$$mL = \frac{1 \text{ mL}}{2 \text{ mg}} \times 5.4 \text{ mg} = 2.7 \text{ mL}$$

| Unit of Measure | Given Quantities | Given Quantity |

The patient should receive 2.7 mL ondansetron (Zofran) intravenously.

Alert!   Certain medications are toxic to infants and children such as chemotherapy drugs and certain antibiotics. You may need to round your answer to the nearest hundredth place instead of the nearest tenth to provide the most accurate dose. Consult the prescribing provider, facility pharmacist, or drug manufacturer for recommendations.

Example 3:   A provider orders ampicillin 200 mg/kg/day, IV, divided every 8 hours. The patient weighs 4.1 kg. Calculate the dosage (mg/dose) of ampicillin the patient should receive. Round the answer to the nearest tenth mg.

Note: Weight-based pediatric dosages may be prescribed in total daily amounts divided into specific time frames, such as every 4 hours or every 8 hours. The doses should be equal in amount.

1. Set up the equation, entering the known quantities for the dosage.

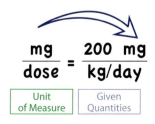

$$\frac{mg}{dose} = \frac{200 \text{ mg}}{kg/day}$$

| Unit of Measure | Given Quantities |

2. Enter the next known quantity—the child's weight.

$$\frac{mg}{dose} = \frac{200\ mg}{kg/day} \times 4.1\ kg$$

<table>
<tr><td>Unit of Measure</td><td>Given Quantities</td><td>Given Quantity</td></tr>
</table>

3. Enter the next set of quantities—the conversion factor changing 1 day into hours.

$$\frac{mg}{dose} = \frac{200\ mg}{kg/\cancel{day}} \times 4.1\ kg \times \frac{1\ \cancel{day}}{24\ hr}$$

<table>
<tr><td>Unit of Measure</td><td>Given Quantities</td><td>Given Quantity</td><td>Conversion Factor (Time)</td></tr>
</table>

Note: Steps 2 and 3 can be done in reverse order. Both *kg* and *day* must be canceled in the first set of given quantities, and it does not matter which is done first.

4. Enter the next set of given quantities—the number of hours between doses.

$$\frac{mg}{dose} = \frac{200\ mg}{kg/\cancel{day}} \times 4.1\ \cancel{kg} \times \frac{1\ \cancel{day}}{24\ \cancel{hr}} \times \frac{8\ \cancel{hr}}{dose}$$

<table>
<tr><td>Unit of Measure</td><td>Given Quantities</td><td>Given Quantity</td><td>Conversion Factor (Time)</td><td>Given Quantities</td></tr>
</table>

5. Solve the equation.

$$\frac{mg}{dose} = \frac{200\ mg}{kg/\cancel{day}} \times 4.1\ \cancel{kg} \times \frac{1\ \cancel{day}}{24\ hr} \times \frac{8\ \cancel{hr}}{dose} = 273.3\ \frac{mg}{dose}$$

<table>
<tr><td>Unit of Measure</td><td>Given Quantities</td><td>Given Quantity</td><td>Conversion Factor (Time)</td><td>Given Quantities</td></tr>
</table>

The nurse should administer 273.3 mg ampicillin every 8 hours to this child.

Alert! A dose received every 8 hours is equal to 3 doses per day, not 8 doses per day.

$$\frac{doses}{day} = \frac{1\ dose}{8\ \cancel{hr}} \times \frac{24\ \cancel{hr}}{1\ day} = 3\ \frac{doses}{day}$$

For example, the equation in Example 3 can be shortened by inserting the number of doses per day $\left(3\ \frac{doses}{day}\right)$ instead of the longer equation $\left(\frac{1\ dose}{8\ \cancel{hr}} \times \frac{24\ \cancel{hr}}{1\ day}\right)$.

$$\frac{mg}{dose} = \frac{200\ mg}{kg/\cancel{day}} \times 4.1\ \cancel{kg} \times \frac{1\ \cancel{day}}{3\ doses} = 273.3\ \frac{mg}{dose}$$

<table>
<tr><td>Unit of Measure</td><td>Given Quantities</td><td>Given Quantities</td><td>Given Quantity</td></tr>
</table>

Example 4: The pharmacy supplies ampicillin in vials containing 50 mg/mL. Using the dosage calculated in Example 3, determine the volume (mL) of medication to be administered intravenously per dose. Round the answer to the nearest tenth mL.

1. Set up the equation, inserting the given quantities for drug concentration.

$$mL = \frac{1\ mL}{50\ mg}$$

| Unit of Measure | Given Quantities |

2. Insert the next given quantity—the dosage of medication determined in Example 3.

$$mL = \frac{1\ mL}{50\ \cancel{mg}} \times 273.3\ \cancel{mg}$$

| Unit of Measure | Given Quantities | Given Quantity |

3. Solve the equation.

$$mL = \frac{1\ mL}{50\ \cancel{mg}} \times 273.3\ \cancel{mg} = 5.5\ mL$$

| Unit of Measure | Given Quantities | Given Quantity |

The patient should receive 5.5 mL ampicillin intravenously, based on a dosage of 273.3 mg.

Example 5: A provider orders vancomycin 40 mg/kg/day, IV, in 6 divided doses. The patient weighs 16.3 kg. Calculate the dosage (mg/dose) of vancomycin to be administered. Round the answer to the nearest tenth mg.

1. Set up the equation using dimensional analysis, inserting the first set of given quantities—the weight-based dosage.

$$\frac{mg}{dose} = \frac{40\ mg}{kg/day}$$

2. Insert the next given quantity—the patient's weight.

$$\frac{mg}{dose} = \frac{40\ mg}{\cancel{kg}/day} \times 16.3\ \cancel{kg}$$

3. Insert the next set of given quantities—the number of doses per day.

$$\frac{mg}{dose} = \frac{40\ mg}{kg/\cancel{day}} \times 16.3\ \cancel{kg} \times \frac{1\ \cancel{day}}{6\ doses} = 108.7\ \frac{mg}{dose}$$

Alert! In this example, the question says that the total daily dosage is to be divided into *6 equal doses*. It does not say *every 6 hours*. No additional calculation is needed to determine the number of doses per day. Read medication labels carefully to avoid making an error in the number of daily doses to administer.

Example 6: The pharmacy supplies vancomycin in vials containing 250 mg/mL. Using the dosage calculated in Example 5, determine the volume (mL) of medication to be administered intravenously per dose. Round the answer to the nearest hundredth mL.

1. Set up the equation, inserting the given quantities for drug concentration.

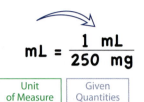

$$mL = \frac{1 \text{ mL}}{250 \text{ mg}}$$

| Unit of Measure | Given Quantities |

2. Insert the next given quantity—the dosage of medication determined in Example 5.

$$mL = \frac{1 \text{ mL}}{250 \text{ mg}} \times 108.7 \text{ mg}$$

| Unit of Measure | Given Quantities | Given Quantity |

3. Solve the equation.

$$mL = \frac{1 \text{ mL}}{250 \text{ mg}} \times 108.7 \text{ mg} = 0.43 \text{ mL}$$

| Unit of Measure | Given Quantities | Given Quantity |

The patient should receive 0.43 mL vancomycin intravenously.

Practice Calculating Dosages for Infants and Children Using Body Weight

(answers on page 394)

Calculate the dosage (mg) and the volume (mL) of medication to be administered per dose. Round answers to the nearest tenth mg and mL.

1. A provider orders cefuroxime (Zinacef) 50 mg/kg/day, PO, every 6 hours in divided doses. The patient weighs 8 kg. The pharmacy supplies cefuroxime (Zinacef) in a suspension containing 125 mg per 5 mL.
   a. mg/dose: _____
   b. mL: _____

2. A provider orders ciprofloxacin (Cipro) 20 mg/kg/day, PO, in 2 divided doses in 24 hours. The patient weighs 44 kg. The pharmacy supplies ciprofloxacin (Cipro) in an oral suspension containing 500 mg per 5 mL.
   a. mg/dose: _____
   b. mL: _____

3. A provider orders ceftriaxone (Rocephin) 75 mg/kg/day, IM, every 12 hours in divided doses. The patient weighs 39 kg. The pharmacy supplies ceftriaxone (Rocephin) in vials containing 500 mg/mL
   a. mg/dose: _____
   b. mL: _____

4. A provider orders acetaminophen (Tylenol) 15 mg/kg, PO, every 6 hours, PRN for a fever. The patient weighs 6.7 kg. The pharmacy supplies acetaminophen (Tylenol) in a suspension containing 100 mg per mL.
   a. mg/dose: _____
   b. mL: _____

5. A provider orders phenytoin (Dilantin) 7 mg/kg/day in 3 divided doses. The patient weighs 37 kg. The pharmacy supplies phenytoin (Dilantin) in a suspension containing 125 mg per 5 mL.
   a. mg/dose: _____
   b. mL: _____

Calculating Dosages for Infants and Children Using Body Surface Area

Calculating drug dosages using body surface area (BSA) is thought to be more accurate than body weight alone. BSA is proportional to an individual's metabolic rate, reflecting a drug's metabolism rate. BSA also correlates well to organ size and fluid compartments within the body, making BSA better than body weight at predicting the effects of drugs (Lack & Stuart-Taylor, (1997). Calculating dosages based on body surface area is covered in Chapter 11, but examples and questions are provided in this chapter as well for additional practice. See Box 18-1 for the BSA formulas.

Example 1: Calculate the BSA for a patient who weighs 28 kg and is 119 cm in height. Round the final answer to the nearest hundredth m².

$$m^2 = \sqrt{\frac{28 \times 119}{3600}}$$

1. Set up the appropriate formula for BSA. Because the height and weight are expressed as metric measures, use *3600* in the denominator.

$$m^2 = \sqrt{\frac{28 \times 119}{3600}} = \sqrt{\frac{3332}{3600}}$$

2. Multiply the numbers in the numerator.

$$m^2 = \sqrt{\frac{3332}{3600}} = \sqrt{0.926}$$

3. Divide the numerator by the denominator.

$$m^2 = \sqrt{0.926} = 0.962 = 0.96 \ m^2$$

4. Find the square root and round the final answer to the nearest hundredth.

This patient's BSA is 0.96 m².

■ Box 18-1 Body Surface Area Formulas

The formula for BSA using pounds (lb) and inches (in):

$$m^2 = \sqrt{\frac{\text{weight (lb)} \times \text{height (in)}}{3131}}$$

The formula for BSA using kilograms (kg) and centimeters (cm):

$$m^2 = \sqrt{\frac{\text{weight (kg)} \times \text{height (cm)}}{3600}}$$

Example 2: A provider orders micafungin (Mycamine), 50 mg/m², IV, daily for the patient in Example 1. Calculate the dosage (mg) to be administered, based on the child's BSA of 0.96 m². Round to the nearest tenth mg.

1. Set up the equation using dimensional analysis, inserting the known quantities—the dosage of medication.

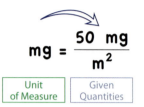

$$mg = \frac{50\ mg}{m^2}$$

| Unit of Measure | Given Quantities |

2. Insert the next given quantity—the patient's BSA.

$$mg = 50\ \frac{mg}{m^2} \times 0.96\ m^2$$

| Unit of Measure | Given Quantities | Given Quantity |

3. Solve the equation.

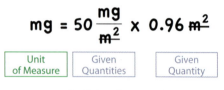

$$mg = 50\ \frac{mg}{m^2} \times 0.96\ m^2 = 48\ mg$$

| Unit of Measure | Given Quantities | Given Quantity |

The nurse should administer 48 mg of micafungin (Mycamine).

Example 3: Calculate the volume (mL) of micafungin (Mycamine) to be administered to the patient, based on the dosage calculated in Example 2. The pharmacy provides micafungin (Mycamine) in a vial containing 50 mg/mL. Round the answer to the nearest hundredth mL.

1. Set up the equation using dimensional analysis and inserting the first set of given quantities—the concentration of the medication.

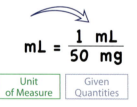

$$mL = \frac{1\ mL}{50\ mg}$$

| Unit of Measure | Given Quantities |

2. Insert the next given quantity—the dosage of micafungin (Micamine) calculated in Example 2.

$$mL = \frac{1\ mL}{50\ mg} \times 48\ mg$$

| Unit of Measure | Given Quantities | Given Quantity |

3. Solve the equation.

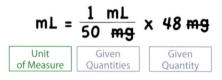
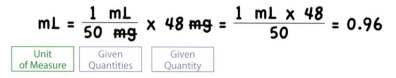

$$mL = \frac{1\ mL}{50\ mg} \times 48\ mg = \frac{1\ mL \times 48}{50} = 0.96$$

| Unit of Measure | Given Quantities | Given Quantity |

The nurse should administer 0.96 mL of micafungin (Mycamine) IV.

Example 4: Calculate the BSA for a patient who weighs 21 lb and is 30 in height. Round the final answer to the nearest hundredth m².

$$m^2 = \sqrt{\frac{21 \times 30}{3131}}$$

1. Set up the appropriate formula. Because the height and weight are expressed in pounds and inches, use *3131* in the denominator.

$$m^2 = \sqrt{\frac{21 \times 30}{3131}} = \sqrt{\frac{630}{3131}}$$

2. Multiply the numbers in the numerator.

$$m^2 = \sqrt{\frac{630}{3131}} = \sqrt{0.201}$$

3. Divide the numerator by the denominator.

$$m^2 = \sqrt{0.201} = 0.448 = 0.45 \ m^2$$

4. Find the square root and round the final answer to the nearest hundredth.

This patient's BSA is 0.45 m².

Example 5: A provider orders vincristine (Oncovin) 1.5 mg/m², IV, once weekly for the patient in Example 4. Calculate the dosage (mg) to be administered, based on the patient's BSA of 0.45 m². Round the answer to the nearest tenth mg.

1. Set up the equation using dimensional analysis. Insert the known quantities—the dosage of medication.

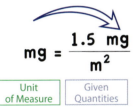

$$mg = \frac{1.5 \ mg}{m^2}$$

Unit of Measure	Given Quantities

2. Insert the next given quantity—the patient's BSA.

$$mg = 1.5 \ \frac{mg}{m^2} \times 0.45 \ m^2$$

Unit of Measure	Given Quantities	Given Quantity

3. Solve the equation.

$$mg = 1.5 \ \frac{mg}{m^2} \times 0.45 \ m^2 = 0.7 \ mg$$

Unit of Measure	Given Quantities	Given Quantity

The nurse should administer 0.7 mg of vincristine (Oncovin).

Example 6: Calculate the volume (mL) of vincristine (Oncovin) to be administered to the patient, based on the dosage calculated in Example 5. The pharmacy provides vincristine (Oncovin) in a vial containing 1 mg/mL. Round the answer to the nearest tenth mL.

1. Set up the equation using dimensional analysis and inserting the first set of given quantities—the concentration of the medication.

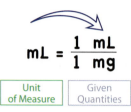

$$mL = \frac{1\ mL}{1\ mg}$$

Unit of Measure	Given Quantities

2. Insert the next given quantity—the dosage of vincristine (Oncovin) calculated in Example 2.

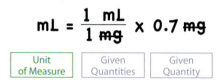

$$mL = \frac{1\ mL}{1\ mg} \times 0.7\ mg$$

Unit of Measure	Given Quantities	Given Quantity

3. Solve the equation.

$$mL = \frac{1\ mL}{1\ mg} \times 0.7\ mg = 0.7\ mL$$

Unit of Measure	Given Quantities	Given Quantity

The nurse should administer 0.7 mL of vincristine (Oncovin) IV.

Practice Calculating Dosages for Infants and Children Using Body Surface Area

(answers on page 395)

Calculate the BSA (m²) for pediatric patients with these weights and heights. Round the final answer to the nearest hundredth m².

1. Weight 8 lb, height 22 in

2. Weight 54 lb, height 38 in

3. Weight 16 kg, height 70 cm

4. Weight 4.6 kg, height 40 cm

5. Weight 33 kg, height 125 cm

Calculate the dosage of medication (mg) based on the patient's BSA and the volume of medication to be administered (mL) per dose. Round the answers to the nearest tenth mg and mL.

6. Cytarabine (Depocyt), 175 mg/m², IV, every 12 hours. The patient's BSA is 0.87 m². The pharmacy supplies cytarabine (Depocyt) in vials containing 20 mg/mL.
   a. mg: _____
   b. mL: _____

7. Busulfan (Myleran), 1.8 mg/m², PO, daily. The patient's BSA is 0.59 m². The pharmacy supplies busulfan (Myleran) in a bottle containing 2 mg in 5 mL.
   a. mg: _____
   b. mL: _____

8. Acyclovir (Zovirax), 250 mg/m², IV, every 8 hours. The patient's BSA is 0.62 m². The pharmacy supplies acyclovir (Zovirax) in vials containing 25 mg/mL.
   a. mg: _____
   b. mL: _____

9. Vinblastine (Velban), 2.5 mg/ m², IV, now. The patient's BSA is 0.73 m². The pharmacy supplies vinblastine (Velban) in vials containing 1 mg/mL.
   a. mg: _____
   b. mL: _____

10. Carboplatin (Paraplatin), 175 mg/ m², IV, once weekly. The patient's BSA is 0.95 m². The pharmacy supplies carboplatin (Paraplatin) in vials containing 150 mg/mL.
    a. mg: _____
    b. mL: _____

Controlling Intravenous Infusions for Children

Extra care must be taken when initiating and monitoring IV therapy in infants and children to avoid accidental fluid overload.

Infusion Pumps

Infusion pumps specifically designated for pediatric use should be used to infuse IV fluids. Pediatric infusion pumps deliver fluids at a PSI that is lower than that needed for adults, which reduces the risk of rapid infiltration and volume overload. Electronic drip controllers are not appropriate for pediatric IV therapy nor should fluids be infused under manual control.

Microdrip tubing

Microdrip tubing is specially calibrated to deliver 60 drops per milliliter. Its small diameter will not allow large volumes of fluid to be delivered to the patient unless great pressure is applied (such as from squeezing the IV bag).

Volume Control Sets

Volumes control sets—sold under the brand names Volutrol, Buretrol, Metriset, and Soluset—are infusion devices that hold small volumes of fluid (up to 150 mL) in a chamber called a burette. See Figure 18-1. The purpose of the volume control set is to limit the amount of fluid that the child receives if the infusion pump malfunctions. To prevent children from receiving an accidental fluid bolus, the burette is filled with no more than two or three times the prescribed hourly flow rate. For example, if the prescribed IV flow rate is 12 mL/hr, the nurse should ensure that no more than 24 to 36 mL of fluid is in the volume control chamber.

Calculating Maintenance IV Fluids for Children

Fluid balance is monitored very carefully in children to avoid overhydration. Accurately monitoring and recording fluid intake and output is a crucial responsibility of a pediatric nurse.

The volume of fluid that a child needs over 24 hours is referred to as *daily maintenance fluid* needs and depends upon the child's weight and current hydration status. For an adequately hydrated child, daily maintenance fluid needs are based on weight (see Table 18-2). Calculating the fluid needs of a dehydrated child is beyond the scope of this book.

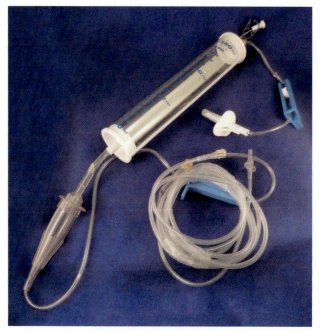

Figure 18-1 Volume Control Set

Table 18-2	**Pediatric Daily Maintenance Fluid Needs for Infants, Toddlers, and Children***
Patient's Weight	Needed Daily Maintenance Fluids
Less than 10 kg	100 mL/kg/day
10 to 20 kg	1000 mL/day + 50 mL/kg/day for each kg over 10
Over 20 kg	1500 mL/day + 20 mL/kg/day for each kg over 20

*this table does not apply to newborns
(Rodgers & Wilson, 2017)

Example 1: A nurse is calculating the daily maintenance fluid needs for an adequately hydrated child who weighs 25 kg. How many mL of fluid will the child need in 24 hours? Round the answer to the nearest whole mL.

1. Refer to Table 18-2 to determine the volume of fluid that this child should receive. The daily maintenance fluid volume for a child weighing 25 kg is 1500 mL/day, plus 20 mL/kg/day for each kg of the child's weight over 20 kg.
2. Calculate the difference between the child's weight and 20 kg.
   Weight difference (kg) = 25 kg − 20 kg = 5 kg
3. Calculate the volume of fluid (mL/day) the child is to receive for the extra 5 kg and add that to the required 1500 mL/day.

Note: Dimensional analysis can be used for only part of the equation.

$$\frac{mL}{day} = \left(\frac{20\ mL}{kg/day} \times 5\ kg \right) + 1500\ \frac{mL}{day}$$

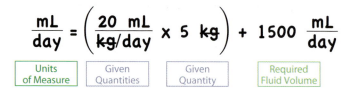

4. Solve the equation.

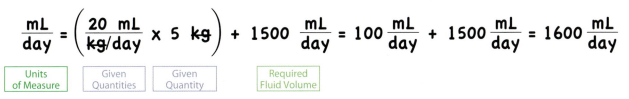

$$\frac{mL}{day} = \left(\frac{20\ mL}{kg/day} \times 5\ kg\right) + 1500\ \frac{mL}{day} = 100\ \frac{mL}{day} + 1500\ \frac{mL}{day} = 1600\ \frac{mL}{day}$$

| Units of Measure | Given Quantities | Given Quantity | Required Fluid Volume |

A child weighing 25 kg requires 1600 mL/day of maintenance fluids.

Example 2:   The provider for the patient in Example 1 wants half the daily maintenance fluid volume to be administered by IV. At what mL/hr flow rate should the nurse set the pump? Round the answer to the nearest tenth mL.

1. Set up the equation using dimensional analysis and inserting the first set of given quantities—the daily maintenance fluid volume needs of the patient.

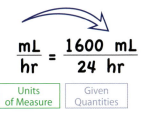

$$\frac{mL}{hr} = \frac{1600\ mL}{24\ hr}$$

| Units of Measure | Given Quantities |

2. Insert the second given quantity—the fraction of fluid ordered by the provider to be administered IV.

$$\frac{mL}{hr} = \frac{1600\ mL}{24\ hr} \times \frac{1}{2}$$

| Units of Measure | Given Quantities | Given Quantity |

Note: You can insert a percentage instead of a fraction for the amount of fluid the provider wants to administer intravenously. See Chapter 3.

$$\frac{mL}{hr} = \frac{1600\ mL}{24\ hr} \times 50\% = \frac{1600\ mL}{24\ hr} \times 0.5$$

3. Solve the equation.

$$\frac{mL}{hr} = \frac{1600\ mL}{24\ hr} \times \frac{1}{2} = \frac{1600\ mL \times 1}{24\ hr \times 2} \times \frac{1600\ mL}{48\ hr} = 33.3\ \frac{mL}{hr}$$

| Units of Measure | Given Quantities | Given Quantity |

The nurse should infuse the ordered IV fluid at 33.3 mL/hour.

Example 3:   A nurse is calculating the daily maintenance fluid needs for an adequately hydrated child who weighs 6 kg. How many mL of fluid will the child need in 24 hours? Round the answer to the nearest whole mL.

1. Refer to Table 8-2 to determine the child's daily maintenance fluid needs. A child weighing 6 kg has a fluid requirement of 100 mL/kg/day.

2. Calculate the volume of fluid (mL/day) the child is to receive.

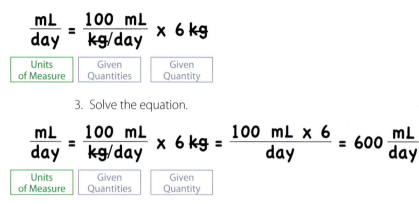

3. Solve the equation.

$$\underbrace{\frac{mL}{day}}_{\substack{\text{Units} \\ \text{of Measure}}} = \underbrace{\frac{100\ mL}{kg/day}}_{\substack{\text{Given} \\ \text{Quantities}}} \times \underbrace{6\ kg}_{\substack{\text{Given} \\ \text{Quantity}}} = \frac{100\ mL \times 6}{day} = 600\ \frac{mL}{day}$$

A child weighing 6 kg requires 600 mL/day of maintenance fluids.

Example 4: The provider for the patient in Example 3 wants all of the daily maintenance fluid volume to be administered by IV. At what mL/hr flow rate should the nurse set the pump? Round the answer to the nearest tenth mL.

1. Set up the equation using dimensional analysis and inserting the first set of given quantities—the daily maintenance fluid volume needs of the child.

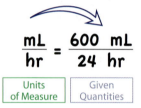

$$\underbrace{\frac{mL}{hr}}_{\substack{\text{Units} \\ \text{of Measure}}} = \underbrace{\frac{600\ mL}{24\ hr}}_{\substack{\text{Given} \\ \text{Quantities}}}$$

2. Insert the second given quantity—the fraction of fluid ordered by the provider to be administered IV. In this example, all of the fluid will be infused intravenously.

Note: No fraction needs to be inserted in this step, although you could enter 1/1 or 100% if you need to provide proof in the equation.

$$\underbrace{\frac{mL}{hr}}_{\substack{\text{Units} \\ \text{of Measure}}} = \underbrace{\frac{600\ mL}{24\ hr}}_{\substack{\text{Given} \\ \text{Quantities}}} \times \underbrace{\frac{1}{1}}_{\substack{\text{Given} \\ \text{Quantity}}}$$

$$\underbrace{\frac{mL}{hr}}_{\substack{\text{Units} \\ \text{of Measure}}} = \underbrace{\frac{600\ mL}{24\ hr}}_{\substack{\text{Given} \\ \text{Quantities}}} \times \underbrace{\frac{1}{1}}_{\substack{\text{Given} \\ \text{Quantity}}} = \frac{600\ mL \times 1}{24\ hr \times 1} = 25\ \frac{mL}{hr}$$

The nurse will infuse the ordered IV fluid at 25 mL/hour.

Example 5: A nurse is calculating the daily maintenance fluid needs for an adequately hydrated child who weighs 13 kg. How many mL of fluid will the child need in 24 hours? Round the answer to the nearest whole mL.

1. Refer to Table 18-2 to determine the volume of fluid that this child should receive. The daily maintenance fluid volume for a child weighing 13 kg is 1000 mL/day, plus 50 mL/kg/day for each kg of the child's weight over 10 kg.

2. Calculate the difference between the child's weight and 10 kg.
   Weight difference (kg) = 13 kg − 10 kg = 3 kg
3. Calculate the volume of fluid (mL/day) the child is to receive for the extra 3 kg and add that to the required 1000 mL/day.

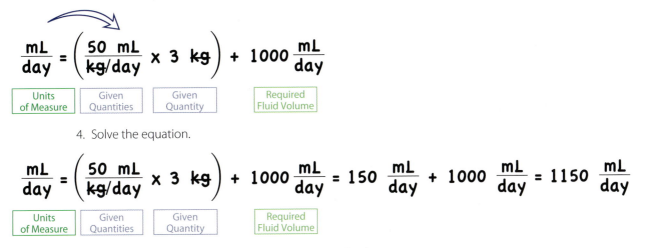

4. Solve the equation.

$$\underset{\substack{\text{Units}\\\text{of Measure}}}{\frac{mL}{day}} = \left(\underset{\substack{\text{Given}\\\text{Quantities}}}{\frac{50\ mL}{kg/day}} \times \underset{\substack{\text{Given}\\\text{Quantity}}}{3\ kg} \right) + \underset{\substack{\text{Required}\\\text{Fluid Volume}}}{1000\ \frac{mL}{day}} = 150\ \frac{mL}{day} + 1000\ \frac{mL}{day} = 1150\ \frac{mL}{day}$$

A child weighing 13 kg requires 1150 mL/day of maintenance fluids.

Example 6: The provider for the patient in Example 5 wants 1/3 of the daily maintenance fluid volume to be administered by IV. At what mL/hr flow rate should the nurse set the pump? Round the answer to the nearest tenth mL.

1. Set up the equation using dimensional analysis and inserting the first set of given quantities—the daily maintenance fluid volume needs of the child.

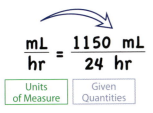

2. Insert the second given quantity—the fraction of fluid ordered by the provider to be administered IV.

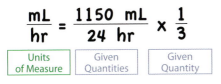

3. Solve the equation.

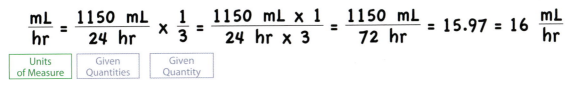

The nurse should infuse the ordered IV fluid at 16 mL/hour.

Practice Calculating Maintenance IV Fluids for Children

(answers on page 396)

Using Table 18-2, calculate these fluid volumes and rates. Assume that the children are adequately hydrated.

a. *Daily maintenance fluid needs (mL). Round the answer to the nearest whole mL.*

b. *IV flow rate (mL/hr). Round the answer to the nearest tenth mL.*

1. Child's weight is 32 kg; ¼ from IV fluids.
   a. Total daily fluid needs (mL): _____
   b. IV flow rate (mL/hr): _____

2. Child's weight is 5 kg; ½ from IV fluids.
   a. Total daily fluid needs (mL): _____
   b. IV flow rate (mL/hr): _____

3. Child's weight is 46 kg; ⅓ from IV fluids.
   a. Total daily fluid needs (mL): _____
   b. IV flow rate (mL/hr): _____

4. Child's weight is 17 kg; 100% from IV fluids.
   a. Total daily fluid needs (mL): _____
   b. IV flow rate (mL/hr): _____

5. Child's weight is 8 kg; ¾ from IV fluids.
   a. Total daily fluid needs (mL): _____
   b. IV flow rate (mL/hr): _____

General Considerations for Pregnant and Lactating Women

A woman taking medications during pregnancy or breastfeeding must consider the impact that the drug has on her body, the fetus, or the nursing infant. Very few drugs are considered completely safe for use during pregnancy and lactation.

Drug Use During Pregnancy

During pregnancy, a woman's body undergoes many changes that can affect how medications are absorbed, distributed, metabolized, and excreted (Table 18-3). However, most concerns about

Table 18-3	**Alteration in Organ Function Related to Pregnancy**	
Organ	**Alterations Related to Pregnancy**	**Effect on Medication Absorption, Distribution, Metabolism, or Excretion**
Heart	Increased blood volume	Dilutes plasma proteins that bind to drugs, leading to higher amounts of free drugs in plasma
	Increased cardiac output	Greater distribution
Gastrointestinal	Increased hydrochloric acid production	Altered absorption of acid-based drugs
	Decreased peristalsis/increased pressure of expanding uterus on stomach/slowed gastric emptying time	Prolonged absorption due to medications taking longer to leave the stomach
	Nausea and vomiting	May not be able to take drugs or drug may be incompletely absorbed due to vomiting
Kidneys	Increased blood flow to kidneys	Increased excretion
	Increased filtration rate of substances	Increased excretion
Liver	Placenta and fetal liver contribute toward metabolism	Increased metabolism of certain drugs

medication use during pregnancy relate to ways in which a medication may affect the fetus. Although the blood supply of the mother and fetus never come into direct contact during a normal pregnancy, many medications can cross the placenta and be distributed throughout the fetus's body, adversely affecting fragile developing organs. Other medications may not cross the placenta but may cause changes in the mother's system that can affect blood flow to the placenta. For example, any substance (such as nicotine or cocaine) that causes constriction of the blood vessels can reduce blood flow to the placenta, thereby affecting the delivery of oxygen and other nutrients to the fetus.

The fetus is at the greatest risk for injury from medications during the first trimester. During that time, fetal organs are undergoing rapid growth and are particularly prone to the harmful effects of drugs. Pregnant women are advised to avoid taking medications during this time unless the benefit of the drug outweighs the risk. For example, an expectant mother who has high blood pressure may need medication to reduce her risk of having a stroke, even though the medication has not been proven to be safe for the developing fetus. The FDA has categorized the risk of drugs based on whether or not the drug has demonstrated a risk to the fetus (see Table 18-4). Obviously, testing medications on pregnant women would be unethical; therefore, the categories provide an educated guess about the actual risk to the fetus.

Drug Use During Lactation

Most drugs can be passed from mother to baby through breast milk. Unfortunately, there is no way to accurately predict how much medication the infant will receive and how it will affect the infant's behavior, growth, or development. The fear of causing harm has caused many women to quit breastfeeding prematurely. Box 18-2 offers general guidelines to reduce the potential risk to infants from maternal medication use.

General Considerations for Aging Adults

Persons aged 65 and older represent an estimated 14.5% of the total population in the United States (U.S. Census Bureau, 2016). They account for one-third of all prescription drug use (National Institute on Drug Abuse, 2016). However, certain medication types can alter an elderly person's cognitive status, leading to increased risk of injuries. For example, narcotic pain medications and sedatives can cause central nervous system depression, which may lead to falls that result in

Table 18-4	FDA Pregnancy Categories	
Pregnancy Category	Definition	Example of Drugs
A	Adequate and well-controlled human studies have failed to demonstrate a risk to the fetus in the first trimester of pregnancy (and there is no evidence of risk in later trimesters).	Folic acid, levothyroxine, prenatal vitamins
B	Animal reproduction studies have failed to demonstrate a risk to the fetus and there are no adequate and well-controlled studies in pregnant women.	Acetaminophen, prednisone, regular insulin
C	Animal reproduction studies have shown an adverse effect on the fetus and there are no adequate and well-controlled studies in humans, but potential benefits may warrant use of the drug in pregnant women despite potential risks.	Codeine, hydralazine, morphine
D	There is positive evidence of human fetal risk based on adverse reaction data from investigational or marketing experience or studies in humans, but potential benefits may warrant use of the drug in pregnant women despite potential risks.	Aspirin (first trimester), epirubicin, tetracycline
X	Studies in animals or humans have demonstrated fetal abnormalities and/or there is positive evidence of human fetal risk based on adverse reaction data from investigational or marketing experience, and the risks involved in use of the drug in pregnant women clearly outweigh potential benefits.	Pravastatin, temazepam, *warfarin*

> **■ Box 18-2 Reducing Potential Risks to Breastfed Infants**
>
> • Avoid medication use when possible.
> • Use topical instead of oral or injectable medications when possible.
> • Use medications that are safe for infants because such medications are generally safe for the breastfeeding mother.
> • Select medications whose use in infants has been well studied.
> • Administer once-daily doses right before the infant's longest sleep period.
> • Have the mother breastfeed the infant immediately before or after the dose is taken when medications are given multiple times daily.
> • Refer to a reliable reference before administering or using medications. Those that are safe in pregnancy are not necessarily safe in lactation.

broken bones or brain injuries. Some diuretics used to control blood pressure may cause confusion in an older adult, resulting in poor judgment and forgetfulness.

Medication use by the elderly is also more likely to result in adverse drug reactions due to several factors:

• Declining organ function that alters how medications are absorbed, distributed, metabolized, and excreted (see Table 18-5 and Box 18-3).
• Low body mass index (BMI) that requires small dosages of some medications.

Table 18-5 Alterations in Organ Function Related to Aging

Organ	Alterations Related to Aging	Effect on Medication Absorption, Distribution, Metabolism, or Excretion
Heart	Decreased cardiac output	Decreased absorption and distribution
Gastrointestinal	Increased pH of stomach secretions (alkaline)	Altered absorption
	Decreased peristalsis/slowed gastric emptying time	Prolonged absorption due to medications taking longer to leave the stomach
Kidneys	Decreased blood flow	Decreased excretion
	Reduced filtration rate of substances	Decreased excretion
	Decreased number of functioning nephrons	Decreased excretion
Liver	Reduced enzyme production	Decreased metabolism
	Decreased blood flow	Decreased metabolism

> **■ Box 18-3 Common Medication Errors Involving Aging Adults**
>
> Data collected by the U.S. Pharmacopeia (2002) showed that harmful medication errors occurred more often in the elderly population than they did in the general population (3.47% versus 1.67%), and that 55% of the fatalities in 2002 from harmful medication errors involved older adults. Errors occurred in all phases of the medication administration process from prescribing to dispensing, administering, monitoring, and documenting. However, the bulk of errors occurred during the administration phase, and most of those errors involved errors of omission. Other common errors included improper dose, unauthorized drug, extra dose, wrong time, and wrong patient. The most common medications implicated in the errors included heparin, insulin, morphine, potassium, and warfarin. The most common cause of the errors was performance deficit (an error that cannot be attributed to any specific cause), followed by not following procedure or protocol, inaccurate transcription of the order, and lack of communication.
>
> Since this report was published, many changes have been instituted in healthcare facilities: use of smart IV pumps, electronic provider order entry, automated dispensing devices, and the medication reconciliation process. Despite these advances, the nurse still needs to be aware that aging adults are a population that suffers greatly from medication errors. By the year 2030, the number of people over the age of 65 is estimated to increase to 20% of the population (Ortman, Velkoff, & Hogan, 2014). Therefore, safety in medication administration will become even more important to avoid injury to the aging adult population.

- Decreased total body water and increased total body fat that affects the distribution of water- and fat-soluble drugs.
- Use of multiple medications (called *polypharmacy*)—including prescription drugs, over-the-counter (OTC) drugs, and dietary supplements—a situation that raises the risk of drug interactions.
- High rate of comorbid illnesses.

There are no special mathematical formulas available to nurses to calculate the proper dosages of medications for seniors. However, providers and/or pharmacists may modify dosages for aged patients based on kidney function. Many drugs are excreted by the kidneys, so adequate kidney function is essential. If a patient's kidney function is poor, smaller dosages are required so that the drug does not accumulate in the body and become toxic. Liver function tests should also be monitored to determine whether the liver can metabolize medications.

Key Points

1. Children are particularly prone to adverse drug reactions because of the immaturity of their organs.
2. Body weight is a quick and convenient method for calculating drug dosages, but it may not accurately reflect age-related variation in drug absorption, distribution, metabolism, excretion, or serum drug levels.
3. Some drugs prescribed for children, such as some anti-infectives or chemotherapy agents, may be prescribed based on body surface area instead of weight.
4. Pediatric-only IV pumps, microtubing, and volume control sets are devices that can help safeguard against accidentally overhydrating children during IV therapy.
5. Many physiological changes occur during pregnancy and place the fetus at risk for the development of birth defects or injury. The fetus is at highest risk of developing injuries from medications during the first trimester.
6. Breastfeeding mothers should take medications right before or right after breastfeeding to reduce the amount of medication that may be transferred to the infant.
7. Aging adults are at risk for adverse drug reactions because of deteriorating organ function and polypharmacy.

References

1. Lack, J.A., & Stuart-Taylor, M.E. (1997). Calculation of drug dosage and body surface area of children. *British Journal of Anaesthesia, 78*, 601-605.
2. National Institute on Drug Abuse. (2016). Misuse of prescription drugs: Older adults. Retrieved from https://www.drugabuse.gov/publications/research-reports/prescription-drugs/trends-in-prescription-drug-abuse/older-adults.
3. Ortman, J.M., Velkoff, V.A., & Hogan, H. (2014). An aging nation: The older population in the United States. Retrieved from https://www.census.gov/prod/2014pubs/p25-1140.pdf.
4. Rodgers, C.C., & Wilson, K.D. (2017). The child with gastrointestinal dysfunction. In M. Hockenberry, D. Wilson, & C. Rodgers (Eds.). *Hockenberry: Wong's Essentials of Pediatric Nursing (10th ed.)*, pp. 689-737. St. Louis: Elsevier.
5. U.S. Census Bureau. (2016). Population estimates program (PEP). Retrieved from http://www.census.gov/quickfacts.
6. U.S. Pharmacopeia. (2002). MEDMARX 2002 annual data report: The quest for quality. Retrieved from http://www.usp.org.

Chapter Post-Test   *(answers in Unit 4)*

Calculations

Calculate the dosage (mg or mcg) and the volume (mL) of medication to be administered per dose. Round the answers to the nearest tenth mcg, mg, and mL.

1. A provider orders amoxicillin (Amoxcil) 25 mg/kg/day, PO, in divided doses every 12 hours. The patient weighs 9.2 kg. The pharmacy provides amoxicillin (Amoxil) in an oral suspension containing 50 mg per mL.
   a. mg/dose: _____
   b. mL: _____

2. A provider orders digoxin (Lanoxin) 6 mcg/kg/day, PO, in divided doses every 12 hours. The patient weighs 23 kg. The pharmacy supplies digoxin (Lanoxin) in an oral suspension containing 0.05 mg per mL.
   a. mcg/dose: _____
   b. mL: _____

3. A provider orders neomycin 15 mg/kg, PO every 4 hours. The patient weighs 27 kg. The pharmacy supplies neomycin in an oral solution containing 125 mg per 5 mL.
   a. mg/dose: _____
   b. mL: _____

4. A provider orders acetaminophen (Tylenol) 10 mg/kg, PO, every 6 hours, PRN for a fever. The patient weighs 4.2 kg. The pharmacy supplies acetaminophen (Tylenol) in an elixir containing 160 mg per 5 mL.
   a. mg/dose: _____
   b. mL: _____

5. A provider orders metoclopramide (Reglan) 0.4 mg/kg/day, PO, in 3 divided doses. The patient weighs 17 kg. The pharmacy supplies metoclopramide (Reglan) in a syrup containing 5 mg per 5 mL.
   a. mg/dose: _____
   b. mL: _____

6. A provider orders cephradine (Velosef) 19 mg/kg/day, PO, in 4 divided doses. The patient weighs 3.8 kg. The pharmacy supplies cephradine (Velosef) in a suspension containing 125 mg per 5 mL.
   a. mg/dose: _____
   b. mL: _____

7. A provider orders cloxacillin (Tegopen) 12.5 mg/kg/day, PO, in 4 divided doses. The patient weighs 23 kg. The pharmacy supplies cloxacillin (Tegopen) in an oral solution containing 125 mg per 5 mL.
   a. mg/dose: _____
   b. mL: _____

8. A provider orders furosemide (Lasix) 2 mg/kg, PO, once daily. The patient weighs 31 kg. The pharmacy supplies furosemide (Lasix) in an oral solution containing 8 mg per mL.
   a. mg/dose: _____
   b. mL: _____

Calculate the BSA (m²) for pediatric patients with these weights and heights. Round the final answer to the nearest hundredth m².

9. Weight 12 pounds, height 25 in

10. Weight 97 pounds, height 58 in

11. Weight 7 pounds, height 20 in

12. Weight 45 pounds, height 32 in

13. Weight 3.5 kg, height 42 cm

14. Weight 24 kg, height 88 cm

15. Weight 18 kg, height 94 cm

16. Weight 9.2 kg, height 60 cm

Calculate the dosage of medication (mg) based on each patient's BSA and the volume of medication to be administered (mL) per dose. Round the answers to the nearest tenth mg and mL.

17. Allopurinol (Zyloprim), 200 mg/m², IV, once daily. The patient's BSA is 0.57 m². The pharmacy supplies allopurinol (Zyloprim) in vials containing 6 mg/mL.
   a. mg: _____
   b. mL: _____

18. Clofarabine (Clolar), 52 mg/m², IV, daily for 5 days. The patient's BSA is 0.23 m². The pharmacy supplies clofarabine (Clolar) in vials containing 1 mg/mL.
   a. mg: _____
   b. mL: _____

19. Nelarabine (Arranon) 650 mg/m², IV, over 2 hours every other day. The patient's BSA is 0.81 m². The pharmacy supplies nelarabine (Arranon) in vials containing 50 mg/mL.
   a. mg: _____
   b. mL: _____

20. Leukovorin, 10 mg/m², IV, once. The patient's BSA is 0.49 m². The pharmacy supplies leukovorin in vials containing 10 mg/mL.
   a. mg: _____
   b. mL: _____

21. Clindamycin (Cleocyn), 87.5 mg/m², IV, every 6 hours. The patient's BSA is 0.77 m². The pharmacy supplies clindamycin (Cleocyn) in vials containing 25 mg/mL.
   a. mg: _____
   b. mL: _____

22. Aminocaproic acid (Amicar), 3000 mg/m², IV, every 12 hours. The patient's BSA is 0.95 m². The pharmacy supplies aminocaproic acid (Amicar) in vials containing 1000 mg/4 mL.
   a. mg: _____
   b. mL: _____

23. Bendamustine (Treanda), 120 mg/m², IV, daily. The patient's BSA is 1.05 m². The pharmacy supplies bendamustine (Treanda) in vials containing 5 mg/mL.
   a. mg: _____
   b. mL: _____

24. Acyclovir (Zovirax), 200 mg/m², IV, every 8 hours. The patient's BSA is 0.34 m². The pharmacy supplies acyclovir (Zovirax) in vials containing 15 mg/mL.
   a. mg: _____
   b. mL: _____

Using Table 18-2, calculate these fluid volumes and flow rates. Assume that the children are adequately hydrated.

a. *Daily maintenance fluid needs (mL). Round to the nearest whole mL.*

b. *IV flow rate (mL/hr). Round to the nearest tenth mL.*

25. Child's weight is 1 kg; 100% from IV fluids.
    a. Total daily fluid needs (mL): _____
    b. IV flow rate (mL/hr): _____

26. Child's weight is 19 kg; 1/2 from IV fluids.
    a. Total daily fluid needs (mL): _____
    b. IV flow rate (mL/hr): _____

27. Child's weight is 63 kg; 1/4 from IV fluids.
    a. Total daily fluid needs (mL): _____
    b. IV flow rate (mL/hr): _____

28. Child's weight is 7 kg; 100% from IV fluids.
    a. Total daily fluid needs (mL): _____
    b. IV flow rate (mL/hr): _____

29. Child's weight is 14 kg; 3/4 from IV fluids.
    a. Total daily fluid needs (mL): _____
    b. IV flow rate (mL/hr): _____

30. Child's weight is 2 kg; 1/2 from IV fluids.
    a. Total daily fluid needs (mL): _____
    b. IV flow rate (mL/hr): _____

31. Child's weight is 43 kg; 1/2 from IV fluids.
    a. Total daily fluid needs (mL): _____
    b. IV flow rate (mL/hr): _____

Multiple Choice

Choose the best answer for each question.

32. The nurse is preparing to administer medication to a 6-month old infant. Which statement regarding immature kidney function in infants is true?
    a. Medications are metabolized faster.
    b. Medications are absorbed slowly.
    c. Medications are excreted slowly.
    d. Medications are excreted rapidly.

33. The purpose of a volume control set is to:
    a. prevent accidental dehydration in children.
    b. limit the volume of fluid the child will receive if the infusion pump malfunctions.
    c. decrease the pressure needed by the infusion pump to overcome venous resistance.
    d. increase the volume of fluid available for infusion.

34. The nurse is teaching a patient about taking medications during pregnancy and breastfeeding. Which statement by the patient indicates that she understands the teaching?
    a. "The greatest risk of injury to my baby is in the first trimester of pregnancy."
    b. "The placenta protects my baby from the medications I am taking."
    c. "I should never take any medications during my pregnancy, no matter what the problem."
    d. "My baby is not affected by any drugs I take while breastfeeding."

35. The elderly are more likely to experience adverse drug reactions because:

    a. They tend to have a higher body mass index than younger adults.

    b. They have an increased amount of body water that affects how medications are distributed throughout the body.

    c. Declining organ function affects how medications are absorbed, distributed, metabolized, and excreted.

    d. They tend to have a decreased amount of body fat compared to younger adults.

Answers to Practice Questions

Calculating Dosages for Infants and Children Using Body Weight

1. a. $\dfrac{mg}{dose} = \dfrac{50\ mg}{kg/day} \times 8\ kg \times \dfrac{1\ day}{24\ hr} \times \dfrac{6\ hr}{dose} = 100\ \dfrac{mg}{dose}$

   b. $mL = \dfrac{5\ mL}{125\ mg} \times 100\ mg = 4\ mL$

2. a. $\dfrac{mg}{dose} = \dfrac{20\ mg}{kg/day} \times 44\ kg \times \dfrac{1\ day}{2\ doses} = 440\ \dfrac{mg}{dose}$

   b. $mL = \dfrac{5\ mL}{500\ mg} \times 440\ mg = 4.4\ mL$

3. a. $\dfrac{mg}{dose} = \dfrac{75\ mg}{kg/day} \times 39\ kg \times \dfrac{1\ day}{24\ hr} \times \dfrac{12\ hr}{dose} = 1462.5\ \dfrac{mg}{dose}$

   b. $mL = \dfrac{1\ mL}{500\ mg} \times 1462.5\ mg = 2.9\ mL$

> **Note:** This dose must be divided into 2 separate injections since the maximum IM dose for a child is 1 mL for infants and small children, and 2 mL for older, larger children.

4. a. $\dfrac{mg}{dose} = \dfrac{15\ mg}{kg/dose} \times 6.7\ kg = 100.5\ \dfrac{mg}{dose}$

> **Alert!** The provider ordered acetaminophen 15 mg/kg, PO, every 6 hours. This means 15 mg/kg per *dose*, not per *day*. Do not divide the calculated dosage any further.

   b. $mL = \dfrac{1\ mL}{100\ mg} \times 100.5\ mg = 1\ mL$

5. a. $\dfrac{mg}{dose} = \dfrac{7\ mg}{kg/day} \times 37\ kg \times \dfrac{1\ day}{3\ doses} = 86.3\ \dfrac{mg}{dose}$

   b. $mL = \dfrac{5\ mL}{125\ mg} \times 86.3\ mg = 3.5\ mL$

Calculating Dosages for Infants and Children Using Body Surface Area

1. $m^2 = \sqrt{\dfrac{8 \times 22}{3131}} = \sqrt{\dfrac{176}{3131}} = \sqrt{0.056} = 0.236 = 0.24\ m^2$

2. $m^2 = \sqrt{\dfrac{54 \times 38}{3131}} = \sqrt{\dfrac{2052}{3131}} = \sqrt{0.655} = 0.809 = 0.81\ m^2$

3. $m^2 = \sqrt{\dfrac{16 \times 70}{3600}} = \sqrt{\dfrac{1120}{3600}} = \sqrt{0.311} = 0.557 = 0.56\ m^2$

4. $m^2 = \sqrt{\dfrac{4.6 \times 40}{3600}} = \sqrt{\dfrac{184}{3600}} = \sqrt{0.051} = 0.225 = 0.23\ m^2$

5. $m^2 = \sqrt{\dfrac{33 \times 125}{3600}} = \sqrt{\dfrac{4125}{3600}} = \sqrt{1.145} = 1.07\ m^2$

6. a. $mg = 175\dfrac{mg}{m^2} \times 0.87\ m^2 = 152.3\ mg$

   b. $mL = \dfrac{1\ mL}{20\ mg} \times 152.3\ mg = \dfrac{1\ mL \times 152.3}{20} = 7.6\ mL$

7. a. $mg = 1.8\dfrac{mg}{m^2} \times 0.59\ m^2 = 1.1\ mg$

   b. $mL = \dfrac{5\ mL}{2\ mg} \times 1.1\ mg = \dfrac{5\ mL \times 1.1}{2} = 2.8\ mL$

8. a. $mg = 250\dfrac{mg}{m^2} \times 0.62\ m^2 = 155\ mg$

   b. $mL = \dfrac{1\ mL}{25\ mg} \times 155\ mg = \dfrac{1\ mL \times 155}{25} = 6.2\ mL$

9. a. $mg = 2.5\dfrac{mg}{m^2} \times 0.73\ m^2 = 1.8\ mg$

   b. $mL = \dfrac{1\ mL}{1\ mg} \times 1.8\ mg = 1.8\ mL$

10. a. $mg = 175\dfrac{mg}{m^2} \times 0.95\ m^2 = 166.3\ mg$

    b. $mL = \dfrac{1\ mL}{150\ mg} \times 166.3\ mg = \dfrac{1\ mL \times 166.3}{150} = 1.1\ mL$

Calculating Maintenance IV Fluids for Children

1. $mL = 1500 \ mL + \left(\dfrac{20 \ mL}{1 \ kg} \times 12 \ kg \right) = 1500 + 240 = 1740 \ mL$

$\dfrac{mL}{hr} = \dfrac{1740 \ mL}{24 \ hr} \times \dfrac{1}{4} = 18.1 \ \dfrac{mL}{hr}$

2. $mL = \dfrac{100 \ mL}{kg} \times 5 \ kg = 500 \ mL$

$\dfrac{mL}{hr} = \dfrac{500 \ mL}{24 \ hr} \times \dfrac{1}{2} = 10.4 \ \dfrac{mL}{hr}$

3. $mL = 1500 \ mL + \left(\dfrac{20 \ mL}{1 \ kg} \times 26 \ kg \right) = 1500 + 520 = 2020 \ mL$

$\dfrac{mL}{hr} = \dfrac{2020 \ mL}{24 \ hr} \times \dfrac{1}{3} = 28.1 \ \dfrac{mL}{hr}$

4. $mL = 1000 \ mL + \left(\dfrac{50 \ mL}{1 \ kg} \times 7 \ kg \right) = 1000 + 350 = 1350 \ mL$

$\dfrac{mL}{hr} = \dfrac{1350 \ mL}{24 \ hr} = 56.3 \ \dfrac{mL}{hr}$

5. $mL = \dfrac{100 \ mL}{kg} \times 8 \ kg = 800 \ mL$

$\dfrac{mL}{hr} = \dfrac{800 \ mL}{24 \ hr} \times \dfrac{3}{4} = 25 \ \dfrac{mL}{hr}$

Unit 3 Post-Test

(answers in Unit 4)

After studying Unit 3, "Special Topics," answer these questions and solve the problems.

Multiple Choice

Choose the best answer for each question.

1. A feeding tube placed directly into the stomach through a small incision is called:
   a. percutaneous endoscopic jejunostomy tube.
   b. percutaneous endoscopic gastrostomy tube.
   c. nasogastric tube.
   d. nasojejunal tube.

2. Which feeding most closely mimics natural mealtimes?
   a. continuous feeding
   b. bolus feeding
   c. cyclic feeding
   d. intermittent feeding

3. Which feeding tube offers the lowest risk of aspiration?
   a. nasogastric tube
   b. nasojejunal tube
   c. orogastric tube
   d. percutaneous endoscopic jejunostomy tube

4. Diabetes mellitus is managed by:
   a. diet, exercise, and meditation.
   b. diet, exercise, and medication.
   c. medication only.
   d. diet and exercise only.

5. The amount of insulin that an individual needs to maintain normal or near-normal blood glucose levels:
   a. is the same for everybody.
   b. depends on the type of diabetes.
   c. varies greatly from person to person.
   d. depends upon the individual's body type.

6. Which type of insulin should be administered 5 to 15 minutes before meals?
   a. NPH insulin (Novolin N)
   b. regular insulin (Humulin R)
   c. insulin glargine (Lantus)
   d. insulin lispro (Humalog)

7. Which type of insulin is rapid-acting?
   a. insulin aspart (NovoLog)
   b. insulin glargine (Lantus)
   c. regular insulin (Humulin R)
   d. insulin detemir (Levemir)

8. A potential serious side effect of heparin is:
   a. sore joints
   b. bleeding
   c. vomiting
   d. constipation

Questions 9 and 10 refer to this scenario:

A provider writes the following sliding-scale insulin order for a patient:

Insulin lispro (Humalog), subcut, before every meal, and at bedtime according to the following fingerstick blood glucose (BG) levels:

BG less than or equal to 150	0 units
BG 151–160	2 units
BG 161–170	4 units
BG 171–180	6 units
BG 181–190	8 units
BG 191–200	10 units
BG over 200	Call provider

9. The nurse obtains a fingerstick blood glucose level before breakfast. It is 108 mg/dL. How many units of insulin lispro should the nurse administer to the patient?
   a. 0 units
   b. 2 units
   c. 4 units
   d. 6 units

10. At lunch, the nurse obtains another fingerstick blood glucose level from the patient. It is now 157 mg/dL. What action should the nurse take?
    a. Administer 0 units of insulin lispro.
    b. Administer 2 units of insulin lispro.
    c. Administer 4 units of insulin lispro.
    d. Call the provider for further orders.

Calculations

Calculate the daily calorie and protein needs for these patients. Assume that the patients require normal amounts of calories (25 cal/kg/day) and protein (0.8 g/kg/day). Round the answers to the nearest whole number.

11. Patient weighs 73 kg.
    a. Calorie needs: _____
    b. Protein needs: _____

12. Patient weighs 65 kg.
    a. Calorie needs: _____
    b. Protein needs: _____

13. Patient weighs 49 kg.
    a. Calorie needs: _____
    b. Protein needs: _____

14. Patient weighs 57 kg.
    a. Calorie needs: _____
    b. Protein needs: _____

15. Patient weighs 81 kg.
    a. Calorie needs: _____
    b. Protein needs: _____

Calculate the volume of formula (mL/day) needed to meet these patients' daily calorie needs. Assume that the patients require normal amounts of calories (25 cal/kg/day). Round the answers to the nearest whole mL.

16. Patient weighs 72 kg. The formula provides 1 calorie per 1 mL.

17. Patient weighs 63 kg. The formula provides 1500 calories per 1 L.

18. Patient weighs 36 kg. The formula provides 240 calories per 240 mL.

19. Patient weighs 85 kg. The formula provides 1000 calories per 1 L.

20. Patient weighs 69 kg. The formula provides 1.5 calories per mL.

Calculate the daily volume of formula (mL/day) needed to meet these patients' protein needs. Assume that the patients require normal amounts of protein (0.8 g/kg/day). Round the answers to the nearest whole mL.

21. Patient weights 41 kg. The formula provides 24 g protein per 240 mL.

22. Patient weighs 83 kg. The formula provides 20 g protein per 240 mL.

23. Patient weighs 75 kg. The formula provides 40 g protein per 480 mL.

24. Patient weighs 50 kg. The formula provides 100 g protein per 1 L.

25. Patient weighs 64 kg. The formula provides 150 g protein 1 L.

Calculate the flow rate (mL/hr) for these enteral feedings. Round the answers to the nearest whole mL.

26. 750 mL over 10 hours

27. 240 mL over 45 minutes

28. 250 mL over 90 minutes

29. 100 mL over 10 minutes

30. 1 L over 24 hours

Calculate the volume of water (mL) to add to the formula to dilute the feeding strength indicated in the question. Round the answers to the nearest whole mL.

31. A formula is to be diluted to one-quarter strength; 300 mL of formula available.

32. A formula is to be diluted to half strength; 480 mL of formula available.

33. A formula is to be diluted to one-third strength; 240 mL of formula available.

34. A formula is to be diluted to three-quarters strength; 240 mL of formula available.

35. A formula is to be diluted to two-thirds strength; 400 mL of formula available.

Draw a line across the syringes to indicate the correct amount of insulin to be administered for each figure.

36. 25 units (Fig. U3PT-1)

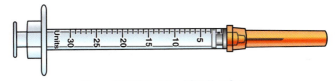

Figure U3PT-1 0.3-mL/30-Unit Syringe

37. 38 units (Fig. U3PT-2)

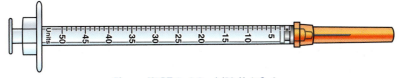

Figure U3PT-2 0.5-mL/50-Unit Syringe

38. 8 units (Fig. U3PT-3)

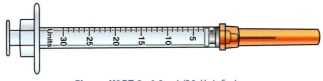

Figure U3PT-3 0.3-mL/30-Unit Syringe

39. 22 units (Fig. U3PT-4)

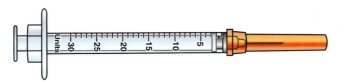

Figure U3PT-4 0.3-mL/30-Unit Syringe

40. 3 units (Fig. U3PT-5)

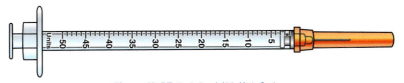

Figure U3PT-5 0.5-mL/50-Unit Syringe

Calculate the volume (mL) of these anticoagulant medications to be administered. Round the answers to the nearest hundredth mL.

41. A provider orders heparin 4500 units, subcut, every 12 hours. The pharmacy supplies heparin in a 1-mL vial containing 5000 units/mL.

42. A provider orders enoxaparin 5000 units, subcut, every 12 hours. The pharmacy supplies enoxaparin in a prefilled syringe containing 1000 units per 0.1 mL.

43. A provider orders heparin 7500 units, subcut, every 12 hours. The pharmacy provides a 5-mL vial of heparin with a concentration of 10,000 units/mL.

44. A provider orders enoxaparin 1.5 mg/kg, subcut, every 12 hours. The patient weighs 69 kg. The pharmacy provides enoxaparin in a 3-mL vial containing 300 mg/mL.

45. A provider orders dalteparin 15,000 IU, subcut, daily. The pharmacy supplies dalteparin in a vial containing 25,000 IU/mL.

Calculate the volume (mL) of the heparin bolus to be administered. Round the answers to the nearest hundredth mL.

46. A provider orders a heparin bolus of 90 units/kg, IV. The patient weighs 85 kg. The pharmacy provides heparin in a concentration of 5000 units/mL.

47. A provider orders a heparin bolus of 5500 units, IV. The pharmacy provides heparin in a vial containing 10,000 units/mL.

48. A provider orders a heparin bolus of 6500 units, IV. The pharmacy supplies heparin in a vial containing 10,000 units/mL.

49. A provider orders a heparin bolus of 70 units/kg, IV. The patient weighs 52 kg. The pharmacy supplies heparin in a vial containing 1000 units/mL.

50. A provider orders a heparin bolus of 80 units/kg, IV. The patient weighs 68 kg. The pharmacy supplies heparin in a vial containing 5000 units/mL.

Calculate the flow rate (mL/hr) for these heparin infusions. Round the answers to the nearest tenth mL.

51. A provider orders a continuous heparin infusion to begin at 13 units/kg/hour. The patient weighs 73 kg. The pharmacy supplies heparin in a premixed bag of 40,000 units in 500 mL 5% dextrose solution.

52. A provider orders a continuous heparin infusion to begin at 16 units/kg/hour. The patient weighs 58 kg. The pharmacy supplies heparin in a premixed bag of 25,000 units in 250 mL 5% dextrose solution.

53. A provider orders a continuous heparin infusion to begin at 20 units/kg/hour. The patient weighs 66 kg. The pharmacy supplies heparin in a premixed bag of 25,000 units in 500 mL 5% dextrose solution.

54. A provider orders a continuous heparin infusion to begin at 17 units/kg/hour. The patient weighs 90 kg. The pharmacy supplies heparin in a premixed bag of 40,000 units in 500 mL 5% dextrose solution.

55. A provider orders a continuous heparin infusion to begin at 33 units/kg/hour. The patient weighs 83 kg. The pharmacy supplies heparin in a premixed bag of 25,000 units in 250 mL 5% dextrose solution.

Calculate the new flow rate (mL/hr) for these heparin infusions. Round the answers to the nearest tenth mL.

56. A patient has a continuous heparin infusion running at 1200 units/hr. The infusion bag contains 25,000 units in 250 mL 5% dextrose solution. The nurse is to decrease the infusion by 150 units/hr.

57. A patient has a continuous heparin infusion running at 1300 units/hr. The infusion bag contains 25,000 units in 250 mL 5% dextrose solution. The nurse is to increase the infusion by 100 units/hr.

Calculate the new flow rate (units/hr) for these heparin infusions. Round the answers to the nearest whole unit.

58. A patient has a continuous heparin infusion running at 9 mL/hr. The nurse is to increase the infusion by 100 units/hr. The infusion bag contains 25,000 units in 250 mL 5% dextrose solution.

59. A patient has a continuous heparin infusion running at 14 mL/hr. The nurse is to decrease the infusion by 200 units/hr. The infusion bag contains 25,000 units in 500 mL 5% dextrose solution.

60. A patient has a continuous heparin infusion running at 12 mL/hr. The nurse is to increase the infusion by 50 units/hr. The infusion bag contains 40,000 units in 500 mL 5% dextrose solution.

Calculate the flow rate (mL/hr) for these secondary intravenous medications. Round the answers to the nearest tenth mL.

61. Nitroprusside is to be infused at 150 mcg/min, IV, continuously. The IV bag contains 25 mg in 100 mL 5% dextrose solution.

62. Eptifibatide is to be infused at 125 mcg/min, IV, continuously. The IV bag contains 250 mg eptifibatide in 200 mL 0.9% sodium chloride solution.

63. Norepinephrine is to be infused at 5 mcg/min, IV, continuously. The IV bag contains 10 mg norepinephrine in 500 mL 5% dextrose solution.

64. Procainamide is to be infused at 100 mcg/min, IV, continuously. The IV bag contains 1 g procainamide in 250 mL 0.9% sodium chloride.

65. Inamrinone is to be infused at 250 mcg/min, IV, continuously. The IV bag contains 250 mg inamrinone in 200 mL 0.9% sodium chloride.

Calculate the flow rate (mL/hr) for these weight-based IV medications. Round the answers to the nearest tenth mL.

66. Dopamine is to be infused at 5 mcg/kg/min, IV, continuously. The patient weighs 75 kg. The IV bag contains 100 mg dopamine in 100 mL 0.9% sodium chloride solution.

67. Esmolol is to be infused at 0.15 mg/kg/min, IV, continuously. The patient weighs 59 kg. The IV bag contains 2 g esmolol in 100 mL 5% dextrose solution.

68. Abciximab is to be infused at 0.2 mcg/kg/min, IV, continuously. The patient weighs 51 kg. The IV bag contains 6 mg abciximab in 500 mL 0.9% sodium chloride solution.

69. Nitroprusside is to be infused at 2 mcg/kg/min, IV, continuously. The patient weighs 64 kg. The IV bag contains 100 mg nitroprusside in 500 mL 5% dextrose solution.

70. Inamrinone is to be infused at 0.02 mg/kg/min, IV, continuously. The patient weighs 88 kg. The IV bag contains 250 mg inamrinone in 100 mL 0.9% sodium chloride.

Calculate the dosage (mcg/min) from the mL/hr flow rate of the IV. Round the answers to the nearest whole mcg/min.

71. An IV of infliximab is infusing at 29 mL/hr. The IV bag contains 125 mg of infliximab in 100 mL 0.9% sodium chloride.

72. An IV of nesiritide is infusing at 8 mL/hr. The IV bag contains 32 mg nesiritide in 250 mL 5% dextrose solution.

73. An IV of tirofiban is infusing at 12 mL/hr. The IV bag contains 50 mg of tirofiban in 500 mL of 0.9% sodium chloride.

74. An IV of octreotide is infusing at 18 mL/hr. The IV bag contains 4 mg of octreotide in 250 mL 0.9% sodium chloride.

75. An IV of lidocaine is infusing at 27 mL/hr. The IV bag contains 2000 mg of lidocaine in 250 mL 0.9% sodium chloride.

Calculate the flow rate range (mL/hr) for these IV infusions. Round the answers to the nearest tenth mL.

76. Begin procainamide, IV, at 0.5 mg/min. The maximum dose is 6 mg/min. The IV bag contains 1 g procainamide in 250 mL 5% dextrose solution.

77. Begin norepinephrine, IV, at 2.5 mcg/min. The maximum dose is 4 mcg/min. The IV bag contains 5 mg norepinephrine in 250 mL 5% dextrose solution.

78. Begin argatroban, IV, at 1.5 mcg/kg/min. The maximum dose is 10 mcg/kg/min. The patient weighs 63 kg. The IV bag contains 250 mg of argatroban in 250 mL 5% dextrose solution.

79. Begin dobutamine, IV, at 2.5 mcg/kg/min. The maximum dose is 10 mcg/kg/min. The patient weighs 59 kg. The IV bag contains 500 mg dobutamine in 500 mL 5% dextrose solution.

80. Begin cisatracurium, IV, at 2 mcg/kg/min. The maximum dose is 12 mcg/kg/min. The patient weighs 80 kg. The IV bag contains 250 mg cisatracurium in 250 mL 5% dextrose solution.

Calculate the dosage (mcg/min) that is currently infusing for these IV medications. Round the answers to the nearest tenth mcg. Indicate whether the dosage currently infusing is within the prescribed range by circling Yes or No.

81. Phenylephrine is infusing at 5.2 mL/hr. The IV bag contains phenylephrine 200 mg in 500 mL 0.9% sodium chloride. The prescribed dosage range is 40 to 60 mcg/min.
    a. mcg/min rate: _____
    b. Is the dosage within prescribed range?
        Yes   No

82. Isoproterenol is infusing at 30 mL/hr. The IV bag contains isoproterenol 2 mg in 250 mL 5% dextrose solution. The prescribed dosage range is 0.5 to 5 mcg/min.
    a. mcg/min rate: _____
    b. Is the dosage within prescribed range?
        Yes   No

83. Diltiazem is infusing at 20 mL/hr. The IV bag contains diltiazem 100 mg in 250 mL 5% dextrose solution. The prescribed dosage range is 84 to 167 mcg/min.
    a. mcg/min rate: _____
    b. Is the dosage within prescribed range?
        Yes   No

84. Conivaptan is infusing at 12 mL/hr. The IV bag contains conivaptan 20 mg in 200 mL 5% dextrose solution. The prescribed dosage range is 13.8 to 26.7 mcg/min.
    a. mcg/min rate: _____
    b. Is the dosage within prescribed range?
        Yes   No

85. Nitroprusside is infusing at 5 mL/hr. The IV bag contains nitroprusside 50 mg in 250 mL 0.9% sodium chloride. The prescribed dosage range is 30 to 60 mcg/min.
    a. mcg/min rate: _____
    b. Is the dosage within prescribed range?
        Yes   No

Calculate the dosage (mg or mcg) and volume (mL) of medication that the nurse should administer per dose for these pediatric patients. Round the answers to the nearest tenth mg and mL.

86. Digoxin 5 mcg/kg/day, PO, in divided doses every 12 hours is ordered for a child weighing 46 kg. The pharmacy supplies digoxin in an oral suspension containing 0.05 mg per mL.
    a. mcg/dose: _____
    b. mL: _____

87. Nafcillin 75 mg/kg/day, IM, in 6 divided doses is ordered for a child weighing 21 kg. The pharmacy supplies nafcillin in a vial containing 250 mg/mL.
    a. mg/dose: _____
    b. mL: _____

88. Neomycin 20 mg/kg, PO, every 4 hours is ordered for a child weighing 31 kg. The pharmacy supplies neomycin in an oral solution containing 125 mg per 5 mL.
  a. mg/dose: _____
  b. mL: _____

89. Acetaminophen 15 mg/kg, PO, every 6 hours, PRN for a fever is ordered for a child weighing 5.8 kg. The pharmacy supplies acetaminophen in an elixir containing 160 mg per 5 mL.
  a. mg/dose: _____
  b. mL: _____

90. Metoclopramide 0.5 mg/kg/day, PO, in 3 divided doses is ordered for a child weighing 22 kg. The pharmacy supplies metoclopramide in a syrup containing 5 mg per 5 mL.
  a. mg/dose: _____
  b. mL: _____

Calculate the dosage (mg) and volume (mL) of medication to be administered per dose based on each child's BSA. Round the answers to the nearest tenth mg and mL.

91. Calculate the dosage of diphenhydramine 50 mg/m^2, PO, once daily, for a child who weighs 22 lb and is 29 in in height. The pharmacy supplies diphenhydramine in a bottle containing 25 mg in 5-mL suspension.
  a. mg/dose: _____
  b. mL: _____

92. Calculate the dosage of gallium 100 mg/m^2, IV, one time, for a child who weighs 112 lb and is 59 in in height. The pharmacy supplies gallium in vials containing 150 mg in 5 mL.
  a. mg/dose: _____
  b. mL: _____

93. Calculate the dosage of caspofungin acetate 70 mg/m^2, IV, once weekly, for a child who weighs 27 kg and is 93 cm in height. The pharmacy supplies caspofungin acetate in vials containing 7 mg/mL.
  a. mg/dose: _____
  b. mL: _____

94. Calculate the dosage of doxorubicin 20 mg/m^2, IV, twice weekly, for a child who weighs 50 kg and is 145 cm in height. The pharmacy supplies doxorubicin in vials containing 2 mg/mL.
  a. mg/dose: _____
  b. mL: _____

95. Calculate the dosage of aminocaproic acid 100 mg/m^2, PO, now, for a child who weighs 19.3 kg and is 82 cm in height. The pharmacy supplies aminocaproic acid in a bottle containing 250 mg/mL suspension.
  a. mg/dose: _____
  b. mL: _____

Calculate the daily maintenance fluid needs (mL/day) and IV flow rate (mL/hr) for these pediatric patients. See Table U3PT-1. Assume the children are adequately hydrated.

Table U3PT-1	Pediatric Daily Maintenance Fluid Needs
Patient's Weight	Needed Maintenance Fluids in 24 Hours
Less than 10 kg	100 mL/kg
10 to 20 kg	1000 mL + 50 mL for each kg over 10
Over 20 kg	1500 mL + 20 mL for each kg over 20

a. Daily maintenance fluid needs (mL). Round to the nearest whole mL.

b. IV Flow rate (mL/hr). Round to the nearest tenth mL.

96. Child's weight is 1 kg; 100% from IV fluids.
   a. Total daily maintenance fluid needs (mL/day): _____

   b. IV flow rate (mL/hr): _____

97. Child's weight is 19 kg; half from IV fluids.
   a. Total daily maintenance fluid needs (mL/day): _____

   b. IV flow rate (mL/hr): _____

98. Child's weight is 12 kg: two-thirds from IV fluids
   a. Total daily maintenance fluid needs (mL/day): _____

   b. IV flow rate (mL/hr): _____

99. Child's weight is 63 kg; one-quarter from IV fluids.
   a. Total daily maintenance fluid needs (mL/day): _____

   b. IV flow rate (mL/hr): _____

100. Child's weight is 4.3 kg: one-third from IV fluids.
   a. Total daily maintenance fluid needs (mL/day): _____

   b. IV flow rate (mL/hr): _____

Comprehensive Post-Test   *(answers in Unit 4)*

After studying all of the chapters, answer these questions.

True or False

1. The metric system is the preferred unit of measure for prescribing and dispensing medication.
True   False

2. The abbreviation μg is not an acceptable abbreviation according to the Institute for Safe Medication Practices.   True   False

3. State boards of nursing are responsible for overseeing the laws that govern a nurse's scope of practice.   True   False

4. A medication should be checked at least 4 times before administering it to a patient.   True   False

5. Nurses taking telephone orders must read back the orders to the provider before hanging up.
True   False

6. Microdrip IV tubing has a drop factor of 30 gtt/mL.   True   False

7. Medications administered through an enteral feeding tube should be diluted with sterile water, not tap water.   True   False

Write the correct notation for these quantities.

8. 453 micrograms

9. 22 milliliters

10. 36 liters

Fill in the Blanks

11. What are the six rights governing medication administration?

_____
_____
_____
_____
_____
_____

12. A provider writes the following medication order for a patient: "Morphine sulfate 2 mg, every 4 to 6 hours, PRN." What information is missing from the order?

_____

Multiple Choice

13. Which agency is responsible for improving patient safety in healthcare facilities through an accreditation and certification process?
   a. the Food and Drug Administration
   b. the Department of Agriculture
   c. the Joint Commission
   d. the Institute for Healthcare Improvement

14. Which of these actions by the nurse is the correct method of verifying patient identity?
   a. The nurse compares the name and date of birth on the patient's armband with the patient's stated name and date of birth.
   b. The nurse compares the patient's room number on the Medication Administration Record with the patient's room number on the door.
   c. The nurse compares the name and date of birth on the Medication Administration Record with the name and date of birth in the patient's chart.
   d. The nurse asks a coworker the name of the patient and compares this to the Medication Administration Record.

15. The purpose of medication reconciliation is to:
   a. ensure that the facility receives payment for all prescribed drugs.
   b. reduce the occurrence of Medicare fraud.
   c. ensure that a current medication list accompanies the patient at all steps in the healthcare process.
   d. increase the workload of nurses and pharmacists.

16. Which type of insulin is long-acting?
   a. insulin glargine (Lantus)
   b. insuline lispro (Humalog)
   c. regular insulin (Humulin R)
   d. insulin aspart (NovoLog)

Matching

Match Column A with the correct measurement unit in Column B.

Column A	Column B
17. International Units _____	a. mEq
18. milliequivalents _____	b. liter, gram, meter
19. household system _____	c. IU
20. metric system _____	d. fluid ounce, pound, mile

Match the abbreviation in Column A with the correct meaning in Column B.

Column A	Column B
21. gtt _____	a. orally, by mouth
22. ad lib _____	b. as needed
23. q _____	c. three times daily
24. PRN _____	d. drop
25. t.i.d. _____	e. every
26. PO _____	f. as desired

Convert These Measures

Do not round the answers.

27. 0.75 mg = _____ mcg

28. 2.015 L = _____ mL

29. 4.3 g = _____ mg

30. 0.76 kg = _____ g

31. 5 tsp = _____ mL

32. 33 lb = _____ kg

33. 2 in = _____ cm

34. 138 cm = _____ in

35. 12 mcg = _____ mg

Medication Labels

Answer these questions for the medication label in Figure CPT-1.

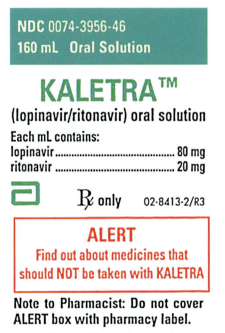

NDC 0074-3956-46
160 mL   Oral Solution

KALETRA™
(lopinavir/ritonavir) oral solution

Each mL contains:
lopinavir .... 80 mg
ritonavir .... 20 mg

℞ only   02-8413-2/R3

ALERT
Find out about medicines that
should NOT be taken with KALETRA

Note to Pharmacist: Do not cover
ALERT box with pharmacy label.

Figure CPT-1 Kaletra Label

36. What is the trade name of this drug?

37. What are the active ingredients of this drug?

38. What form this drug come in?

39. What is the total volume (mL) of medication in this container?

Volumes

Draw a line across the syringes at the volume indicated for each figure.

40. 0.56 mL (Fig. CPT-2)

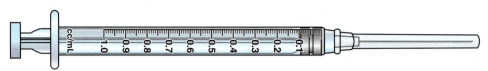

Figure CPT-2 1-mL Syringe

41. 1.6 mL (Fig. CPT-3)

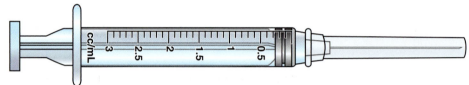

Figure CPT-3 3-mL Syringe

42. 3.4 mL (Fig. CPT-4)

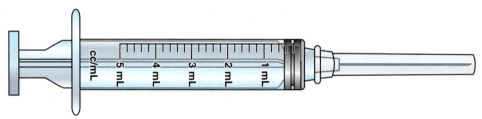

Figure CPT-4 5-mL Syringe

43. 6 units (Fig. CPT-5)

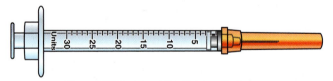

Figure CPT-5 0.3-mL/30-Unit Insulin Syringe

44. 62 units (Fig. CPT-6)

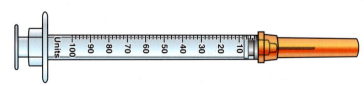

Figure CPT-6 1-mL/100-Unit Insulin Syringe

Calculations

Calculate the dosage (mg) and volume (mL) of medication that the nurse should administer for these liquid medications. Round the answers to the nearest tenth mg and mL.

45. A provider orders amoxicillin suspension 250 mg, by mouth, every 6 hours, for 7 days. The pharmacy provides amoxicillin suspension in bottles containing 500 mg in 5 mL.

46. A provider orders dicyclomine syrup 15 mg, by mouth, three times daily. The pharmacy supplies dicyclomine syrup in a concentration of 10 mg in 5 mL.

Calculate the number of tablets that the nurse should administer for these oral medications. Round the answers to the nearest ½ tablet.

47. A provider orders pioglitazone 15 mg, by mouth, once daily. The pharmacy supplies pioglitazone in tablets containing 30 mg.

48. A provider orders meloxicam 15 mg, by mouth, once daily. The pharmacy supplies meloxicam in tablets containing 7.5 mg.

Calculate the volume (mL) of medication that the nurse should administer for these parenteral medications. Round the answer to the nearest tenth mL.

49. A provider orders peginterferon Alpha-2b 100 mcg, subcut, once weekly for 1 year. The pharmacy supplies peginterferon Alpha-2b in vials containing 50 mcg in 0.5 mL.

50. A provider orders cyanocobalamin 200 mcg, IM, once monthly. The pharmacy supplies cyanocobalamin in vials containing 1000 mcg in 1 mL.

51. A provider orders phytonadione 10 mg, subcut, once weekly. The pharmacy supplies phytonadione in ampules containing 10 mg in 1 mL.

52. A provider orders leuprolide 7.5 mg, IM once monthly. The pharmacy supplies leuprolide in vials containing 5 mg in 1 mL.

Answer these questions for the medication label in Figure CPT-7.

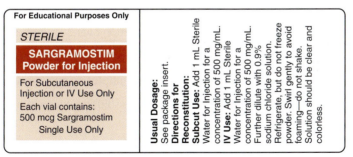

Figure CPT-7 Simulated Sargramostim Label

53. What is the total amount (mcg) of sargramostim in the vial?

54. How much diluent is added to the vial for subcutaneous injections?

55. How should the powdered medication be stored?

56. How should this medication be mixed?

57. If a provider ordered 400 mcg of sargramostim, subcut, how many mL should the nurse administer after reconstitution?

Calculate the BSA (m²) for these weight and height combinations. Round the answers to the nearest hundredth m².

58. weight 200 lb, height 75 in

59. weight 18 lb, height 27 in

60. weight 67 kg, height 156 cm

61. weight 73 kg, height 170 cm

Calculate the dosages (units and mg) of these medications based on body weight (kg).

62. A provider orders epoeitin 25 units/kg, subcut, 3 times per week. The patient weighs 39 kg. How many units of epoetin should the nurse administer per dose?

63. A provider orders pancuronium 0.12 mg/kg, IV, every 30 minutes as needed to maintain paralysis. The patient weighs 65 kg. How many mg of pancuronium should the nurse administer per dose?

Calculate dosage (mg) of these medications based on BSA (m²). Round the answers to the nearest tenth mg.

64. A provider orders docetaxel 75 mg/m², IV, now. The patient weighs 84 kg and is 183 cm in height.

65. A provider orders mitoxantrone 10 mg/m², IV, every 12 hours. The patient weighs 152 lb and is 68 in in height.

Calculate the flow rates (mL/hr) for these IV fluids. Round the answers to the nearest whole mL.

66. Infuse 250 mL over 30 minutes.

67. Infuse 500 mL over 8 hours.

68. Infuse 750 mL over 6 hours.

69. Infuse 1 L over 12 hours.

Calculate the flow rates (mL/hr) for these secondary IV medications. Round the answers to the nearest tenth mL.

70. Infuse cefipime 1 g diluted in 100 mL 0.9% sodium chloride solution over 30 minutes using an infusion pump.

71. Infuse nafcillin 0.5 g diluted in 50 mL 0.9% sodium chloride solution over 45 minutes using an infusion pump.

72. Infuse gentamicin 28 mg diluted in 8 mL D₅W solution over 30 minutes using a syringe pump.

73. Infuse ondansetron 4 mg diluted in 10 mL 0.9% sodium chloride solution over 5 minutes using a syringe pump.

Calculate the flow rate (gtt/min) for these IV fluids. Round the answers to the nearest whole gtt.

74. A provider orders 1 L of lactated Ringer's solution to be infused over 8 hours. The IV tubing has a drop factor of 20 gtt/mL.

75. A provider orders 500 mL of 0.9% sodium chloride solution to be infused over 2 hours. The IV tubing has a drop factor of 15 gtt/mL.

76. A provider orders 250 mL of D₅W solution to be infused over 1 hour. The IV tubing has a drop factor of 10 gtt/mL.

Calculate the ending times for these IV fluids infusing in mL/hr.

77. An IV is infusing at 75 mL/hr with 250 mL of fluid left in the bag. The current time is 0740.

78. An IV is infusing at 125 mL/hr with 900 mL of fluid left in the bag. The current time is 1735.

Calculate the ending times for these IV fluids infusing in gtt/min.

79. An IV is infusing at 40 gtt/min with 400 mL of fluid left in the bag. The IV tubing has a drop factor of 60 gtt/mL. The current time is 0120.

80. An IV is infusing at 30 gtt/min with 250 mL of fluid left in the bag. The IV tubing has a drop factor of 20 gtt/mL. The current time is 1505.

Calculate the flow rate (mL/hr) for these enteral feedings. Round the answer to the nearest whole mL.

81. 480 mL of formula is to be infused over 2 hours

82. 1 L of formula is to be infused over 18 hours

Calculate the volume (mL) of water to add to the enteral formula to make the dilute feeding strength indicated in the question. Round the answer to the nearest whole mL.

83. A formula is to be diluted to three-quarters strength. There is 240 mL of formula available.

84. A formula is to be diluted to half strength. There is 200 mL of formula available.

Calculate the volume (mL) of heparin or low molecular weight heparin (LMWH) the nurse should administer for these subcutaneous injections. Round the answers to the nearest hundredth mL.

85. A provider orders heparin 7000 units, subcut, every 12 hours. The pharmacy provides heparin in a vial containing 10,000 units per mL.

86. A provider orders dalteparin 125 IU/kg, subcut, once daily. The patient weighs 52 kg. The pharmacy provides dalteparin in a prefilled syringe with a concentration of 10,000 IU per 0.4 mL.

Calculate the flow rate (mL/hr) for these heparin infusions. Round the answers to the nearest tenth mL.

87. A provider orders a continuous heparin infusion to begin at 16 units/kg/hr. The patient weighs 80 kg. The pharmacy supplies heparin in a premixed bag containing 25,000 units in 250 mL D_5W solution.

88. A patient has a continuous heparin infusion running at 1250 units/hr. The infusion bag hanging has 25,000 units heparin in 500 mL D_5W solution.

Calculate the flow rate (units/hr) for these heparin infusions. Round the answers to the nearest whole unit.

89. An intravenous pump is infusing heparin at a rate of 11.3 mL/hr. The infusion bag hanging contains 25,000 units of heparin in 500 mL D_5W solution.

90. An intravenous pump is infusing heparin at a rate of 7.1 mL/hr. The infusion bag hanging contains 40,000 units heparin in 250 mL D_5W solution.

Calculate the flow rate (mL/hr) for these medications infusing in mcg/min. Round the answers to the nearest tenth mL.

91. A provider orders isoproterenol to be infused at a rate of 3 mcg/min. The pharmacy supplies isoproterenol in an infusion bag containing 1 mg in 250 mL 0.9% sodium chloride solution.

92. A provider orders abciximab to be infused at a rate of 10 mcg/min. The pharmacy supplies abciximab in an infusion bag containing 7.2 mg in 250 mL 0.9% sodium chloride solution.

Calculate the dosage (mcg/min) for these medications infusing in mL/hr. Round the answers to the nearest tenth mcg.

93. An infusion of octreotide is infusing at 12 mL/hr. The infusion bag contains 2 mg octreotide in 250 mL 0.9% sodium chloride solution.

94. An infusion of infliximab is infusing at 28 mL/hr. The infusion bag contains 250 mg infliximab in 500 mL 0.9% sodium chloride solution.

Calculate the flow rate range (mL/hr) for these medications infusing in mcg/min. Round the answers to the nearest tenth mL.

95. Begin a nitroglycerin infusion at 2 mcg/min. The maximum dose is 15 mcg/min. The infusion bag contains 25 mg in 250 mL D_5W solution.

96. Begin a norepinephrine infusion at 1 mcg/min. The maximum dose is 4 mcg/min. The infusion bag contains 5 mg in 250 mL.

Calculate the flow rate range (mL/hr) for these medications infusing in mcg/kg/min. Round the answers to the nearest tenth mL.

97. Begin an argatroban infusion at 3 mcg/kg/min. The maximum dose is 10 mg/kg/min. The patient weighs 71 kg. The infusion bag contains 250 mg argatroban in 250 mL D_5W solution.

98. Begin a dobutamine infusion at 1.5 mcg/kg/min. The maximum dose is 12 mcg/kg/min. The patient weighs 68 kg. The infusion bag contains 500 mg dobutamine in 250 mL D_5W solution.

Calculate the dosage of medication (mg) based on the child's BSA and the volume (mL) of medication to be administered per dose. Round the answers to the nearest tenth mg and mL.

99. Acyclovir, 200 mg/m², IV, every 12 hours. The child's BSA is 0.83 m². The pharmacy supplies acyclovir in vials containing 50 mg/mL.
   a. mg: _____
   b. mL: _____

100. Carboplatin 150 mg/m², IV, once daily. The child's BSA is 1.03 m². The pharmacy supplies carboplatin in vials containing 125 mg/mL.
   a. mg: _____
   b. mL: _____

Test Answers

Arithmetic Skills Assessment Answers

1. 115
2. 9648
3. 11,098
4. 4180
5. 24
6. 228
7. 2968
8. 543
9. 40
10. 105
11. 920
12. 49,364
13. 22
14. 5
15. 21.75
16. 48.4
17. $1\frac{1}{4}$
18. $1\frac{7}{24}$
19. $10\frac{2}{45}$
20. 11
21. $\frac{1}{3}$

22. $\frac{4}{9}$
23. $\frac{7}{8}$
24. $17\frac{11}{14}$
25. $\frac{5}{18}$
26. $1\frac{11}{21}$
27. $5\frac{5}{8}$
28. $4\frac{1}{6}$
29. $1\frac{1}{5}$
30. 6
31. $1\frac{11}{14}$
32. $3\frac{13}{40}$
33. 4.7
34. 93.2
35. 1.51
36. 832.782
37. 0.2
38. 0.75

39. 1.75
40. 328.21
41. 0.6
42. 65.6
43. 98.4
44. 330.0024
45. 11
46. 3.5
47. 5.075
48. 416
49. 21.1
50. 73.5
51. 152.79
52. 3.085
53. 0.4
54. $63\frac{3}{5}$
55. $8\frac{17}{100}$
56. 0.25
57. 0.892
58. $\frac{23}{1000}$
59. 0.009
60. 56%

Answers to Chapter 1 Post-Test

1. 10
2. 40
3. 173
4. 4945
5. 30,804
6. 2
7. 49

8. 654
9. 1752
10. 26,507
11. 72
12. 77
13. 299
14. 1428

15. 6080
16. 2
17. 3
18. 38
19. 10
20. 52

Answers to Chapter 2 Post-Test

1. $\frac{1}{2}$
2. $\frac{5}{8}$
3. $\frac{2}{3}$
4. $1\frac{1}{4}$
5. $\frac{5}{6}$
6. $\frac{14}{15}$
7. $1\frac{1}{10}$
8. $1\frac{1}{6}$
9. $3\frac{13}{16}$

10. $1\frac{11}{21}$
11. $\frac{5}{9}$
12. $\frac{7}{12}$
13. $1\frac{1}{3}$
14. $\frac{5}{6}$
15. $1\frac{3}{4}$
16. $\frac{1}{3}$
17. $\frac{2}{3}$
18. $1\frac{2}{9}$

19. $2\frac{25}{28}$
20. $1\frac{59}{96}$
21. 2
22. $2\frac{1}{2}$
23. $1\frac{2}{13}$
24. $12\frac{4}{7}$
25. $1\frac{11}{15}$

Answers to Chapter 3 Post-Test

1. 7
2. 42
3. 99.0 *or* 99
4. 75.5
5. 107.23
6. 10.9
7. 16.61
8. 107.232
9. 16.792
10. 133.705
11. 0.3
12. 3.04
13. 43.48
14. 0.671
15. 3.6954
16. 0.8
17. 12.75
18. 53.89
19. 141.642
20. 0.29025
21. 9.2
22. 1.7
23. 4.5
24. 8.15
25. 0.38
26. 56.3%
27. 42.9%
28. 5.34
29. $\dfrac{9}{100}$
30. 80%

Answers to Chapter 4 Post-Test

1. 100 bags
2. 16 lattes
3. 73 hours
4. 200 cookies
5. 125 pounds
6. 15 $\dfrac{\text{gallons}}{\text{day}}$
7. $25,200
8. 96 $\dfrac{\text{doses}}{\text{bottle}}$
9. 72 $\dfrac{\text{beats}}{\text{minute}}$
10. 48 days
11. 4000 cookies
12. 350 $\dfrac{\text{miles}}{\text{day}}$
13. 5.8 hours
14. $43.45 per student
15. 1300 pieces
16. 320 grams
17. 1 $\dfrac{\text{min}}{\text{stop}}$
18. 18 $\dfrac{\text{miles}}{\text{hour}}$
19. $700
20. 440 $\dfrac{\text{stops}}{\text{day}}$
21. $577.78 per month
22. 150 $\dfrac{\text{milliliters}}{\text{bottle}}$
23. 2 $\dfrac{\text{oz}}{\text{slice}}$
24. 100 days
25. 93,600 $\dfrac{\text{beats}}{\text{day}}$

Answers to Chapter 5 Post-Test

1. False
2. False
3. True
4. True
5. True
6. 6.1 gm
7. 412 mgm
8. 6 mLs
9. 8 k
10. 0.09 mcgs
11. 4 ou
12. 42 mg
13. 3 c
14. 700 mcg
15. 35.4 mm
16. 12 L
17. 7 tsp
18. 55 g
19. 4 fl oz or 4 oz
20. 1000 mg
21. 1 kg
22. 2.2 lb
23. 5 mL
24. 1 mg
25. 1000 m
26. 1 cm
27. 1 c
28. 2.5 cm
29. 1 m
30. 454 g
31. 10 mm
32. 1000 kg
33. 1 g
34. 30 cm
35. 1 fl oz

Answers to Chapter 6 Post-Test

1. 1.2 cm
2. 0.432 mg
3. 9.926 L
4. 6.27 m
5. 8.264 g
6. 15 mL
7. 730 g
8. 0.0456 g
9. 1,300,000 mg
10. 450,000 cm
11. 7900 mg
12. 3200 mm
13. 5220 mcg
14. 0.00985 kg
15. 0.067 L
16. 2.7 kg
17. 4 in
18. 180 mL
19. 360 mL
20. 55 lb
21. 240 cm
22. 17,272.7 g
23. 20 oz
24. 2.6 fl oz
25. 6 tsp
26. 270 mL
27. 75 mL
28. 66 in
29. 96.8 lb
30. 10 mL

Answers to Chapter 7 Post-Test

1. a	13. c	25. q
2. b	14. b	26. b
3. c	15. a	27. c
4. d	16. False	28. o
5. b	17. False	29. h
6. d	18. True	30. a
7. c	19. False	31. m
8. b	20. i	32. f
9. a	21. d	33. l
10. c	22. n	34. e
11. d	23. g	35. j
12. c	24. k	36. p

Answers to Chapter 8 Post-Test

1. a	5. d	8. True
2. d	6. a	9. False
3. c	7. c	10. a, b, c, d
4. b		

Answers to Chapter 9 Post-Test

1. False
2. True
3. True
4. False
5. True
6. Thyroidex
7. levothyroxine sodium
8. tablets
9. 125 mcg/tablet or 0.125 mg/tablet
10. between 20°C to 25°C (68°F to 72°F)

11. Expectesin
12. guaifenesin
13. 100 mg/5 mL or 20 mg/mL
14. oral syrup
15. 100 mL
16. furosemide
17. 40 mg in 4 mL or 10 mg in 1 mL
18. IV and IM
19. 4 mL
20. single dose

21. 6.9 mL
22. 10 mL
23. 2 capsules
24. 3 tablets
25. 2 1/2 tablets
26. 3.1 mL
27. 7.5 mL
28. 15 mL
29. 1/2 tablet
30. 15 mL

31.

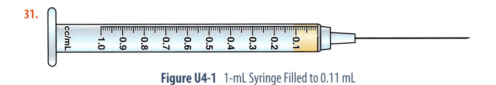

Figure U4-1 1-mL Syringe Filled to 0.11 mL

32.

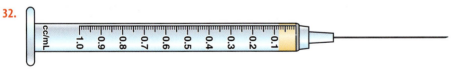

Figure U4-2 1-mL Syringe Filled to 0.08 mL

33.

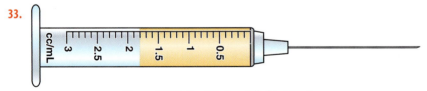

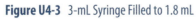

Figure U4-3 3-mL Syringe Filled to 1.8 mL

34.

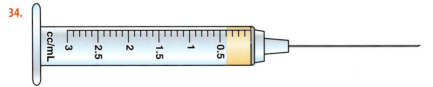

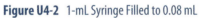

Figure U4-4 3-mL Syringe Filled to 0.4 mL

35.

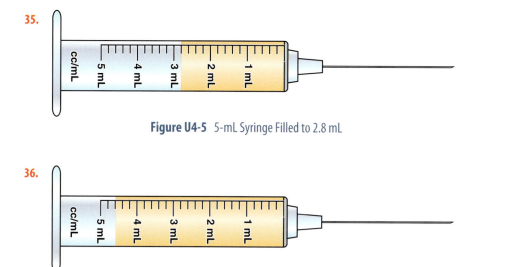

Figure U4-5 5-mL Syringe Filled to 2.8 mL

36.

Figure U4-6 5-mL Syringe Filled to 4.6 mL

37. 1.5 mL   40. 1 mL   43. 0.4 mL
38. 0.5 mL   41. 3.8 mL   44. 0.5 mL
39. 0.7 mL   42. 2 mL   45. 0.7 mL

Answers to Chapter Post Test

Answers to Chapter 10 Post-Test

1. 5 mL
2. 2.5 mL
3. 2.5 mL
4. 10 mL
5. 1.5 mL
6. 1 g
7. 250 to 500 mg IM or IV every 4 to 6 hours
8. 5.7 mL
9. 10 mL
10. 250 mg/1.5 mL
11. 100 mg/mL
12. until the solution is clear
13. for one week
14. 1.8 mL
15. 5 mL
16. 2 g
17. 3 to 4 g IM every 6 to 8 hours
18. 4 mL 0.9% sodium chloride solution
19. No
20. 1 g/2.5 mL
21. until well dissolved
22. 2.5 mL
23. 1.3 mL
24. a, d
25. a

Answers to Chapter 11 Post-Test

1. 35 mg
2. 13 mg
3. 2100 units
4. 11,250 mcg
5. 4.7 mL
6. 0.7 mL
7. 2.4 mL
8. 1.4 mL
9. 5.2 mL
10. 0.6 mL
11. 1.68 m²
12. 1.7 m²
13. 2.11 m²
14. 1.59 m²

15. 2.19 m²
16. 1.72 m²
17. 2.01 m²
18. 2.25 m²
19. 1.81 m²
20. 1.5 m²
21. a. 134 mg
    b. 5.4 mL
22. a. 118 mg
    b. 11.8 mL
23. a. 179 mg
    b. 3.6 mL
24. a. 525 mg
    b. 10.5 mL

25. a. 20 mg
    b. 10 mL
26. a. 686 mg
    b. 6.9 mL
27. a. 77 mg
    b. 1.5 mL
28. a. 24 units
    b. 4 mL
29. a. 278 mg
    b. 13.9 mL
30. a. 17 mg
    b. 1.7 mL

Answers to Chapter 12 Post-Test

1. d
2. c
3. d
4. a
5. c
6. b
7. d
8. b
9. a

10. c
11. d
12. c
13. a
14. b
15. b
16. a
17. b
18. False

19. False
20. True
21. False
22. True
23. True
24. True
25. True

Answers to Chapter 13 Post-Test

1. 64 mL/hr
2. 165 mL/hr
3. 333 mL/hr
4. 163 mL/hr
5. 150 mL/hr
6. 67 mL/hr
7. 33 mL/hr
8. 125 mL/hr
9. 67 mL/hr
10. 200 mL/hr
11. 120 mL/hr
12. 50 mL/hr
13. 90 mL/hr
14. 48 mL/hr
15. 45 mL/hr
16. 3 hr 20 min; ending at 1120

17. 8 hr 20 min; ending at 0350
18. 3 hr 39 min; ending at 0439
19. 6 hr 40 min; ending at 1140
20. 2 hr; ending at 1400
21. 33 gtt/min
22. 42 gtt/min
23. 36 gtt/min
24. 21 gtt/min
25. 42 gtt/min
26. 13 gtt/min
27. 53 gtt/min
28. 8 gtt/min
29. 28 gtt/min
30. 30 gtt/min

31. 2 hr 1 min; ending at 1831
32. 1 hr 23 min; ending at 0623
33. 14 hr 35 min; ending at 1335
34. 8 hr 20 min; ending at 0920
35. 4 hr 10 min; ending at 1840
36. 125 mL/hr
37. 31 gtt/min
38. 0500
39. 125 mL infused; 875 mL remaining
40. 250 mL infused; 750 mL remaining

41. 375 mL infused; 625 mL remaining
42. 500 mL infused; 500 mL remaining
43. 625 mL infused; 375 mL remaining
44. 750 mL infused; 250 mL remaining
45. 875 mL infused; 125 mL remaining
46. 1000 mL infused; 0 remaining

47.

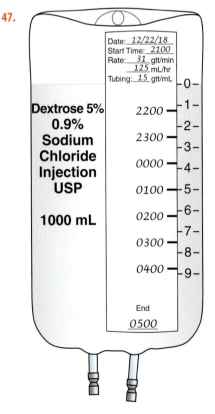

Figure U4-7 Completed time tape

Answers to Chapter 14 Post-Test

1. d
2. d
3. c
4. b
5. a
6. c
7. b
8. c
9. a, c, d
10. a, d
11. calories/day = 2350; protein/day = 75 g/day
12. calories/day = 1455; protein/day = 47 g/day
13. calories/day = 1550; protein/day = 50 g/day
14. calories/day = 2210; protein/day = 71 g/day
15. calories/day = 1900; protein/day = 61 g/day
16. 1700 mL/day

17. 755 mL/day
18. 1290 mL/day
19. 1033 mL/day
20. 1293 mL/day
21. 60 mL/hr
22. 117 mL/hr
23. 800 mL/hr (13 mL/min)
24. 56 mL/hr
25. 200 mL/hr
26. 360 mL/hr (6 mL/min)
27. 200 mL/hr
28. 100 mL/hr
29. 720 mL/hr (12 mL/min)
30. 267 mL/hr
31. 720 mL water
32. 960 to 975 mL water (depending on the method of calculation)
33. 720 mL water
34. 148 to 150 mL water
35. 133 mL water

Answers to Chapter 15 Post-Test

1. d
2. b
3. c
4. a
5. d

6. b
7. b
8. a
9. d
10. d

11. b
12. c
13. d
14. a
15. c

Answers to Chapter Post Test

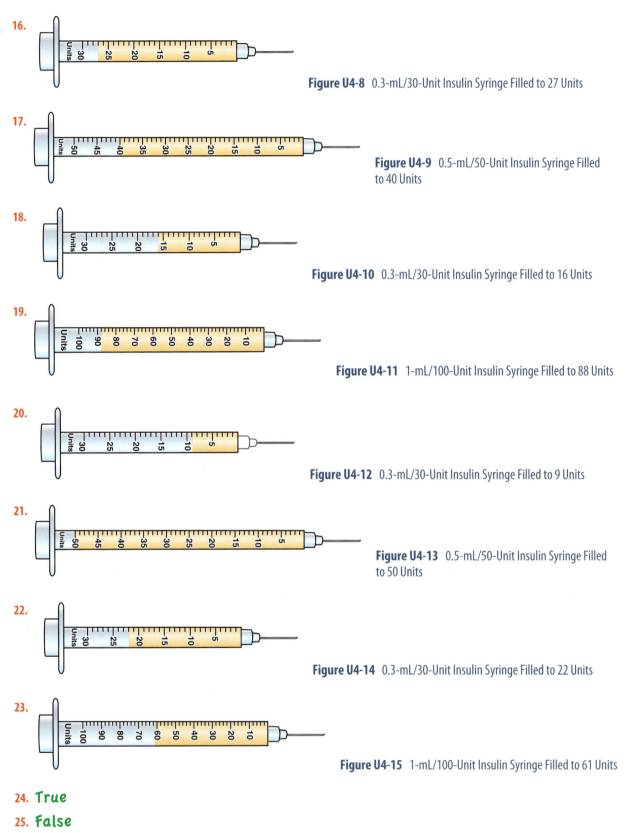

16.

Figure U4-8 0.3-mL/30-Unit Insulin Syringe Filled to 27 Units

17.

Figure U4-9 0.5-mL/50-Unit Insulin Syringe Filled to 40 Units

18.

Figure U4-10 0.3-mL/30-Unit Insulin Syringe Filled to 16 Units

19.

Figure U4-11 1-mL/100-Unit Insulin Syringe Filled to 88 Units

20.

Figure U4-12 0.3-mL/30-Unit Insulin Syringe Filled to 9 Units

21.

Figure U4-13 0.5-mL/50-Unit Insulin Syringe Filled to 50 Units

22.

Figure U4-14 0.3-mL/30-Unit Insulin Syringe Filled to 22 Units

23.

Figure U4-15 1-mL/100-Unit Insulin Syringe Filled to 61 Units

24. True

25. False

Answers to Chapter 16 Post-Test

1. a
2. d
3. b
4. True
5. True
6. 0.8 mL
7. 0.65 mL
8. 0.24 mL
9. 0.4 mL
10. 1.3 mL

11. 3.7 mL
12. 0.6 mL
13. 1.5 mL
14. 17.6 mL/hr
15. 9.5 mL/hr
16. 16.7 mL/hr
17. 12.4 mL/hr
18. 10 mL/hr
19. 13.6 mL/hr
20. 10.6 mL/hr

21. 11 mL/hr
22. Current rate = 1080 units/hr. New rate = 1280 units/hr
23. Current rate = 485 units/hr. New rate = 285 units/hr
24. Current rate = 1010 units/hr. New rate = 810 units/hr
25. Current rate = 712 units/hr. New rate = 812 units/hr

Answers to Chapter 17 Post-Test

1. 52.5 mL/hr
2. 120 mL/hr
3. 22.5 mL/hr
4. 66.7 mL/hr
5. 45 mL/hr
6. 11.2 mL/hr
7. 13.5 mL/hr
8. 15 mL/hr
9. 7.2 mL/hr
10. 22.5 mL/hr
11. 26.8 mL/hr
12. 19.2 mL/hr
13. 2 mL/hr
14. 15.3 mL/hr
15. 76.5 mL/hr

16. 30.6 mL/hr
17. 2 mL/hr
18. 18.5 mL/hr
19. 8.9 mL/hr
20. 27.7 mL/hr
21. 17.1 mg/min
22. 0.3 mg/min
23. 26.7 mg/min
24. 2 mg/min
25. 0.6 mg/min
26. 2.9 mcg/min
27. 21 mcg/min
28. 533.3 mcg/min
29. 15.7 mcg/min
30. 4.3 mcg/min

31. 22.5 to 90 mL/hr
32. 9 to 12 mL/hr
33. 8.1 to 32.4 mL/hr
34. 8.4 to 42.2 mL/hr
35. 12.1 to 40.2 mL/hr
36. 20 mcg/min-within range
37. 10 mcg/min-not within range
38. 133.3 mcg/min-within range
39. 66.7 mcg/min-within range
40. 7000 mcg/min-within range

Answers to Chapter 18 Post-Test

1. 115 mg/dose
   2.3 mL
2. 69 mg/dose
   1.4 mL
3. 105 mg/dose
   16.2 mL
4. 42 mg/dose
   1.3 mL
5. 2.3 mg/dose
   2.3 mL
6. 18.1 mg/dose
   0.7 mL
7. a. 71.9 mg/dose
   b. 2.9 mL
8. a. 62 mg/dose
   b. 7.8 mL
9. 0.31 m²
10. 1.34 m²
11. 0.21 m²
12. 0.68 m²

13. 0.2 m²
14. 0.77 m²
15. 0.69 m²
16. 0.39 m²
17. a. 114 mg
    b. 19 mL
18. a. 12 mg
    b. 12 mL
19. a. 526.5 mg
    b. 10.5 mL
20. a. 4.9 mg
    b. 0.5 mL
21. a. 67.4 mg
    b. 2.7 mL
22. a. 2850 mg
    b. 11.4 mL
23. a. 126 mg
    b. 25.2 mL
24. a. 68 mg
    b. 4.5 mL

25. a. 100 mL/day
    b. 4.2 mL/hr
26. a. 1450 mL/day
    b. 30.2 mL/hr
27. a. 2360 mL/day
    b. 24.6 mL/hr
28. a. 700 mL/day
    b. 29.2 mL/hr
29. a. 1200 mL/day
    b. 37.5 mL/hr
30. a. 200 mL/day
    b. 4.2 mL/hr
31. a. 1960 mL/day
    b. 40.8 mL/hr
32. c
33. b
34. a
35. c

Unit 1 Post-Test Answers

1. 207.6
2. 0.9
3. $\frac{32}{35}$
4. 44
5. 0.799
6. 4.5 hours
7. 2.28
8. $\frac{1}{2}$
9. 34.61
10. $\frac{123}{1000}$
11. $\frac{8}{15}$
12. 6241
13. 17,967.6 feet
14. 45.9
15. $\frac{2}{3}$
16. 0.2979

17. 75.3%
18. $2\frac{5}{8}$
19. $\frac{9}{14}$
20. 50%
21. 80
22. $\frac{551}{1000}$
23. 547 dimes
24. 184.8
25. 70.301
26. 2
27. $\frac{17}{500}$
28. $1\frac{1}{2}$
29. 0.92
30. 1318
31. $\frac{13}{25}$

32. 354
33. 6.789
34. $3\frac{5}{6}$
35. 9
36. 6.7
37. $116.02
38. $1\frac{31}{40}$
39. 0.375
40. 57,287
41. 14.603
42. $1\frac{1}{8}$
43. 7130
44. No, the elevator can only hold a maximum of 9 people who weigh an average of 160 pounds each.
45. 15

Unit 2 Post-Test Answers

1. 7.0 mg
2. 1.34 gm
3. 8.26 Ltr
4. 78 L
5. 440 mcg
6. 80 kg
7. 19 g
8. 10 fl oz
9. 0.082 mg

10. 2.01 L
11. 0.865 g
12. 154 mL
13. 20 g
14. 4000 mg
15. 2,102,000 mcg
16. 0.000915 kg
17. 0.085 L
18. 3.7 kg

19. 4.8 in
20. 60 mL
21. 25 mL
22. 112.2 lb
23. 45 cm
24. 1181.8 g
25. 2.6 fl oz
26. 6 tsp
27. True

28. **True**
29. **True**
30. **False**
31. **True**
32. **a**
33. **b**
34. **c**
35. **d**
36. **b**
37. **a**
38. **d**
39. **b**

40. **d**
41. **a**
42. **b**
43. **e**
44. **i**
45. **g**
46. **f**
47. **b**
48. **h**
49. **a**
50. **d**
51. **c**

52. **dopamine HCl**
53. **200 mg/5mL or 40 mg/mL**
54. **5 mL**
55. **single dose**
56. **1 g/2 mL or 0.5 g/mL**
57. **single dose**
58. **2 mL**
59. **IM or IV**
60. **10 mL**
61. **5 mL**
62. **15 mL**

63.

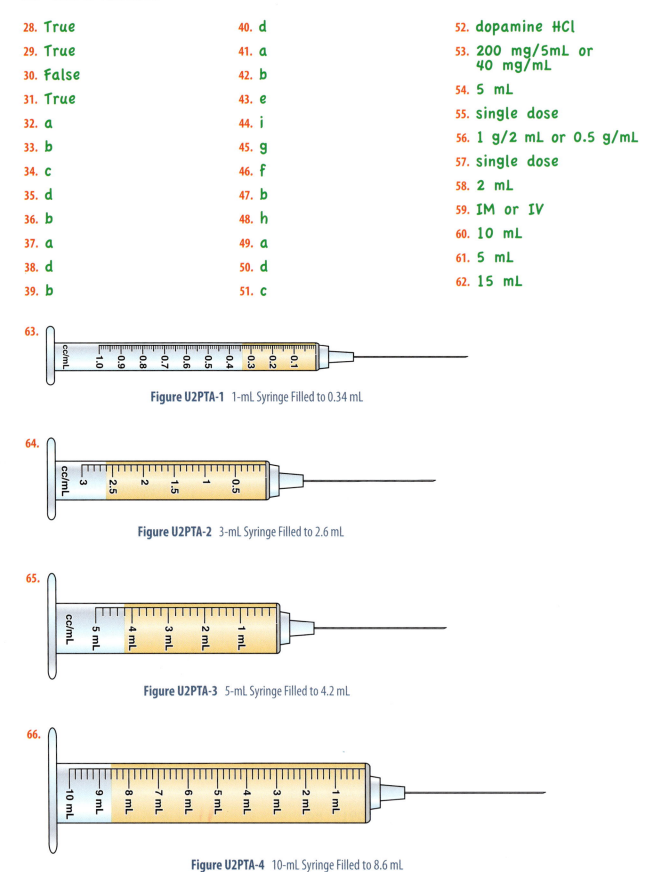

Figure U2PTA-1 1-mL Syringe Filled to 0.34 mL

64.

Figure U2PTA-2 3-mL Syringe Filled to 2.6 mL

65.

Figure U2PTA-3 5-mL Syringe Filled to 4.2 mL

66.

Figure U2PTA-4 10-mL Syringe Filled to 8.6 mL

67. 0.33 mL
68. 1.5 mL
69. 3 mL
70. 2.5 mL
71. 5 mL
72. 10 mL
73. 1 g
74. 500 mg to 1 g every 6 to 8 hours
75. 3.5 mL of sterile water for injection
76. 250 mg/mL
77. 3 mL

78. 10 mg
79. 2600 units
80. 4500 mcg
81. 2.08 m²
82. 1.61 m²
83. 1.98 m²
84. 1.61 m²
85. 106.3 mg, 4.3 mL
86. 49.1 mg, 4.9 mL
87. 333 mL/hr
88. 133 mL/hr
89. 200 mL/hr

90. 100 mL/hr
91. 33 mL/hr
92. 100 mL/hr
93. 1139
94. 0210
95. 31 gtt/min
96. 42 gtt/min
97. 44 gtt/min
98. 1750
99. 1046
100. 0431

Unit 3 Post-Test Answers

1. b
2. b
3. d
4. b
5. c
6. d
7. a
8. b
9. a
10. b
11. a. 1825 cal/day
    b. 58 g protein/day
12. a. 1625 cal/day
    b. 52 g protein/day

13. a. 1225 cal/day
    b. 39 g protein/day
14. a. 1425 cal/day
    b. 46 g protein/day
15. a. 2025 cal/day
    b. 65 g protein/day
16. 1800 mL/day
17. 1050 mL/day
18. 900 mL/day
19. 2125 mL/day
20. 1150 mL/day
21. 328 mL/day
22. 797 mL/day
23. 720 mL/day

24. 400 mL/day
25. 341 mL/day
26. 75 mL/hr
27. 320 mL/hr
28. 167 mL/hr
29. 600 mL/hr
30. 42 mL/hr
31. 900 mL
32. 480 mL
33. 480–487 mL
34. 80 mL
35. 197–200 mL

36.

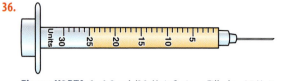

Figure U3PTA-1   0.3-mL/30-Unit Syringe Filled to 25 Units

37.

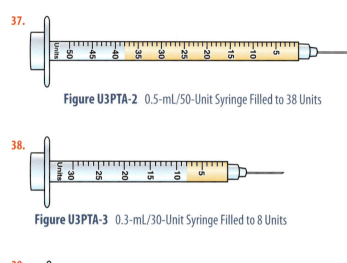

Figure U3PTA-2   0.5-mL/50-Unit Syringe Filled to 38 Units

38.

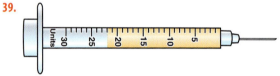

Figure U3PTA-3   0.3-mL/30-Unit Syringe Filled to 8 Units

39.

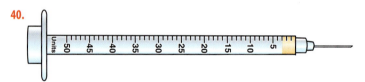

Figure U3PTA-04   0.3-mL/30-Unit Syringe Filled to 22 Units

40.

Figure U3PTA-05   0.5-mL/50-Unit Syringe Filled to 3 Units

41. 0.9 mL	51. 11.9 mL/hr	61. 36 mL/hr
42. 0.5 mL	52. 9.3 mL/hr	62. 6 mL/hr
43. 0.75 mL	53. 26.4 mL/hr	63. 15 mL/hr
44. 0.35 mL	54. 19.1 mL/hr	64. 1.5 mL/hr
45. 0.6 mL	55. 27.4 mL/hr	65. 12 mL/hr
46. 1.53 mL	56. 10.5 mL/hr	66. 22.5 mL/hr
47. 0.55 mL	57. 14 mL/hr	67. 26.6 mL/hr
48. 0.65 mL	58. 1000 units/hr	68. 51 mL/hr
49. 3.64 mL	59. 500 units/hr	69. 38.4 mL/hr
50. 1.09 mL	60. 1010 units/hr	70. 42.2 mL/hr

71. 604 mcg/min
72. 17 mcg/min
73. 20 mcg/min
74. 5 mcg/min
75. 3600 mcg/min
76. 7.5 to 90 mL/hr
77. 7.5 to 12 mL/hr
78. 5.7 to 37.8 mL/hr
79. 8.9 to 35.4 mL/hr
80. 9.6 to 57.6 mL/hr
81. a. 34.7 mcg/min
    b. No
82. a. 4 mcg/min
    b. Yes
83. a. 133.3 mcg/min
    b. Yes
84. a. 20 mcg/min
    b. Yes

85. a. 16.7 mcg/min
    b. No
86. a. 115 mcg/dose
    b. 2.3 mL
87. a. 262.5 mg/dose
    b. 1.1 mL
88. a. 620 mg/dose
    b. 24.8 mL
89. a. 87 mg/dose
    b. 2.7 mL
90. a. 3.7 mg/dose
    b. 3.7 mL
91. a. 22.5 mg/dose
    b. 4.5 mL
92. a. 145 mg/dose
    b. 4.8 mL

93. a. 58.8 mg/dose
    b. 8.4 mL
94. a. 28.4 mg/dose
    b. 14.2 mL
95. a. 66 mg/dose
    b. 0.3 mL
96. a. 100 mL/day
    b. 4.2 mL/hr
97. a. 1450 mL/day
    b. 30.2 mL/hr
98. a. 1100 mL/day
    b. 30.6 mL/hr
99. a. 2360 mL/day
    b. 24.6 mL/hr
100. a. 430 mL/day
    b. 6 mL/hr

Comprehensive Post-Test Answers

1. True
2. True
3. True
4. False
5. True
6. False
7. True
8. 453 mcg
9. 22 mL
10. 36 L
11. right patient, right medication, right dose, right time, right route, right documentation
12. route

13. c
14. a
15. c
16. a
17. c
18. a
19. d
20. b
21. d
22. f
23. e
24. b
25. c
26. a

27. 750 mcg
28. 2015 mL
29. 4300 mg
30. 760 g
31. 25 mL
32. 15 kg
33. 5 cm
34. 55.2 in
35. 0.012 mg
36. Kaletra
37. lopinavir and ritonavir
38. oral solution
39. 160 mL

40.

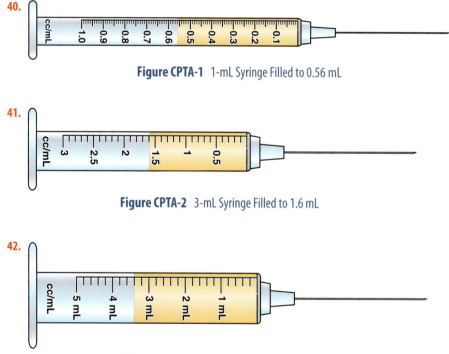

Figure CPTA-1 1-mL Syringe Filled to 0.56 mL

41.

Figure CPTA-2 3-mL Syringe Filled to 1.6 mL

42.

Figure CPTA-3 5-mL Syringe Filled to 3.4 mL

43.

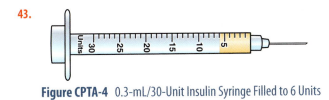

Figure CPTA-4 0.3-mL/30-Unit Insulin Syringe Filled to 6 Units

44.

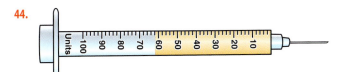

Figure CPTA-5 1-mL/100-Unit Insulin Syringe Filled to 62 Units

45. 2.5 mL

46. 7.5 mL

47. 1/2 tablet

48. 2 tablets

49. 1 mL

50. 0.2 mL

51. 1 mL

52. 1.5 mL

53. 500 mcg

54. 1 mL sterile water for injection

55. In the refrigerator—do not freeze.

56. Mix by swirling gently to avoid foaming. Do not shake.

57. 0.8 mL

58. 2.19 m²

59. 0.39 m²

60. 1.7 m²

61. 1.86 m²

62. 975 units

63. 7.8 mg

64. 155.3 mg

65. 18.2 mg

66. 500 mL/hr

67. 63 mL/hr

68. 125 mL/hr

69. 83 mL/hr

70. 200 mL/hr

71. 66.7 mL/hr

72. 16 mL/hr

73. 120 mL/hr

74. 42 gtt/min

75. 63 gtt/min

76. 42 gtt/min

77. infusion time of 3 hr, 20 min; end time of 1100

78. infusion time of 7 hr, 12 min; tend time of 0047

79. infusion time of 10 hr; end time of 1120

80. infusion time of 2 hr, 47 min; end time of 1752

81. 240 mL/hr

82. 56 mL/hr

83. 80 mL

84. 200 mL

85. 0.7 mL

86. 0.26 mL

87. 12.8 mL/hr

88. 25 mL/hr

89. 565 units/hr

90. 1136 units/hr

91. 45 mL/hr

92. 20.8 mL/hr

93. 1.6 mcg/min

94. 233.3 mcg/min

95. 1.2 to 9 mL/hr

96. 3 to 12 mL/hr

97. 12.8 to 42.6 mL/hr

98. 3.1 to 24.5 mL/hr

99. a. 166 mg

   b. 3.3 mL

100. a. 154.5 mg

   b. 1.2 mL

Appendix A
Calculators

Using a Handheld Calculator

A simple calculator with a square-root function is perfectly adequate for calculating dosage-related problems. The use of programmable calculators may be prohibited during dosage calculation examinations in your health program, and the National Council Licensure Examinations (NCLEX-PN and NCLEX-RN) does not allow test-takers to bring handheld calculators into the exam. However, a drop-down calculator on the computer is available for dosage-related questions on the NCLEX exam.

Make sure to practice using your calculator until you understand how to enter mathematical functions accurately. Calculating the wrong dosage is easy if mathematical operations ($\times$, $\div$, $+$, $-$, or $\sqrt{\ }$) are entered in the wrong order.

Practice 1

Calculate the answers to these problems using a handheld calculator.

1. 5×6

2. $100.68 + 47$

3. $34 + (79 \times 23)$

4. $(99 \div 3.3) - 1.1$

5. $\dfrac{1}{3} \times \dfrac{3}{5}$

6. Find the square root of 14.44.

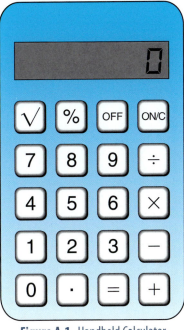

Figure A-1 Handheld Calculator

Using a Drop-Down Calculator

Drop-down calculators on computers may be operated in two ways: You can (1) use the mouse to select the numbers and functions or (2) use the keyboard keypad. If you use the mouse, carefully enter numbers and functions so they register properly. Always double-check to make sure you made the proper entries.

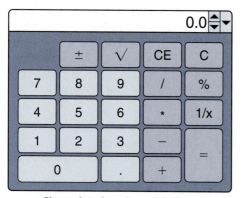

Figure A-2 Drop-Down Calculator

See answers to Practice Questions on page 441.

Practice 2

Calculate the answers to these problems using a drop-down calculator on a computer.

1. $438 \div 16$
2. 92×51
3. $729 - (4 \times 38)$
4. $\dfrac{5}{6} \div \dfrac{2}{3}$
5. $\dfrac{3}{5} \div 2$
6. Find the square root of 39.0625.

Appendix B
Roman Numerals

Using Roman Numerals

For hundreds of years, medications were prescribed using the apothecary system of measurement, which utilized Roman numerals to designate the quantity of a medicine's weight or liquid volume. The Roman numeral system of notation uses the letters I, V, X, L, C, D, and M to represent quantities. Combinations of these letters are used to denote other whole numbers. See Table B-1.

Reading Roman Numerals

Roman numerals are read from left to right; the largest number in the first position and descending numbers to the right. Each number is added to the first.

Example 1:　The Roman numeral II = 1 + 1 = 2

Example 2:　The Roman numeral XVI = 10 + 5 + 1 = 16

Example 3:　The Roman numeral MDCI = 1000 + 500 + 100 + 1 = 1601

Example 4:　The Roman numeral CCCLVIII = 100 + 100 + 100 + 50 + 5 + 1 + 1 + 1 = 358

Note:　To shorten the length of a Roman numeral, only three consecutive I's are used in a row. So, rather than write IIII to denote the number 4, or VIIII to represent 9, a smaller number is placed before the bigger number to signal the need to subtract the smaller number from the larger number. Therefore, the number 4 is written as IV, and the number 9 is written as IX.

Table B-1	Equivalents of Roman Numerals and Arabic Numerals
Roman Numerals	**Arabic Numerals**
I	1
V	5
X	10
L	50
C	100
D	500
M	1000

Example 5:   The Roman numeral XIX = 10 + (10 − 1) = 19

Example 6:   The Roman numeral CXLI = 100 + (50 − 10) + 1 = 141

Example 7:   The Roman numeral DCXCVIII = 500 + 100 + (100 − 10) + 5 + 1+1+1 = 698

Example 8:   The Roman numeral MDXCIX = 1000 + 500 + (100 − 10) + (10 − 1) = 1599

Appendix C
The 24-Hour Clock

Using the 24-Hour Clock

Most healthcare facilities use the 24-hour clock (also known as military time) for documentation purposes. The advantage of the 24-hour clock is eliminating confusion as to whether 3:00 is 3:00 *a.m.* or 3:00 *p.m.* Converting from conventional time to the 24-hour clock is easy, although it takes practice to become proficient:

1. Times up to and including noon stay the same, except for adding a leading *0* for times before 10:00 a.m. For example, 4:15 a.m. becomes 0415. Notice that the colon is omitted, and adding *a.m.* or *p.m.* after the time is unnecessary. Noon (12:00 p.m.) becomes 1200 in military time.

2. For times after noon, add 12 to the hour in the time but do not change the minutes. For example, to change 5:43 p.m. into military time, add 12 to the 5, so 5:43 p.m. becomes 1743. Midnight (12:00 a.m.) can be written in military time as either 0000 or 2400, although 12:05 a.m. in military time is typically stated as 0005, not 2405.

3. Adding hours and minutes to military time involves simple addition, remembering that the clock has 24 hours/day and 60 minutes/hour. For example, add 8 hours and 17 minutes to the time 17:53 (5:53 p.m.).
   a. Calculate the new time in hours new time (hours) = 1700 (current time in hours) + 8 hours = 2400 + 1 additional hour over 24 hours = 0100 (1:00 a.m.).
   b. Calculate the new time in minutes new time (minutes) = 53 (current time in minutes) + 17 min = 70 minutes, or 1 hour, 10 minutes.
   c. Add the hours and minutes together new time = 0100 + 1 hour, 10 minutes = 0210 (2:10 a.m.).

See Figure C-1 and Table C-1.

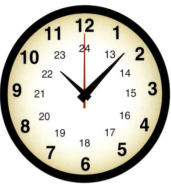

Figure C-1 24-Hour Clock

Table C-1	Converting Conventional Time Into Military Time
Conventional Time	**24-Hour Clock**
12:00 a.m. (midnight)	0000 or 2400
1:00 a.m.	0100
2:00 a.m.	0200
3:00 a.m.	0300
4:00 a.m.	0400
5:00 a.m.	0500
6:00 a.m.	0600
7:00 a.m.	0700
8:00 a.m.	0800
9:00 a.m.	0900
10:00 a.m.	1000
11:00 a.m.	1100
12:00 p.m. (noon)	1200
1:00 p.m.	1300
2:00 p.m.	1400
3:00 p.m.	1500
4:00 p.m.	1600
5:00 p.m.	1700
6:00 p.m.	1800
7:00 p.m.	1900
8:00 p.m.	2000
9:00 p.m.	2100
10:00 p.m.	2200
11:00 p.m.	2300

Practice

Change these conventional times to military time.

1. 3:25 a.m.
2. 3:25 p.m.
3. 7:58 a.m.
4. 7:58 p.m.
5. 12:38 a.m.
6. 12:38 p.m.
7. 5:44 a.m.

8. 5:44 p.m.
9. 2:02 a.m.
10. 2:02 p.m.
11. 9:17 a.m.
12. 9:17 p.m.
13. 10:29 a.m.
14. 10:29 p.m.

See answers to Practice Questions on Page 441.

References

1. Bankhead, R., Boullata, J., Brantley, S., Corkins, M., Guenter, P., Krenitsky, J., Lyman, B., Metheny, N.A., Mueller, C., Robbins, S., & Wessel, J. (2009). A.S.P.E.N. Enteral nutrition practice recommendations. *Journal of Parenteral and Enteral Nutrition, 33*(122), 122–167. doi: 10.1177/0148607108330314

2. Ernst, F.R., & Grizzle, A.J. (2001). Drug-related morbidity and mortality: Updating the cost-of-illness model. *Journal of the American Pharmaceutical Association, 41*(2), 192–199.

3. Hirsh, J., Bauer, K.A., Donati, M.B., Gould, M., Samama, M.M., & Weitz, J.I. (2008). Parenteral anticoagulants. *Chest, 133*, 141S–159S. doi:10.1378/chest.08-0689

4. Institute for Safe Medication Practices. (2016). FDA and ISMP lists of look-alike drug name sets with recommended tall man letters. Retrieved from http://www.ismp.org

5. James, J.T. (2013). A new, evidence-based estimate of patient harms associated with hospital care. *Journal of Patient Safety, 9*(3), 122–128.

6. The Joint Commission. (2018). Accreditation Program: Hospital. Chapter: 2018 National Patient Safety Goals. *National Patient Safety Goals Manual*. Retrieved from http://www.jointcommission.org

7. Kohn, L.T., Corrigan, J.M., and Donaldson, M.S. (Eds.). (2000). *To err is human: Building a safer health system*. Washington, DC: National Academy Press.

8. Lack, J.A., & Stuart-Taylor, M.E. (1997). Calculation of drug dosages and body surface area of children. *British Journal of Anaesthesia, 78*, 601–605.

9. Mosteller, R.D. (1987). Simplified calculation of body surface area. *The New England Journal of Medicine, 317*(17), 1098 (letter).

10. National Coordinating Council for Medication Error Reporting and Prevention. (2018) What is a medication error? Retrieved from http://www.nccmerp.org

11. National Institute on Drug Abuse. (2016). Misuse of prescription drugs: Older adults. Retrieved from https://www.drugabuse.gov/publications/research-reports/prescription-drugs/trends-in-prescription-drug-abuse/older-adults.

12. Ortman, J.M., Velkoff, V.A., & Hogan, H. (2014). An aging nation: The older population in the United States. Retrieved from https://www.census.gov/prod/2014pubs/p25-1140.pdf.

13. Phillips, J., Beam, S., Brinker, A., Holquist, C., Honig, P., Lee, L.Y., et al. (2001). Retrospective analysis of mortalities associated with medication errors. *American Journal of Health-System Pharmacists, 58*(19), 1824–1829.

14. U.S. Census Bureau. (2016). Population estimates program (PEP). Retrieved from http://www.census.gov/quickfacts.

15. U.S. Pharmacopeia. (2002). MEDMARX 2002 annual data report: The quest for quality. Retrieved from http://www.usp.org.

Appendix Answers

Appendix A - Practice 1

1. 30
2. 147.68
3. 1851
4. 28.9
5. 0.2
6. 3.8

Appendix A - Practice 2

1. 27.375
2. 4692
3. 577
4. 1.25
5. 0.3
6. 6.25

Appendix C Answers

1. 0325
2. 1525
3. 0758
4. 1958
5. 0038
6. 1238
7. 0544
8. 1744
9. 0202
10. 1402
11. 0917
12. 2117
13. 1029
14. 2229

Index

Page numbers followed by "b" indicate boxes or boxed elements; "f," figures; "t," tables.